PUBLIC HEALTH ASPECTS OF DIAGNOSIS AND CLASSIFICATION OF MENTAL AND BEHAVIORAL DISORDERS

Refining the Research Agenda for DSM-5 and ICD-11

PUBLIC HEALTH ASPECTS OF DIAGNOSIS AND CLASSIFICATION OF MENTAL AND BEHAVIORAL DISORDERS

Refining the Research Agenda for DSM-5 and ICD-11

Edited by

Shekhar Saxena, M.D.
Patricia Esparza, Ph.D.
Darrel A. Regier, M.D., M.P.H.
Benedetto Saraceno, M.D.
Norman Sartorius, M.D., Ph.D.

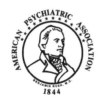

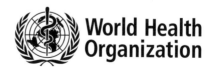

American Psychiatric Association
Arlington, Virginia

World Health Organization
Geneva, Switzerland

If you would like to buy between 25 and 99 copies of this or any other American Psychiatric Publishing title, you are eligible for a 20% discount; please contact Customer Service at appi@psych.org or 800-368-5777. If you wish to buy 100 or more copies of the same title, please e-mail us at bulksales@psych.org for a price quote.

Manufactured in the United States of America on acid-free paper
16   15   14   13   12   5   4   3   2   1
First Edition

Typeset in Adobe's Frutiger and AGaramond.

Published on behalf of the World Health Organization by

American Psychiatric Publishing
a Division of American Psychiatric Association
1000 Wilson Boulevard
Arlington, VA 22209-3901
www.appi.org

Library of Congress Cataloging-in-Publication Data
Public health aspects of diagnosis and classification of mental and behavioral disorders :
refining the research agenda for DSM-5 and ICD-11 / edited by Shekhar Saxena...[et al.]. —
1st ed.
   p. ; cm.
Includes bibliographical references and index.
ISBN 978-0-89042-349-3 (pbk. : alk. paper)
  I. Saxena, Shekhar. II. American Psychiatric Association. III. World Health Organization.
  [DNLM: 1. Diagnostic and statistical manual of mental disorders. 2. International statistical classification of diseases and related health problems. 11th revision. 3. Mental Disorders—classification. 4. Mental Disorders—diagnosis. 5. Public Health. WM 141]
   616.89'075—dc23   2012002597

British Library Cataloguing in Publication Data
A CIP record is available from the British Library.

CONTENTS

CONTRIBUTORS

Margarita Alegría
Director, Center for Multicultural Mental Health Research, Cambridge Health Alliance and Harvard Medical School, Somerville, Massachusetts

Francesco Amaddeo
Professor of Psychiatry, Section of Psychiatry and Clinical Psychology, Department of Public Health and Community Medicine, University of Verona, Verona, Italy

Paul S. Appelbaum
Professor of Psychiatry and Director, Division of Psychiatry, Law, and Ethics, Department of Psychiatry, College of Physicians and Surgeons of Columbia University; and Elizabeth K. Dollard Professor of Psychiatry, Medicine, and Law, Columbia Law School, New York, New York

Julio Arboleda-Flórez
Emeritus Professor, Departments of Psychiatry and of Community Health Sciences and Epidemiology; Director, QUEEN'S/PAHO/WHO Regional Research & Training Program in Psychiatric and Behavioural Epidemiology, Queen's University, Kingston, Ontario, Canada

Bruce Arroll
Professor and Elaine Gurr Chair in General Practice, Department of General Practice and Primary Health Care, University of Auckland, Auckland, New Zealand

Angelo Barbato
Senior Scientist, Epidemiology and Social Psychiatry Unit, Mario Negri Institute, Milano, Italy

Hugo Barrionuevo
Psychiatrist, Master on Health Economy and Management; Associate Director, Hospital Interzonal Especializado José A.Esteves de Buenos Aires; Director, Maestría en Gestión de Servicios de Salud Mental, Universidad ISALUD; President, Instituto de Gestión y Políticas en Salud Mental (IGESAM), Venezuela, Argentina

Aksel Bertelsen
Psychiatrist, Department of Clinical Medicine, Centre for Psychiatric Research, Aarhus University Hospital, Risskov, Denmark

Richard J. Bonnie
Harrison Foundation Professor of Medicine and Law, Professor of Psychiatry and Neurobehavioral Sciences, and Director, Institute of Law, Psychiatry and Public Policy; Professor of Public Policy, Frank Batten School of Leadership and Public Policy, University of Virginia School of Law, Charlottesville, Virginia

Michel Botbol
President, Association of WPA French Member Societies; Consultant, Judicial Protection of the Youth Direction at the French Ministry of Justice, Paris, France

Daniel H. Chisholm
Department of Mental Health and Substance Abuse, Non-communicable Diseases and Mental Health, World Health Organization, Geneva, Switzerland

John Cooper

Frank deGruy III
Woodward Chisholm Professor and Chair, Department of Family Medicine, University of Colorado School of Medicine, Aurora, Colorado

Horst Dilling

Christopher Dowrick
Professor of Primary Medical Care, University of Liverpool, Liverpool, United Kingdom

Patricia Esparza
Research Professor and Clinical Psychologist, Psychology and Counseling Department, Webster University, Bellevue, Switzerland

Michael B. First
Professor of Clinical Psychiatry and Research Psychiatrist, New York State Psychiatric Institute, Mailman School of Public Health, Columbia University, New York, New York; Associate, Forensic Panel Consultant on ICD-11 Revision, World Health Organization

Sandra Fortes
Associate Professor, Mental Health and Psychological Medicine, School of Medical Sciences, University of Rio de Janeiro State, Rio de Janeiro, Brazil

Linda Gask
Professor of Primary Care Psychiatry, University of Manchester, School of Community Based Medicine, Manchester, United Kingdom

Howard H. Goldman
Professor, Department of Psychiatry, University of Maryland School of Medicine, Baltimore, Maryland

Dante Grana
Medical Director, Fundacion Red de Vida; President, Fundacion Avedis Donabedian Argentina, Buenos Aires, Argentina

Rafia Gubash
Professor, Community and Epidemiological Psychiatry, and Past President, Arab Gulf University, Manama, Bahrain

Walter Gulbinat
Manager, Global Network for Research in Mental and Neurological Health, Lichtenstein, Germany

Oye Gureje
Professor, Department of Psychiatry, College of Medicine, University of Ibadan, Ibadan, Nigeria

Deborah Hasin
Professor of Clinical Public Health, Columbia University, New York, New York

Gerhard Heinze

Helen Herrman
Professor of Psychiatry, Orygen Youth Health Research Centre, Centre for Youth Mental Health, The University of Melbourne; Director, World Health Organization Collaborating Centre in Mental Health, Melbourne, Victoria, Australia

John P. Hirdes
Professor, School of Public Health and Health System, University of Waterloo, Waterloo, Ontario, Canada

Fritz Hohagen
Professor, Department of Psychiatry and Psychotherapy, University Medical Center Schleswig-Holstein, Lübeck, Germany

Marcela V. Horvitz-Lennon
Physician Scientist, RAND Corporation, Pittsburgh, Pennsylvania

Clemens Hosman
Professor of Mental Health Promotion and Prevention of Mental Disorders, Maastricht University (Department of Health Promotion) and Radboud University Nijmegen (Department of Clinical Psychology), the Netherlands; Director, Prevention Research Centre, Radboud University, Nijmegen, The Netherlands

Teh-wei Hu
Professor Emeritus of Health Economics, University of California Berkeley School of Public Health, Berkeley, California

Tae-Yeon Hwang

Robert Jakob
Medical Officer, ICD Classifications and Terminology, World Health Organization, Geneva, Switzerland

Aleksandar Janca
Head, School of Psychiatry and Clinical Neurosciences, The University of Western Australia, Crawley, Western Australia, Australia

Eva Jané-Llopis
Head, Chronic Disease and Wellness, World Economic Forum, Geneva, Switzerland

Marianne Kastrup
Director, National Centre for Transcultural Psychiatry, Psychiatric Center Copenhagen, Rigshospitalet University Clinic, Copenhagen, Denmark

David A. Katerndahl
The Dr. Mario E. Ramirez Distinguished Professor, Department of Family and Community Medicine, University of Texas Health Science Center at San Antonio, San Antonio, Texas

Cille Kennedy
Policy Analyst, U.S. Department of Health and Human Services, Washington, D.C.

Michael S. Klinkman
Professor, Department of Family Medicine, University of Michigan Medical School; Chair, Wonca International Classification Committee, Department of Family Medicine, Ann Arbor, Michigan

Nobuko Kobayashi

Norbert Konrad
Professor of Forensic Psychiatry, Institute of Forensic Psychiatry, Charite–University Medecine, Berlin, Germany

Alexander Kornetov

Nenad Kostanjek

Itzhak Levav

Oliver Lewis

Venos Mavreas

Janet Meagher
Divisional Manager of Inclusion, Psychiatric Rehabilitation Australia; Representative, Consumers' Health Forum of Australia, Redfern, NSW, Australia

María Elena Icaza Medina-Mora
Chief Director, Instituto Nacional de Psiquiatria Ramon de la Fuente, Department of Epidemiology & Psychosocial Research, Calzada Mexico-Xochimilco, Mexico

Alberto Minoletti
Associate Professor of Mental Health Policy and Services, School of Public Health, Faculty of Medicine, University of Chile; Former Director, Mental Health Department, Ministry of Health, Chile

Malik Mubbashar
Vice Chancellor, University of Health Sciences, Punjab, Lahore, Pakistan

Srinivasa Murthy
Professor of Psychiatry (Retired), National Institute of Mental Health and Neurosciences, Bangalore, India

William E. Narrow
Associate Director, Division of Research, and Associate Director, American Psychiatric Institute for Research and Education, American Psychiatric Association, Arlington, Virginia; Research Director, DSM-5 Task Force

David M. Ndetei
Professor of Psychiatry, University of Nairobi; Director, Africa Mental Health Foundation (AMHF), Nairobi, Kenya

Inger Nilsson

Frank G. Njenga
Past President, Kenya Psychiatric Association, Nairobi, Kenya

Olabisi Odejide
Professor of Psychiatry, College of Medicine, University of Ibadan, Nigeria

Edgardo Perez
Homewood Health Center, Guelph, Ontario, Canada; Clinical Professor of Psychiatry, University of Toronto, McMaster University and University of Ottawa; Adjunct Professor, School of Public Health and Health Systems, University of Waterloo, Guelph, Ontario, Canada

Robert M. Plovnick
Director, Department of Quality Improvement and Psychiatric Services, American Psychiatric Association, Arlington, Virginia

Svetlana V. Polubinskaya
Chief Research Officer, Institute of State and Law, Russian Academy of the Sciences, Moscow, Russia

Darrel A. Regier
Executive Director, American Psychiatric Institute for Research and Education; Director, Division of Research, American Psychiatric Association, Arlington, Virginia; and Vice-Chair, DSM-5 Task Force

David Reiss
Affiliated Scientist, Oregon Social Learning Center, Eugene, Oregon

Genevra Richardson
Professor of Law, King's College, London, United Kingdom

Diana Rose
Reader in User-Led Research, Head of Section and Co-director, Service User Research Enterprise (SURE), Health Services and Population Research, Institute of Psychiatry at King's College London, London, United Kingdom

Khalid Saeed
Regional Advisor Mental Health and Substance Abuse, Division of Health Promotion and Protection, World Health Organization, Regional Office for the Eastern Mediterranean Region, Cairo, Egypt

Benedetto Saraceno
Professor of Psychiatry and Director of WHO Collaborating Center on Mental Health of the University of Geneva, Switzerland

Norman Sartorius
President, Association for the Improvement of Mental Health Programmes (AMH), Geneva, Switzerland

Shekhar Saxena
Director, Department of Mental Health and Substance Abuse, World Health Organization, Geneva, Switzerland

Liz Sayce

Pratap Sharan
Professor, Department of Psychiatry, All India Institute of Medical Sciences, New Delhi, India

Shona Sturgeon
Immediate Past President, World Federation for Mental Health, Department of Social Development, University of Cape Town, Rondebosch, Republic of South Africa

Carlos Téllez

Graham Thornicroft
Professor of Community Psychiatry and Head, Health Service and Population Research Department; Consultant Psychiatrist and Director of Research and Development, South London and Maudsley NHS Foundation Trust, Institute of Psychiatry at King's College London, London, United Kingdom

Francisco Torres-Gonzalez
Senior Researcher, Centro Investigación Biomédica en Red de Salud Mental (CIBERSAM), Faculty of Medicine, Granada University, Granada, Spain

Pichet Udomratn
Songklanagarind University Hospital , Department of Psychiatry, Faculty of Medicine, Prince of Songkla University, Songkhla, Thailand

Bedirhan Üstün
Coordinator, Classification, Terminology and Standards, Health Statistics and Informatics, World Health Organization, Geneva, Switzerland

Martti Virtanen
Nordic Centre for Classifications in Health Care, Uppsala, Sweden

Jerome C. Wakefield
University Professor, Professor of Social Work, and Professor of Psychiatry, New York University; Research Professor, Institute for Social and Psychiatric Initiatives, Bellevue, New York, New York

Mitchell G. Weiss
Titular Professor, University of Basel, Swiss Tropical and Public Health Institute, Department of Epidemiology and Public Health, Basel, Switzerland

Liu Xiehe

Disclosure of Competing Interests

The following contributors to this book have indicated financial interests in or other affiliations with a commercial supporter, a manufacturer of a commercial product, a provider of a commercial service, a nongovernmental organization, and/or a government agency, as listed below:

Bruce Arroll—The author is a member of the educational committee for Pharmac, the New Zealand government purchasing agency for medications.

David A. Katerndahl—The author owns stock in Abbott Laboratories.

Michael S. Klinkman—The author is a co-inventory of a medical quality management software application (Cielo Clinic) licensed through the University of Michigan Office of Technology Transfer. As one of the inventors of the software, the author has received royalties from Cielo for external sales. The author received stock options from CieloMedSolutions. The author served as a member of the Cielo Medical Advisory Board but received no compensation for this role.

Darrel A. Regier—The author, as Director of American Psychiatric Institute for Research and Education, oversees all federal and industry-sponsored research and research training grants in APIRE but receives no external salary funding or honoraria from any government or industry.

Norman Sartorius—The author has participated as a speaker or chairperson in symposium organized by Eli Lilly and Lundbeck. The author has served as a consultant to Eli Lilly, Lundbeck, and Servier.

The following contributors to this book do not have any conflicts of interest to disclose:

Margarita Alegría
Julio Arboleda-Flórez
Daniel H. Chisholm
Frank deGruy III
Christopher Dowrick
Patricia Esparza
Linda Gask
Howard H. Goldman
Oye Gureje
Helen Herrman
Marcela V. Horvitz-Lennon
Teh-wei Hu
William E. Narrow
Diana Rose
Khalid Saeed
Benedetto Saraceno

Shekhar Saxena
Graham Thornicroft

FOREWORD

Darrel A. Regier
Shekhar Saxena

This monograph presents technical reviews presented in the World Health Organization–American Psychiatric Institute for Research and Education (WHO-APIRE) conference "Public Health Aspects of Diagnosis and Classification of Mental Disorders." This conference was one in a series of conferences organized by APIRE collectively entitled *The Future of Psychiatric Diagnosis: Refining the Research Agenda.* The organization of these conferences was facilitated by a grant from the National Institutes of Health to APIRE and WHO.

The conference was organized by APIRE and WHO and had the objective of reviewing the available evidence and experience on public health implications of diagnosis and classification of mental disorders. This material is relevant for the ongoing development of the fifth edition of *Diagnostic and Statistical Manual of Mental Disorders* (DSM-5) and the mental and behavioral disorders chapter of the 11th edition of *International Classification of Diseases* (ICD-11). The conference was chaired by Benedetto Saraceno, M.D., and Norman Sartorius, M.D., Ph.D. The steering committee included, besides the chairs, Darrel A. Regier, M.D., M.P.H., Shekhar Saxena, M.D., and Graham Thornicroft, Ph.D., F.R.C.Psych.

The preparation of the conference included formation of international Conference Expert Groups (CEGs) around a series of relevant topics. The CEGs were asked to prepare background papers based on a review of literature, personal knowledge, and experience of the members. The topics of the background papers were selected for their relevance to the theme of the conference and on the expectation that sufficient material would be available internationally on the topic. These included topics such as the public health implications of defining mental disorders, service user and carer perspectives, disease prevention, delivery of mental health treatment in

A working paper for the WHO/APIRE conference held in Geneva, Switzerland, September 2007, was the basis for this chapter. The authors wish to thank Drs. L. Kirmayer, J. Orley, and N. Rose for their very useful comments on early versions of that working paper.

primary care, economic aspects, statistical aspects, forensic aspects, disability and diagnosis, and education and training aspects. The background papers prepared by the CEGs were discussed in the conference and subsequently revised. Especially valuable was the contribution of chairs of other conferences in this series. Additional material was also added after a selective search of more recent literature. This monograph is a collection of this material, edited for consistency and ease of understanding for broader audiences.

The WHO has always considered the global public health perspective to be important to the revision of diagnoses and classification systems for mental disorders. Public health needs and applications must be considered in the process of revision as well as reflected in the content and use of the diagnoses and classification systems. These applications include uniform recording and reporting of individual- as well as population-level health and disease data. Diagnosis and classification systems for mental disorders also need to be appropriate and usable in a variety of settings and by a variety of health personnel, leading to improvement of quality and quantity of care provided to persons with mental and behavioral disorders in all regions of the world.

The WHO and the American Psychiatric Association believe that this monograph will be useful to the advisory groups, task forces, and working groups for the revision of DSM-5, ICD-11, and future classifications. It is also expected to be useful for researchers in the area of diagnosis and classification and more generally in public health. This monograph will likely lead to generations of more research findings in areas that are particularly deficient in evidence.

INTRODUCTION

Public Health and the Classification of Mental Disorders

Norman Sartorius

Itzhak Levav

Jerome C. Wakefield

Mitchell G. Weiss

We should precede any discussion about a classification of mental disorders and its uses with an acknowledgment of the significant difference between psychiatry and programs for the mental health of populations. *Psychiatry* is a medical discipline, the main tasks of which are treatment of mental disorders and advocacy for prevention of the disorders and the promotion of mental health. *Mental health programs* are agglomerates of activities taken jointly by all the social sectors concerned—health, social welfare, education, labor, and others—that aim at prevention of mental disorders, improvement of human relationships, appropriate consideration of psychosocial aspects of health and development, and many other objectives in addition to the organization of health services for the mentally ill and their families.

In this introduction, we focus on mental disorders and the contribution that psychiatry can make to their classification within the framework of public health efforts to reduce disease and disability in the population at large. A detailed consideration of interrelations between the introduction of a classification of mental disorders and the development of mental health programs would surpass the frame of this introduction; therefore, we do not attempt such an endeavor here.

Most definitions of *public health* refer to the prevention and treatment of "disease," and a generally accepted definition of *diseases* helps in the planning of health services, the design of preventive interventions in the rehabilitation of people with disabilities, and the promotion of health. The problem with focusing public health action in psychiatry is that in the field of psychiatry, no conditions correspond to the nosological class of "diseases" because the conditions do not satisfy criteria that allow listing of a condition as a disease.[1]

---

[1]The nosological requirements to name a condition a disease include a statement of an established cause of its pathogenesis, clinical symptoms, and natural history and outcome.

ICD-10 (World Health Organization 1992) used the term *disorder* for conditions whose treatment is considered the principal task of psychiatry. Admittedly, this term is imprecise and creates problems of denotation and connotation when translated into the working languages of the World Health Organization (WHO) and other languages. However, there is a long tradition of using this term to refer to mental disorders, both in the medical sense in which normal human functioning is disturbed and to contrast such conditions with states that are normal responses to difficult circumstances. For example, *disorder* was already the term of choice for mental pathology in various entries of Samuel Johnson's *Dictionary of the English Language,* published in 1755. In October 1844, in the second issue of the *American Journal of Insanity* (later to morph into the *American Journal of Psychiatry*), the editor, Amariah Brigham, published an essay, "The Definition of Insanity," that begins, "By Insanity is generally understood some disorder of the faculties of the mind" (Brigham 1844, p. 97). The bibliography notes that Dr. Henry Johnson (1843) had published a book, *On the Arrangement and Nomenclature of Mental Disorders,* just the year before. The *Diagnostic and Statistical Manual of Mental Disorders* (DSM) of the American Psychiatric Association has used this title since the first edition in 1952. The advantage of using the term *disorder* is that it covers all sorts of medically relevant failures of normal functioning, including diseases and consequences of traumatic injuries.

Mental disorders are defined for various purposes by many actors—by the medical profession, governments (and their different sectors), the general population, social scientists, insurance companies, industries, various "interest groups," individuals who have mental health problems, and families who have a member with such problems. There is substantial, although by no means complete, agreement between the definitions made by the different actors as to the most severe forms of mental disorder. Agreement is less clear for less severe forms of disorder. We would expect such differences because each group approaches the task of delineating the domain of mental disorder with its own goals in mind. Furthermore, although there is continuity of descriptions (though not of their names) of some disorders (e.g., bipolar illness) through the ages, definitions and descriptions of mental disorders have changed considerably over time, and there is rarely a synchrony between the changes made by the groups mentioned previously. Despite differences, the similarities in underlying intuitions about major groups are sufficiently similar to allow a dialogue, in general terms, even if there is much disagreement about the definition of disorders subsumed under larger headings.

The medical and the legal professions have supported the notions that medical diagnoses of mental disorders are the best definitions of mental disorders and that all concerned should accept them as such. These definitions refer to symptoms and signs as well as to the course of development of the disorder and include instructions about ways of searching for symptoms, signs, and other features of a condition. There is general agreement that symptoms and information about the clinical course of the condition over time should enter into the definition of the disorder. There is a considerable debate about using information about the level of functioning in social roles when making the diagnosis. Social functioning depends, to a large extent, on the environment and the people surrounding the person with a problem. Finding employment, for example, depends on the technical capacity and personality of the individual who seeks it, on the situation in the labor market, and on the levels of prejudice prevailing in society. Functioning in other social roles is similarly dependent on the personality and capacity of the individual and other factors. The ICD has avoided use of the level of social functioning as a criterion for a diagnosis because an international classification has to be suitable for use in a variety of countries, and the norms of performance in social roles and expectations about such performance may differ significantly from one setting to another. DSM-IV (American Psychiatric Association 2000) includes level of functioning on a separate axis rather than making it a criterion for an Axis I disorder.

One could argue that all definitions of mental disorders have the same value and that there is no justification for primacy of the medical professions' definition of mental disorder. The way in which a group of people belonging to a particular cultural group label abnormalities of behavior allows communication about the disorder among members of the group and thus satisfies the main purpose of use of a defining label. Car insurance companies often define and give a label to a particular health state based on its consequence in terms of impairment or likely disability—thus grouping the damage to visual acuity that follows an accident with other impairments that produce a similar loss of function.

It is possible to list numerous other intragroup uses of definitions of disorders, and it is probable that these definitions survive because they serve the purpose of communication within the group. For a variety of reasons, the classifications of some of these groups may gain wider use or acceptance for some time before being replaced by classifications produced by others.

There are, however, serious disadvantages to the position that each group should have its own definitions of mental disorders. Such a situation makes communication among those who are concerned with mental disorders difficult, especially across institutions or social domains that must, in an overall public health system, be in continuous communication. Absence of a set of definitions of mental disorders, based on the best of evidence and on consensus between stakeholders, might open the way to abuse of psychiatry (and medicine). A government could decide that a certain type of activity (that goes against the state) is irrational and therefore a mental disorder. It also then could request placement of an individual with such behavior into an institution created to house people with mental disorder. A cultural or subcultural group may deny treatment access to people with mental disorders or expel them under the belief that such behavior is not the consequence of an illness but malevolence or lack of willingness to adjust to cultural norms.

Thus, although it is important to understand the ways in which different stake-holders in the field of mental health speak about mental disorder, it also is necessary to strive for acceptance of a scientifically based system of diagnosis and definition of morbid state. Such a system will allow communication among medical professionals and scientists as well as the planning of measures to help affected individuals and society as a whole.

At the same time, however, acceptance of a medically based system of diagnosis and definitions is not eternal; the system needs periodic revision and improvements, taking into account not only the advances of science and the accumulation of experience but also the opinions of persons who have mental disorders and those who care for these individuals. Many terms used have terrible connotations and stigmatize individuals who are labeled by such terms;[2] other terms are no more than sophisticated jargon that could well be replaced by ordinary words rather than remain hidden behind Latin or Greek words. The development of a structure that will allow equitable consideration of the evidence as well as of the experience, opinions, and needs of all of the stakeholders is clearly a major challenge that must be faced without delay.

The system of diagnosis and definitions of mental disorders are not immune to influences that have no basis in science but reflect vested or declared interests of various groups in society. Thus, producers of devices that change sleep patterns might wish to see a particular sleep pattern declared a medical disorder because that would allow prescription of the use of such devices as well as reimbursement of their cost and increased sales. Producers of a particular drug that could deal with a specific problem might try to influence the bodies revising the diagnostic criteria and the classifications in order to give a specific diagnostic label to such a problem and thus define it as a separate disorder.[3] Social groups that feel wronged by the existence of a diagnostic term might fight to remove such a term from the nomenclature of diseases and from the list of accepted diagnoses.[4] Groups of patients might also request removal of a disorder from one chapter of the classification and placement elsewhere.[5] Political and social pressures might also facilitate, or lead

---

[2]Through a joint effort of the Japanese Society of Psychiatry and Neurology and several groups of families and users of psychiatric services, the term *schizophrenia* has been removed from legal and medical language in Japan.

[3]The introduction of a medication shown to be effective in panic disorder influenced, at least in part, the subsequent introduction of panic disorder as a separate category into most classifications of mental disorders.

[4]For example, it was for this reason that the American Psychiatric Association removed homosexuality from classification of mental disorders.

[5]The history of placement of the diagnosis "chronic fatigue syndrome" in the classification illustrates this kind of effort.

to, the introduction of a diagnostic label into practice and into the system of classification.[6]

The definitions of mental disorders,[7] as well as changes in their definitions, have a variety of consequences for individuals who have mental health problems, their families, the organization and evaluation of health services, the financing of mental health care, and the government, with its various social sectors, ranging from health to education, social welfare, and labor. This is particularly true for the boundary between mental disorders and problems of living but also holds for the distinction among disorders.

For the individuals concerned, the definition of disorders makes the difference between having problems and having a diagnosis of a mental disorder. The latter might entitle individuals to care, change their relationships with their families, lead to receiving sickness benefits, and change their perceptions of themselves. It also might mean stigmatization, rejection by family and community, loss of employment, and blocking of career paths.

For the family of an afflicted individual, the definition of a disorder and the consequent labeling of the member's mental health problems as a mental disorder also has important implications. This distinction may lead to a feeling of guilt about things done or not done; sometimes it might lead to a decision to hide the person with the problem or to chase him or her away to reduce the stigmatization of the family that persists in most countries of the world. In some instances, the stress of having a family member with a mental disorder may lead to severe damage to family relations—transmission of culture, care for sick or elderly members, upbringing of children, contribution to the community, and economic productivity. Many of these consequences are due to the stigma attached to mental disorders, not to the act of defining a disorder: unfortunately, however, stigma of mental illness is still omnipresent, and it is not possible to disentangle the impact of this stigma from the act of defining the disorder.

For science, also, definition of mental disorders based on their medical diagnosis has numerous consequences. The definition of disorders will guide epidemiological studies that aim to discover causes, course, and outcomes of mental disorders. Definitions will also have a major impact on the composition of groups of individuals participating in biological and psychopharmacological research and on interpretation of findings from these scientific studies.

---

[6]The introduction of posttraumatic stress disorder as a category of the classification exemplifies such a situation.

[7]It is important to remember that consequences of the labels subsumed under the title "mental disorder" differ to a significant degree: thus, the label *schizophrenia* has very different consequences from the label *anxiety disorder*.

The definitions of mental disorders have direct consequences for public health action. Definitions affect the estimation of needs for service and the evaluation of performance of mental health and general health care services. In disaster situations, the definition of mental disorders may determine how much of often-limited resources will be reserved for professional psychiatric interventions and how much will be used to provide direct material help to those affected. Definitions will also affect economic analyses and estimation of burden of disease—calculations that have been gaining in importance in recent years. They have a direct influence on the level of priority given to mental health programs at national and local levels.

It is useful to remember that the relation between prevalence of mental disorders—dependent on methods of investigation and definitions of mental disorders—and estimation of needs for services is not simple. There are diseases and disorders for which health systems have no effective and acceptable intervention; people with such disorders might need social services or other help from society, but estimations of health-service needs should not include them. Similarly, people who have symptoms of a mental disorder but who do not wish to receive mental health care, having found a way to cope with their problems without the intervention of health services, may also be excluded from the measurement of unmet needs for mental health services.[8] Estimations of needs for health care (or other services) must also take into account the fact that people seek help when a medical condition causes distress and/or disability and that distressed people may not necessarily have a diagnosable disorder, in terms of the prevailing operational classifications.

Definitions of mental disorders will also have a direct impact on financial arrangements for mental health care. Definition will determine which interventions insurance schemes will or will not pay for, which often makes the difference between individuals receiving care and not receiving it.

Finally, definitions of mental disorders have a significant impact on education and training of health personnel. Health workers receive training that should enable them to deal with medically defined disorders: in most instances, their education pays little, if any, attention to teaching about ways of dealing with other problems that patients might have. In their practices, health workers often will have to spend much of their time dealing with problems that do not amount to a disorder or that have only indirect links to the diseases that their patients have. The workers often will try to avoid dealing with such problems in order to concentrate on what they can diagnose as an illness with a specific treatment. Health care workers are thus more likely to take mental health problems seriously if they see them as a mental disorder.

---

[8]It is questionable whether it is useful in such cases to make the diagnosis of a mental disorder and record it, but this may negate efforts to develop better interventions.

This is not how things should be; health workers should give attention to the treatment of diseases and the support of their patients in any way possible. Yet the introduction of operational definitions contained in current classification systems—which were undoubtedly a great step forward in scientific terms—also meant that subthreshold conditions (i.e., conditions that do not meet criteria of a disorder) receive little attention. However, the subthreshold conditions might cause just as much distress and disability as conditions that do meet criteria for a disorder and may well be worthy of intervention. The biases in the present system and specifically the possibility of receiving greater attention and help if a condition is classified as a disorder tempt practitioners, and sometimes those seeking help, to medicalize conditions despite the consequences that this might have on the choice of intervention and on an individual's life. Thus, the process of defining mental disorders must go hand-in-hand with devotion to serve all those who require help, regardless of whether they have a medically defined disorder or other problems that endanger or affect their health.

Because definitions of mental disorders have so many consequences for affected individuals, those who care for them, their communities, and society as a whole, it is important to base the definition process on available scientific evidence, careful conceptual and theoretical analysis, and an examination of experience. Adherence to these principles may ensure protection of both the classification and definitions of mental disorders and of the interests of all stakeholders—including patients and their families—from untoward commercial, political, and personal influences.

References

American Psychiatric Association: Diagnostic and Statistical Manual of Mental Disorders, 4th Edition, Text Revision. Washington, DC, American Psychiatric Association, 2000

Brigham A (ed): Definition of insanity: nature of the disease, article 1. The American Journal of Insanity 1:97–115, 1844

Johnson H: On the Arrangement and Nomenclature of Mental Disorders: A Prize Essay, to which the Society for the Improvement of the Condition of the Insane awarded the prize of twenty guineas, March, 1843. London, Longmans, 1843

World Health Organization: The ICD-10 Classification of Mental and Behavioral Disorders: Clinical Descriptions and Diagnostic Guidelines. Geneva, World Health Organization, 1992

PREFACE

WHO Perspectives on Stakeholder Involvement in Revision of the Diagnosis and Classification of Mental Disorders

Benedetto Saraceno

The World Health Organization (WHO) defines a *classification* as a system of categories of morbid entities assigned according to an established set of criteria. WHO classifications provide the framework for the organization's vital role in collating and interpreting mortality and morbidity information from 192 member countries. In addition, WHO classifications serve important functions in enabling communication between health professionals and among those professionals, their patients, and the health systems in which they work. WHO classifications also serve other sectors, including health policy makers and payers of health care services, judicial systems, and governments. Classifications also make possible comparative clinical and epidemiological studies and facilitate the training of health professionals across countries and cultures.

Because of their broad importance, WHO considers that classifications should be designed in consultation and, where possible, collaboration with stakeholders. I have enumerated the most important direct stakeholders in WHO classifications. It is partly WHO's responsibility to these stakeholders that differentiates WHO's position in relation to the *International Classification of Diseases* (ICD) revision from the position of the American Psychiatric Association with regard to the *Diagnostic and Statistical Manual of Mental Disorders* (DSM).

The first direct stakeholder group to which WHO considers itself accountable consists of governments of WHO member countries. These governments have specific interests in ICD for three main reasons. First, governments are asked to report morbidity and mortality statistics to WHO according to the ICD classification. Second, governments want health classification to reflect their particular perspectives and priorities for health care. For example, governments may not share the assumption that categories of mental illness are both culturally universal and adequately defined by existing categories. In spite of repeated calls for more attention to the interaction of culture and psychiatric diagnosis, the dominant psychiatric establishment has generally not viewed attention to culture as essential to developing a body of universal knowledge. An increasing inclination to frame psychiatry as exclusively based on the biological underpinnings of mental disorders has exacerbated this tendency. WHO views attention to the cultural framework to be a key element in developing future classifications and diagnostic criteria. Third, governments are interested in the ICD because diagnostic classification provides a large part of the framework that defines a government's obligations to provide free or subsidized health care services, social services, and disability benefits to its citizens. For example, currently there is a discussion in many countries about parity between mental health benefits and benefits for other medical and surgical conditions. People are more likely to have access to mental health services if a precise, valid, and clinically useful classification system is available.

For the mental disorders classification within ICD, WHO recognizes the users of mental health services and their family members as a second direct stakeholder group. This group has increasingly aligned itself with the disability-rights movement, adopting the motto of "Nothing about us without us," rejecting what they see as medical paternalism, and demanding to be consulted about decisions that affect their lives. The ICD revision process must encompass substantive and serious opportunities for participation of this group, not just symbolic and ritualistic gestures. This will raise a variety of issues in relation to the divergent perspectives and priorities and representativeness of different individuals and advocacy organizations; the compatibility of their views with the professional model of mental health care; and the conflicts of interest that may characterize some of these organizations based on their having been established and funded by the pharmaceutical industry. Meaningful collaboration will not be an easy process, but it is a necessary one.

The third important group of direct stakeholders in the revision of the ICD mental health classification consists of health care professionals. Psychiatrists are not the only professionals involved in the diagnosis and classification of mental disorders. This stakeholder group also includes other mental health professionals such as psychologists, social workers, nurses, other physician groups (most especially primary care physicians), and lay health care workers who deliver most of the primary and mental health care in some developing countries. Until now, psychiatry as a profession has occupied an exclusive and privileged position in creation and revision of the diagnostic classification for mental disorders. WHO's view is that other professional groups also should have a meaningful and proportionate role in the process. Geographic and linguistic diversity need to be addressed carefully in creating mechanisms for such participation, because it is generally professionals from wealthier, usually Anglophone, countries who can most easily participate. Another influence the process must address seriously is that of the pharmaceutical industry on other groups of professionals. To avoid undue influence it will be necessary to strengthen scrutiny of possible conflicts of interest among participants involved in revision of the classification of mental disorders and diagnostic criteria.

The same level of participation will not be necessary for every stakeholder. Participation may be conceptualized in terms of four levels: 1) informing, 2) listening, 3) soliciting advice, and 4) working in partnership. Of course, every process of revising diagnostic criteria and classification has its own specificities. Those who initiate such a process have a responsibility to consider carefully the appropriate and necessary level of involvement for each category of stakeholder.

1

SERVICE USER AND CARER STAKEHOLDER PERSPECTIVES ON THE PUBLIC HEALTH ASPECTS OF DIAGNOSIS AND CLASSIFICATION OF MENTAL ILLNESSES

Diana Rose
Graham Thornicroft
Nobuko Kobayashi
Oliver Lewis
Janet Meagher
Inger Nilsson

In this chapter, we discuss a series of key issues relating to psychiatric diagnoses (and their implications) that are important for two particular stakeholder groups: service users/consumers and family members/carers. We address these themes from the point of view of the stakeholder groups. Although these groups are the

---

The quotations in this chapter are from Thornicroft G: *Shunned: Discrimination Against People With Mental Illness.* Oxford, UK, Oxford University Press, 2006.

primary intended beneficiaries of treatment and care, relatively few scientific reports represent their views directly. Many researchers have taken a stakeholder
point of view into account (Entwistle et al. 1998) in relation to particular treatments (Castle et al. 2002; Rose et al. 2005); needs for care (Beeforth and Wood
2001; Leese et al. 1998); types of psychiatric services (Dickey and Wagenaar 1994;
Lester et al. 2003; O'Toole et al. 2004; Okin et al. 1983; Rose 2001; Shepherd et
al. 1995); and employment (Dalgin and Gilbride 2003), but this is less often the
case for diagnosis and classification (Sartorius 1988; Tylee 1999; Wasow 1983).

Currently, we have no consensus on relevant terminology. The terms *service user,*
consumer, client, survivor, and *person with mental illness* are commonly used in the
relevant literature, whereas *patient* is still common in many clinical contexts. In
this chapter, we use *service user/consumer,* which is an unsatisfactory hybrid that we
nonetheless hope is clear to the reader (Rose 2001; Rose and Lucas 2006; Rose et
al. 2002, 2006).

> The issue of stigma against mental illness sometimes feels like the worst
> part about it. I find that nearly every day I find myself lying or dodging ques-
> tions to cover up my history of manic depression in an attempt to avoid the
> stigma that I perceive I'd encounter otherwise. I tend to explore what people
> think of it "under cover" when I get the chance. For example, if I've just met
> someone who is talking about a person they know who had a mental illness,
> I won't let on that I have suffered, but instead I'll try to find out what they
> genuinely think about it. I do this because I need to know who is prejudiced
> and to keep in touch with what people think generally.
>
> Robert

Help Seeking in Relation to Diagnosis

There is evidence that information in the public domain about diagnoses can have
a profound effect on individuals seeking help for mental health problems. We consider here the example of young people who have features of mental disorder. Most
such young people do not seek help (Bailey 1999; Kessler et al. 2005; Sawyer et
al. 2001; Weiss 1994; Zachrisson et al. 2006). Yet indicators of mental illnesses
among children and adolescents are common, affecting about 10% of young people (Bilenberg et al. 2005; Ford et al. 2003). The rates for some mental disorders,
including suicide, are increasing (Costello et al. 2006; McClure 2001). Up to half
of young people who fail to complete secondary school have mental illness (Stoep
et al. 2003). Those who have such illness more often turn to friends and family for
help than to health professionals (Evans et al. 2005; Jorm et al. 2000).

Teenagers seek help less often than do adults (Oliver et al. 2005). As few as 4%
of young people with a mental illness seek help from a family doctor (Potts et al. 2001),

and consultation rates are especially low among young men (Biddle et al. 2004). We argue that the stigma against mental illness is a powerful (and potentially reversible) contributory factor toward the reluctance of many young people to seek help for mental illness.

Research on help seeking has paid particular attention to the confidentiality of health care, young people's knowledge about services, and the accessibility of those services (Booth et al. 2004). However, such factors do not explain fully the very low rates of consultation among young people who are mentally ill (Tyssen et al. 2004; Zwaanswijk et al. 2003). Recent work has focused attention on whether young people know enough to allow them to identify mental illness in themselves or their peers correctly (so-called mental health literacy; Burns and Rapee 2006), as well as on their emotional/attitudinal responses (and associated stigma) toward people with mental illness and treatments of mental illness, as potential explanatory factors for help seeking or help avoidance (Angermeyer et al. 1999).

In relation to knowledge about mental illness, it is clear that there are striking knowledge gaps (Gasquet et al. 1997; Hinshaw and Cicchetti 2000; Secker et al. 1999). For example, in Scotland most children do not know what to do if they have a mental health problem or what to recommend to a friend with mental health difficulties. Only 1% mentioned school counseling, 1% nominated help lines, 4% recommended talking with friends, and 10% said that they would turn to a doctor, but more than one-third (35%) were unsure where to find help (Braunholtz et al. 2004).

There is also fairly strong evidence that negative emotions and attitudes act as barriers to care. Compared with adults, young people have less favorable attitudes toward people with mental illness (Stuart and Arboleda-Flórez 2001). Conversely, young people with mental illness may be exposed to higher levels of stigma than adults (Thara and Srinivasan 2000). Commonly, young people feel that mental illness is embarrassing (Barney et al. 2006) and should be handled privately; people with these views tend to seek help less often (Chew-Graham et al. 2003; Corrigan et al. 2005; Gould et al. 2004).

Attributions for the cause of the condition are also important. Young people who believe that mental illnesses are the responsibility of the person affected are more likely to react to people who are mentally ill with anger, pitilessness, or avoidance (Corrigan et al. 2005). Therefore, there are grounds to consider that stigma may be one important factor in reducing help seeking for mental illnesses, for example, by causing people to avoid the embarrassment of receiving a diagnosis (Chew-Graham et al. 2003; Hugo et al. 2003; Saldivia et al. 2004).

A recent study investigated whether accurate recognition and labeling of mental illness diagnoses are associated with better help-seeking preferences in young people ages 12–25 years (Wright et al. 2007). After being shown a vignette of a young person with either depression or psychosis, each participant was asked what he or she thought was wrong with the person in the vignette, how long the person should wait to get help, and what form of help the person should seek. Results showed that the young people who correctly labeled the disorder were also those who most often identified help-seeking and treatment options. Within the public domain, there is both widespread ignorance and misinformation about mental disorders. A series of popular "myths," examples of which are given below, are still commonplace (Hegner 2000; Jones and Hayward 2004; Social Exclusion Unit 2004):

- Schizophrenia means a split personality.
- All "schizophrenics" are violent and dangerous.
- People with serious mental illness are completely disabled.
- Schizophrenia means you can never do anything with your life.
- Schizophrenia represents a form of creative "inner journey."
- People with mental illness are lazy and not trying.
- It's all the fault of their genes.
- People with mental illness cannot work.
- They are incapable of making their own decisions.
- There's no hope for people with mental illnesses.
- Mental illnesses cannot affect me.
- Mental illness is the same as mental retardation.
- Once people develop mental illnesses, they will never recover.
- Mental illnesses are brought on by a weakness of character.
- Psychiatric disorders are not true medical illnesses like diabetes.
- Mental illness is the result of bad parenting.
- Depression results from a personality weakness or character flaw, and people who are depressed could just snap out of it if they tried hard enough.
- Depression is a normal part of the aging process.
- If you have a mental illness, you can will it away, and being treated for a psychiatric disorder means you have in some way "failed" or are weak.

However, we do not know if such low levels of accurate information about people with a diagnosis of mental illnesses are consistent among different countries and cultures. Information here is sparse (Thornicroft 2006), but several points are clear. First, there is no known country, society, or culture in which people with a mental illness diagnosis are considered to have the same value and to be as acceptable as people who do not have mental illness. Second, the quality of information that we have is relatively poor, with very few comparative studies between countries or over time. We do, however, need to distinguish between sparse information and wrong or misinformation (myths). Third, there do seem to be clear links among popular understandings of the meaning of a diagnosis of mental illness, people's willingness to seek help, and whether they feel able to disclose their problems (Littlewood 1998). The core experiences of shame (to oneself and one's family) and blame (from others) are common everywhere in studies of stigma, but to differing extents. In comparisons with people with other conditions, such as visual impairment, people with a diagnosis of mental illness were more, and in some cases far more, stigmatized (Lai et al. 2001; Lee et al. 2005), and mental illnesses were considered the "ultimate stigma" (Falk 2001). Finally, rejection and avoidance of people with a diagnosis of mental illness appear to be universal phenomena.

Avoidance of Help Seeking for Fear of Receiving a Psychiatric Diagnosis

Although research findings lead us to expect that up to a third of the population will have a clear-cut mental illness each year, in every country studied, two-thirds or more (70%) of people who are mentally ill go fully untreated (Kessler et al. 2005). This situation is true even in countries with the best resources: in the United States, almost a third (30.5%) of the population is affected by mental illness each year; nevertheless, 67% of these individuals do not receive formal treatment (Kessler et al. 2005). Similarly, across Europe, mental illness affects 27% of the population each year (Wittchen and Jacobi 2005), of whom 74% receive no treatment (Alonso et al. 2007). By comparison, only 8% of people with diabetes mellitus do not receive care (Alonso et al. 2007). We would argue that one factor in avoiding help seeking is the fear of receiving a psychiatric diagnosis. A linked issue may be a reluctance on the part of people who suspect they may have a mental illness to present for assessment because they might be prescribed medication they wish to avoid (Jaycox et al. 2006).

> Nobody knows what it feels like, nobody.
>
> Robert

Diagnosis and Service Users/Consumers

DETERMINING HOW ACCEPTABLE DIAGNOSES ARE TO SERVICE USERS/CONSUMERS

Very few reports in the literature consider diagnoses from the point of view of service users/consumers. One important dimension is whether users consider the diagnostic process to be one of simple allocation of a label or one of negotiation. One study found that when the process was considered one of negotiation, the person was more satisfied with his or her care. Indeed, although researchers have explored these issues in detail in relation to treatment for forms of cancer (Cox et al. 2006; Fallowfield and Jenkins 2004, 2006), so far such issues have been largely ignored in relation to mental disorders, except for Alzheimer's disease (Bamford et al. 2004).

I can't have schizophrenia because I'm not a violent person.

Leroy

RECEIVING A NEGATIVE LABEL VERSUS NAMING A PERSONAL PROBLEM

A person with mental illness may perceive receiving a diagnosis as the naming of something fearful and previously without meaning, thus "containing" a fearful process. On the other hand, the diagnosis can be seen as a pernicious label. For example, in one study people with a diagnosis of personality disorder were asked about their reactions to the diagnosis. On some occasions, people found the diagnosis helpful in making sense of experiences that previously made no sense and thereby giving a name to a personal problem; on other occasions, they found the diagnosis unhelpful and stigmatizing.

These two reactions may be different for different diagnoses. For example, depression may be a more acceptable diagnosis than schizophrenia or personality disorder (Crisp 2004). Furthermore, we should not forget that the relationship between mental health professional and service user is not equal in the diagnostic process.

ASSESSING SERVICE USERS'/CONSUMERS' EXPERIENCES OF BEING (RE)DIAGNOSED

It is common for a service user/consumer to be given one (or several) diagnoses at one time and for these diagnoses to be changed at another time. For example, the average time from onset to a diagnosis of bipolar disorder is more than 10 years (Berk et al. 2007). Prior to this, service users/consumers most often receive diagnoses of either unipolar depression or personality disorder (or both). Once again, receiving a new diagnosis can be a relief that the problem is finally clearly understood, especially when the new diagnosis is a better "match" to the service user's subjective experience. However, it also is possible that the service user will be very confused by these multiple and changing diagnoses.

USING DIAGNOSTIC TERMS FOR SICKNESS CERTIFICATIONS

When people with mental illness require sickness certification by a doctor for a period of absence from work, it is common for them to encourage the doctor to avoid using any term that refers specifically to mental illness. In this case, a generic term such as *stress* may be preferred. Declaring a more severe diagnosis may assist the person with mental illness gain welfare benefits on a more secure long-term basis. Some studies show, for example, that almost half of all sickness certificates are because of mental disorders (Shiels et al. 2004); in fact, not as many mental disorders are clearly identified as reasons for work absence because medical practitioners may be complicit in seeking to avoid potentially stigmatizing reactions to a clear-cut diagnostic term (Haldorsen et al. 1996). Indeed, mental illness predicts a longer period of certification than most physical disorders (Dunner et al. 2001), and there appear to be growing requirements for sickness certification in some countries (Hensing et al. 2006).

Advantages and Disadvantages of Having or Accepting a Diagnosis

A series of positive consequences can follow the acceptance—or at least the partial or provisional acceptance—of a diagnosis by a person with mental distress. The person can access information about that condition, for example, its features, associations, treatment, and prognosis, and test how far this information matches his or her own experience. The primary diagnosis may also bring relief from worry that the problem was some other condition. A clear diagnosis may allow a person to gain access to self-help groups of people with the condition and find mutual support there: for example, on how to self-manage the disorder (Mueser et al. 2006), how to self-assess progress (Salyers et al. 2007), or how to cope with impairments in everyday life that are consequent upon the condition (Mueser and Gingerich 2005). Agreement on a diagnosis can also allow a person to seek referral to treatment centers specializing in treatment of this particular condition. Diagnosis can offer a rationale for experiences and confusions and, if dealt with carefully, can assist a move to acceptance and self-directed rehabilitation and recovery.

One of the disadvantages of receiving a diagnosis is the association of mental illness with violence (Thornicroft 2006). However, this association is gradually changing for those with common mental disorders and seems to apply more to diagnoses such as paranoid schizophrenia. Such a diagnosis might be devastating for a person. Interestingly, Lakoff (2006) found that when patients presented with psychotic symptoms, psychiatrists in the Argentine Republic always began with a diagnosis of bipolar disorder because they thought this less stigmatizing than a diagnosis of schizophrenia.

A further set of concerns revolves around implications for treatability/untreatability: the belief that the course of the illness will be chronic and the worry, often reinforced by doctors, that there is a strong likelihood of recurrence after a first episode (Repper and Perkins 2003). Once again, such concerns are more likely for a particular range of mental health problems and are not always assuaged by mental health professionals.

There may be a concern about genetic transmission to children, which is likely to be particularly frightening if the person already has children. Those who do not may be persuaded that they should not (Phelan et al. 2006). Genetic counseling may be complicit with this, and of course many geneticists, and some researchers, believe that psychotic illnesses are inherited.

There are further worries about a loss of human rights, for example, through incapacity determinations and compulsory treatments (Amnesty International 2000). This is particularly the case for coercive measures such as seclusion and control and restraint in some countries, mechanical and pharmacological restraints in others, and the use of "cage beds" in some Eastern European countries (Bartlett et al. 2006). We need to ask serious questions about the "therapeutic" validity and value of such measures. Concern about the effects of stigma and discrimination are realistic. Forms of discrimination in financial services, such as taking out loans; in buying insurance; in travel, such as restrictions posed by visas; and in employment and occupation all affect people with psychiatric diagnoses. Are diagnoses helpful at all in these situations, or do we need to address the associated discrimination directly?

Finally, service users/consumers often receive poor care for physical ailments. "Diagnostic overshadowing" means that physical problems are seen through the lens of the psychiatric diagnosis, leading to underinvestigation and undertreatment (Coghlan et al. 2001; Disability Rights Commission 2006; Druss 2000). This overshadowing can lead to higher mortality rates from physical disorders for people with concurrent physical disorders.

Self-Stigmatization Following Diagnosis

A very important consequence of diagnosis is that some people with mental illness come to see this not as one feature of their lives but as the defining aspect of their core identity (Corrigan 2005), sometimes called a "master status" (Smart and Wegner 2000). This definition is encouraged by the common use in medical and research writings of terms such as "schizophrenics" or "depressives," whereas it would be unacceptable to refer to people with heart disease as "cardiacs." The progression from seeing oneself as having a particular condition (along with many other characteristics and attributes) to being identified essentially by the disorder is a crucial step, because these labels confer a lower social value on people to whom they stick (Biernat and Dovidio 2000; Dovidio et al. 2000; Smart and Wegner 1999, 2000) both in the person's own eyes and in the estimation of others.

Thus, not only do others tend to attach a lower social value to people they know to have a diagnosis of mental illness but also people with a diagnosis of mental illness can perform worse if their diagnosis is revealed to others or if they believe this to be true. In a series of studies, students with a history of psychiatric treatment were asked to undertake tests of intellectual performance. In some of the tests, others knew their diagnosis in the group. In other tests, their medical history was concealed. Results showed that students who revealed their psychiatric history did worse on the reasoning test than did those who concealed their mental health status (Quinn et al. 2004).

> I have a friend who is very stigmatizing when he talks about people with mental illness. For this reason I hide my problem. I know that if he knew about me he would break up our friendship.
>
> Alex

One interesting example of the link between diagnosis and self-stigmatization is the association between having a diagnosis of an eating disorder and self-esteem. Although eating disorders are sometimes described in relation to low self-esteem (Geller et al. 2002; Polivy and Herman 2002; Steinberg and Shaw 1997), other studies show that people who are overweight show few or no differences in self-esteem compared with those of normal weight (Miller and Downey 1999). Another example refers to African Americans, a group for whom there is clear evidence of widespread discrimination (Williams 1999), yet available evidence indicates that, if anything, levels of self-esteem are higher among African Americans than among people in the United States of European descent (Gray-Little and Hafdahl 2000). This suggests that the relations between core ingredients of stigma and discrimination are not fixed, but vary according to their social and cultural context.

In short, the social identity of people with mental illness can be influenced by a person's own sense of what it means to have a mental illness, by expected discriminatory reactions of others, and by the actual reactions of others. Combinations of these factors can lead to material poverty (Estroff 1985), social marginalization (Dear and Wolch 1992), and reduced social participation (Social Exclusion Unit 2004).

Evidence we have discussed in this chapter leads to the following conclusions:

1. The experience of mental illness may depend on the mix of several factors at the same time.
2. An intervention for one particular aspect—for example, control (Fogarty 1997), self-esteem (Link et al. 2001), or acceptance, rejection, or denial (Camp et al. 2002; Pyne et al. 2001) of the diagnosis—may have consequences in other domains (e.g., in employment).
3. Such experiences may vary in different places or at different times and thus may be changeable (Corrigan 2005; Estroff et al. 2004).

The International Study of Discrimination and Stigma Outcomes (INDIGO), in 28 countries across the world, conducted face-to-face interviews with 736 people with a clinical diagnosis of schizophrenia. The main purpose of the study was to assess anticipated and experienced discrimination. Several questions related to the name of the condition. In reply to the question "Do you know what diagnosis your doctor has made?," 83% answered yes; to the question "Do you agree with the diagnosis?," 72% agreed, 17% disagreed, and 10% were unsure. When asked "How much has it been an advantage or disadvantage for you to have the specific diagnosis of schizophrenia?," 54% reported disadvantage, 26% reported advantage (e.g., in directing them to information on the condition, to a self-help group, or to assistance with housing or welfare benefits), and 18% reported no difference. Therefore, most people given, or offered, this diagnosis saw it, on balance, as a negative rather than a positive attribute (Thornicroft et al. 2007).

Reactions to Being Offered a Diagnosis

On receiving a diagnosis, some service users/consumers simply deny it. Often this is because of social stigma attached to psychiatric diagnoses, as discussed earlier. Service users/consumers may feel that accepting a diagnosis is just too much to bear and thus may bury the very idea that such a label has been attached to them. Rejection of a diagnosis is a stronger form of denial. The diagnosis may be seen as unwelcome, even as an affront. Rejection of the diagnosis then may lead to rejection of the psychiatric profession and unwillingness to comply with suggested treatment. Once again, there may be differences between different diagnoses, with people who are given the more serious diagnoses being most likely to reject them. People with mental health problems are part of the society in which they live, so it is unsurprising that they share in societal beliefs and feelings.

Changing Diagnostic Terms

In a unique move undertaken to reduce social rejection, the name for schizophrenia was changed in Japan. Following a decade of pressure from family member groups, including Zenkaren, the name for this condition was changed from *seishin bunretsu byo* (split-mind disorder) to *togo shiccho sho* (integrative disorder) (Desapriya and Nobutada 2002; Takizawa 1993). With the previous term, only 20% of people with this condition were told the diagnosis by their doctors (Goto 2003; Kim and Berrios 2001; Mino et al. 2001). There are indications, from service users/consumers and family members, that the new term is seen as less stigmatizing and more often discussed openly. This is consistent with work in the Federal Republic of Germany suggesting that giving the label "schizophrenia" has a significant and negative effect on public perceptions (Angermeyer and Matschinger 2005).

The Treatment Gap

It is important to put the use of psychiatric diagnoses within the wider context of how far these conditions are treated or neglected. Although each year up to 30% of the population worldwide has some form of mental illness, at least two-thirds of these people receive no treatment. This undertreatment occurs even in countries with the best resources (Kohn et al. 2004). In the United States, for example, 31% of the population is affected by mental illness every year, but 67% of these individuals are not treated (Kessler et al. 2005). Moreover, in Europe mental illness affects 27% of people every year; 74% receive no treatment (Wittchen and Jacobi 2005). The proportions of people with mental illness who are treated are far lower in low- and middle-income countries. For example, a recent worldwide survey found that the proportion of respondents receiving mental health care over 12 months was as low as 1.6% in the Federal Republic of Nigeria and that in most of the 17 countries studied, only a minority of people with severe disorder received treatment (Wang et al. 2007).

A World Health Organization (WHO) review of 37 studies across the world found the proportions of people untreated for particular conditions were as follows: schizophrenia, 32.2%; depression, 56.3%; dysthymia, 56.0%; bipolar disorder, 50.2%; panic disorder, 55.9%; generalized anxiety disorder, 57.5%; obsessive-compulsive disorder, 57.3%; and alcohol abuse and dependence, 78.1% (Kohn et al. 2004; Wittchen and Jacobi 2005; World Health Organization 2005). Indeed, in one particular study of depressed people in St. Petersburg, Russia, only 3% were treated (Simon et al. 2004), both because of the low level of coverage of services and because of demand-limiting factors such as the need for out-of-pocket payments to afford treatment.

In our view, two contributory factors toward this degree of neglect are 1) the reluctance of many people to seek help for mental illness–related problems because of the anticipated stigma, should they be diagnosed; and 2) the reluctance of many people who do have a diagnosis of mental illness to advocate for better mental health care for fear of shame and rejection if they disclose their condition (Kohn et al. 2004).

Multiple Perspectives on What Is Evidence in Relation to Diagnosis

Recently, there has been a rapid growth in the involvement of service users/ consumers in the conducting of research and the debate over what constitutes evidence (Rose et al. 2006). Over the past 5 years, service-user research has "grown wings and begun to fly" (Strategies for Living 2003). One example of such research is the Review of Consumers' Perspectives on Electro-Convulsive Therapy (Rose et al. 2003). This study was commissioned by the Department of Health in England alongside a meta-analysis of trials of the effectiveness and safety of the treatment. The two empirical researchers on the project had experienced electroconvulsive therapy (ECT) themselves; the team also included a psychiatrist and a psychologist whose roles were to help with analysis and reporting.

This review relied on existing materials and used 26 papers written by clinical academics and 9 authored by consumers or in collaboration with consumers. In addition, 139 "testimonies," or firsthand accounts, of receiving ECT were gathered; most of these were in electronic form, mainly from the Internet. The scientific papers reported much higher levels of satisfaction with ECT than did either the user-led research or the testimonies. A standard response to this finding is that the user-led research and testimonies relied on biased sampling. However, because the user-researchers on the project not only had experienced the treatment but also had experienced being in the hospital and being interviewed as to whether this treatment had helped, it seemed to them that other explanations were at least as plausible.

The academic articles that reported the highest levels of satisfaction had a very particular methodology. Satisfaction interviews were conducted as soon as treatment ended, or even during treatment, and the interviewer was the treating doctor, who asked a few simple questions. From the personal experience of the researchers they considered that, under these circumstances, users would not want to complain or might not tell the truth, either to avoid more treatments or simply to get rid of the doctor who was asking yet more questions! Therefore, it was argued that these academic papers were overestimating user satisfaction with ECT. This use of personal experience led to novel results, in contrast to previously received psychiatric wisdom.

One critique of the evidence-based medicine approach is that the biomedical model on which it is based is not fully applicable to mental health; unlike other areas of medicine, in psychiatry, diagnosis is not disease. Therefore, the use of nomothetic (group-level) designs, such as randomized controlled trials, in preference to idiographic (individually focused) methodologies neglects the importance of differing individual experiences and meanings of mental health problems. In some more economically developed nations, consumer involvement in research is beginning to become more common.

Perspectives of Carers

The research reviewed previously was conducted by service users/consumers themselves. Carers have conducted no comparable research. In addition, few studies have considered what kind of evidence carers favor or how they would prioritize the content of research. However, carers and their priorities have been subjects of research by professionals. Here, studies have been conducted on the issues most salient to carers. Several recurrent themes emerged, namely, a sense of loss of expected future of the affected relative; concerns for their own mental health, especially in terms of anxiety and depression; financial worries; the need for respite breaks; a clear requirement for information and advice on the psychiatric condition, its cause, and future treatment and care options; and fear for a future when they can no longer provide care (Berry et al. 1997; Lefley 1989; Perlick et al. 1999, 2004).

During the past 20 years, we increasingly have recognized that not only are people with mental illness the butt of limited understanding, prejudiced attitudes, and discriminatory behavior but their family members are as well. In 1989, almost 500 members of the National Alliance for the Mentally Ill in 20 U.S. states were surveyed about their experiences. They expressed very clear and consistent views. Almost all identified stigma as a key problem for their mentally ill relatives. They said that the most common effects of stigma on their relatives were damage to self-esteem, difficulty making and keeping friends, difficulty finding a job, and reluctance to admit mental illness. In terms of the worst effects that family members experienced themselves, the most serious problems were lowered self-esteem and damaged family relationships. Family members gave mental health professionals mixed reviews. Although not generally viewed as contributing to stigma, professionals were seen as generally unhelpful in dealing with stigma (Wahl and Harman 1989).

How does stigma affect families? One study in the United States examined this question among 156 parents and spouses of people who had been admitted to a psychiatric hospital for the first time. Although most family members did not see themselves as being shunned by others, half did say that they tried to hide the fact of hospital admission. Family members with more education or whose relative had been unwell recently reported more avoidance by others (Phelan et al. 1998).

Most reports on effects on family members refer to families with a person diagnosed as having schizophrenia (like most of the literature on stigma). An exception is a study with more than 500 family members in New York that compared the views of families of people diagnosed with major depression, schizophrenia, or bipolar disorder (Struening et al. 2001). Interestingly, no differences emerged between these three groups, but experience of ignorance and prejudice was the rule rather than the exception. About half of family members agreed with the following statements:

- Most people in my community would rather not be friends with families who have mentally ill relatives living with them.
- Most people look down on families who have a mentally ill member living with them.
- Most people believe their friends would not visit them as often if a member of the family were hospitalized with serious mental illness.
- Most people would rather not visit families with a member who is mentally ill.

The study concluded that both people with mental illness and their families feel devalued by their predicaments. In other words, a family's reputation was lower because of the presence of a family member with a diagnosis of mental illness.

Developing a Multiple-Perspectives Paradigm

From the preceding discussion, we can see that it is not so much that these stakeholder groups take differing views on which evidence to prioritize but rather that the epistemological status of evidence is now often disputed (Wakefield 2005). Service user–led or –controlled studies are more often within qualitative scientific traditions, whereas practitioner-led research more often is quantitative. In part, this reflects a long-standing ambivalence about the nature of evidence that is reflected in its very definition, being both 1) available facts, circumstances, etc., indicating whether a thing is true or valid (permanently true); and 2) in law, information tending to prove a fact or proposition, statements or proofs admissible as testimony in a law court. Indeed, it is this contestability and contestation that are progressively introducing a need to develop an integrative paradigm that can interrelate differing forms of knowledge to contribute to a more satisfactory evidence base.

Even within an empirical paradigm, approaches are available that directly incorporate more than one perspective. Partly randomized preference trials, for example, can compare two or more treatment conditions when treatment preferences of service users/consumers are taken into account. These trials allow preferred treatment options to be provided; randomization, then, is applied only to those people who have expressed no clear treatment preference. This design allows both treatment effects and preference effects to be estimated in the analyses (Chamberlin 2005; Rose et al. 2003).

A related approach within the empirical tradition is to rate, separately, the views of staff and service users/consumers and to make explicit comparisons, for example, as to what extent needs are met or unmet. In one study in London, for example, an epidemiologically representative group of 137 service users/consumers with an ICD-10 (World Health Organization 1992) diagnosis of a functional psychotic disorder was assessed cross-sectionally by users themselves and by staff (Slade et al. 1998) using the Camberwell Assessment of Need (Slade et al. 1999). Yet another approach to including several perspectives simultaneously includes arrangements such as joint crisis plans, crisis cards, and advanced directives that aim to achieve agreement between staff and service users/consumers on the future-care plan (Flood et al. 2006; Henderson et al. 2004). In relation to diagnosis, specifically, this approach suggests that a full assessment of experienced symptoms of mental illness is based on full disclosure by the service user/consumer made in the context of a strong and trusting therapeutic relationship. In this case, a service user is likely to disclose more information if the user feels his or her perspective is taken seriously by the clinician (Bindman et al. 2005).

The central tension we have identified is between differing paradigms for understanding mental disorder that lead to contradictory methodologies for scientific inquiry. For example, these paradigmatic differences underpin recent debate on the scientific importance of individual case studies. How can these tensions and contradictions be managed, if not resolved? We propose that work continue to build what we refer to as a "multiple perspectives" paradigm to integrate these varied sources of evidence. In the meanwhile, we propose increasing service user access to setting research questions, developing a wider range of interventions assessed, creating and consolidating structures to develop service user and carer research, and using research designs that actively take account of service-user preferences. These steps can be taken in a context where it is necessary to admit that the overall evidence base is relatively weak in mental health; there is a predominance of quantitative over qualitative evidence; research questions are usually set by researchers and policy makers; and there is rarely qualitative-quantitative cross-fertilization of ideas or research methods. Meanwhile, in conceptual and methodological work, it is now timely to extend current early approaches to multimethods research so as to more firmly ground it in a nascent paradigm that values multiple perspectives on evidence in mental health (Thomas et al. 2004).

In this chapter, we have focused narrowly on views and interests of service users/consumers and family members/carers, but of course a far wider range of stakeholders have interests in current and new diagnostic systems. As the WHO Department of Mental Health and Substance Abuse has argued, the wider range of people and organizations concerned with diagnostic systems for mental illnesses will include governments and their policy implementation agencies, the whole range of professionals and practitioners active in the field of mental health, those creating products and services used in the treatment of people with mental illness, and professionals within the criminal justice system and the field of occupational health and medicine. For each of these constituencies, the challenge arises of how to meaningfully engage them in the process of revising the diagnostic and classification systems.

> The next time that you call someone strange, "nutter," "psycho," "weirdo," silently or not, consider what it would be like to be in their shoes. Try and empathize. One day you might be in a similar position. How would you want society to treat you then? I used to be extremely sensitive when I heard people I know use words like those above. Everyone is entitled to his or her beliefs and opinions, but how to challenge those when you believe that they are wrong is an area that needs further work. We don't realize how damaging the language we use can be sometimes. I questioned someone that I knew about this, asking them if they thought the same about me, as I my-

self have mental health problems. The response was "No, you are different." I ask myself, why is it different? They know me, have grown up with me, and have seen how I have been affected by my life experiences. Apply this to a stranger, and where is the difference? Ignorance is not bliss, it is just ignorance.

Martina

Recommendations

In writing this chapter, it has become clear to us that many of the issues we raise have little formal scientific evidence base—for example, whether adopting a negotiating approach to communication about diagnoses is in fact beneficial. The stigma and discrimination of people given a diagnosis of schizophrenia can be grave and adversely influence their quality of life as well as the course and outcome of the condition (Sartorius and Schulze 2005; Thornicroft 2006). In other domains of medicine, there are numerous examples of name changes intended to make a condition "more speakable," for example, Hansen's disease ("leprosy") or Down syndrome ("mongolism"), the name of which has been changed repeatedly over the past century without clear data on whether this has been beneficial (Jain et al. 2002). These debates were rarely illuminated by evidence. We therefore have identified key recommendations on current action, on how to strengthen the evidence base on public health implications of diagnostic and classificatory systems, and on implementation of these systems.

Concerning what can be done, given current knowledge, we recommend that developers of the new system of classification of mental disorders take into account the following concerns:

- New classifications should not be "totalizing." In other words, mental health professionals should not assume that a diagnosis of mental disorder should be used as the essential defining feature of a person (so-called master identity).
- Clinicians should be given guidance on assisting service users/consumers to recognize fully their assets and the positive aspects of their lives when a diagnostic consultation takes place.
- Each diagnosis should contain "criteria" that state that the diagnosis "does not preclude X," where X is a positive attribute (such as being able to marry or work); this will strengthen the previous recommendation.
- The new diagnostic manual should contain a chapter explaining to clinicians how psychiatric diagnoses, especially those that may be severely disabling, may have profoundly stigmatizing effects. Guidance should be provided on how this knowledge should be woven into any consultation in which a diagnosis is given or discussed, along with references to resources that can assist individuals and families in coping with stigmatizing reactions from others.

- A short, user-friendly version of any new diagnostic manual should be prepared so that service users/consumers know what their doctor is talking about. A loose-leaf format would enable a service user to be given the information relevant to the diagnosis he or she has been assigned. Knowledge should not be esoteric.
- A variety of stakeholders should be involved in the process of revision, particularly consumers/users of mental health services. Efforts should be made to inform these stakeholders about the ICD and DSM revision processes, and their responses should be taken seriously.
- A training program should be developed to educate clinicians and others involved in the health care system about how the process of diagnosis can affect consumers/users of mental health services and about sensitive and appropriate ways to manage communication about diagnosis.
- Ethical principles related to the diagnosis of mental disorders should be compiled for inclusion in the front of the classification (e.g., warnings against misuse of the diagnosis, use of person-first language, avoiding the use of diagnoses as names).

For the future, research is needed to clarify

- Whether changing the names and diagnostic terms applied to conditions changes their degree of stigmatization (Lieberman and First 2007), for example, the implications of renaming manic depression as bipolar disorder. It is notable that when diagnostic terms have been changed, such as the renaming of schizophrenia in Japan, the proportion of such people who were told the name of their condition reportedly increased from 8% to 60% (Kim and Berrios 2001).
- Whether there is a need for a greater understanding by mental health professionals of explanatory models of health and the differences between the paradigms of the staff making and giving diagnoses and the people receiving these diagnoses (Cox et al. 2006).
- The effects of different methods of giving/offering diagnoses, the comprehensibility of different rationales for the diagnosis, and how far these are accepted by service users/consumers.
- The implications of involvement of service users/consumers as active participants in a negotiation process and whether such a process changes the acceptability to service users/consumers of receiving a diagnosis.
- The consequences of involving service users/consumers in policy decisions stemming from different diagnoses, for example, in relation to welfare benefits or access to driving licenses. This will include developing methods to properly sample representative views across target groups of service users/consumers, such as User-Focused Monitoring (Rose et al. 1998), or samples of people treated by mental health services (Thornicroft et al. 2007)
- The extent to which receiving a diagnosis is experienced as an empowering or a dis-empowering process by services users/consumers.

- The extent to which diagnostic information should be tailored to the needs of each person in terms of rationale and implications for care.
- Whether decision-aid methods assist in the communication of diagnoses, for example, materials available from the Internet that set out evidence-based treatment options for each particular condition.
- Key aspects of how diagnoses can be offered by professionals and practitioners in ways that are relevant and acceptable to service users/consumers in high-, medium-, and low-resource settings (Lancet Global Mental Health Group 2007; Saxena et al. 2007).
- The effect of giving opportunities to engage carers and family members in information sharing at the time of diagnosis, as well as the proper and practical limits of confidentiality.

Conclusions

In this chapter, we presented evidence that many people with mental illness are faced with forms of discrimination that have the effect of promoting social exclusion. These processes appear to be active in every country where they have been studied. Discrimination can be effected both by others against a person with mental illness (e.g., by not hiring a person for a job) and by the person with mental illness (e.g., in deciding not to apply for a job while expecting rejection); the latter has been described as self-stigma or anticipated discrimination. One consequence of the widespread cultural acceptance of these processes of social exclusion is that many people with possible mental illness are reluctant to present for assessment and treatment, fearing a diagnosis of mental illness. Another consequence is that mental health care, as a whole, has been subjected to what may be called "structural" discrimination, namely, levels of resource investment far lower than the scale necessary to respond to actual prevalence levels of mental disorders. The net result is that, worldwide, at least 75% of people with mental disorders are untreated. We argue that the series of steps discussed in our recommendations will make a contribution toward reducing the harm that follows from stigmatization and discrimination.

References

Alonso J, Codony M, Kovess V, et al: Population level of unmet need for mental healthcare in Europe. Br J Psychiatry 190:299–306, 2007

Amnesty International: Ethical Codes and Declarations Relevant to the Health Professions, 4th Revised Edition. London, Amnesty International, 2000

Angermeyer MC, Matschinger H: Labeling—stereotype—discrimination: an investigation of the stigma process. Soc Psychiatry Psychiatr Epidemiol 40:391–395, 2005

Angermeyer MC, Matschinger H, Riedel-Heller SG: Whom to ask for help in case of a mental disorder? Preferences of the lay public. Soc Psychiatry Psychiatr Epidemiol 34:202–210, 1999

Bailey S: Young people, mental illness and stigmatisation. Psychiatr Bull 23:107–110, 1999

Bamford C, Lamont S, Eccles M, et al: Disclosing a diagnosis of dementia: a systematic review. Int J Geriatr Psychiatry 19:151–169, 2004

Barney LJ, Griffiths KM, Jorm AF, et al: Stigma about depression and its impact on help-seeking intentions. Aust N Z J Psychiatry 40:51–54, 2006

Bartlett P, Lewis O, Thorold O: Mental Disability and the European Convention on Human Rights: International Studies in Human Rights. Leiden, The Netherlands, Martinus Nijhoff, 2006

Beeforth M, Wood H: Needs from a user perspective, in Measuring Mental Health Needs, 2nd Edition. Edited by Thornicroft G. London, Royal College of Psychiatrists, 2001, pp 190–199

Berk M, Dodd S, Callaly P, et al: History of illness prior to a diagnosis of bipolar disorder or schizoaffective disorder. J Affect Disord 103:181–186, 2007

Berry D, Szmukler G, Thornicroft G: Living with Schizophrenia: The Carers' Story. Brighton, UK, Pavilion Publishing for Department of Health, 1997

Biddle L, Gunnell D, Sharp D, et al: Factors influencing help seeking in mentally distressed young adults: a cross-sectional survey. Br J Gen Pract 54:248–253, 2004

Biernat M, Dovidio J: Stigma and stereotypes, in The Social Psychology of Stigma. Edited by Heatherton TF, Kleck RE, Hebl MR, et al. New York, Guilford, 2000, pp 88–125

Bilenberg N, Petersen DJ, Hoerder K, et al: The prevalence of child-psychiatric disorders among 8–9-year-old children in Danish mainstream schools. Acta Psychiatr Scand 111:59–67, 2005

Bindman J, Reid Y, Szmuckler G, et al: Perceived coercion at admission to psychiatric hospital and engagement with follow-up: a cohort study. Soc Psychiatry Psychiatr Epidemiol 40:160–166, 2005

Booth ML, Bernard DE, Quine S, et al: Access to health care among Australian adolescents: young people's perspectives and their sociodemographic distribution. J Adolesc Health 34:97–103, 2004

Braunholtz S, Davidson S, King S: Well? What do you think? The Second National Scottish Survey of Public Attitudes to Mental Health, Mental Well-Being and Mental Health Problems. Edinburgh, Scotland, Scottish Executive, 2004. Available at: http://www.scotland.gov.uk/Publications/2005/01/20506/49612. Accessed January 30, 2012.

Burns JR, Rapee RM: Adolescent mental health literacy: young people's knowledge of depression and help seeking. J Adolesc 29:225–239, 2006

Camp DL, Finlay WM, Lyons E: Is low self-esteem an inevitable consequence of stigma? An example from women with chronic mental health problems. Soc Sci Med 55:823–834, 2002

Castle D, Morgan V, Jablensky A: Antipsychotic use in Australia: the patients' perspective. Aust N Z J Psychiatry 36:633–641, 2002

Chamberlin J: User/consumer involvement in mental health service delivery. Epidemiologica e Psichiatria Sociale 14:10–14, 2005

Chew-Graham CA, Rogers A, Yassin N: "I wouldn't want it on my CV or their records": medical students' experiences of help-seeking for mental health problems. Med Educ 37:873–880, 2003

Coghlan R, University of Western Australia, Department of Public Health, et al: Duty to care: physical illness in people with mental illness. Perth, Department of Public Health, Centre for Health Services Research, University of Western Australia, 2001

Corrigan PW: Dealing with stigma through personal disclosure, in On the Stigma of Mental Illness: Practical Strategies for Research and Social Change. Edited by Corrigan PW. Washington, DC, American Psychological Association, 2005, pp 257–280

Corrigan PW, Lurie BD, Goldman HH, et al: How adolescents perceive the stigma of mental illness and alcohol abuse. Psychiatr Serv 56:544–550, 2005

Costello EJ, Foley DL, Angold A: 10-year research update review: the epidemiology of child and adolescent psychiatric disorders, II: developmental epidemiology. J Am Acad Child Adolesc Psychiatry 45:8–25, 2006

Cox A, Jenkins V, Catt S, et al: Information needs and experiences: an audit of UK cancer patients. Eur J Oncol Nurs 10:263–272, 2006

Crisp AH: Every Family in the Land: Understanding Prejudice and Discrimination Against People With Mental Illness, Revised Edition. London, Royal Society of Medicine Press, 2004

Dalgin RS, Gilbride D: Perspectives of people with psychiatric disabilities on employment disclosure. Psychiatr Rehabil J 26:306–310, 2003

Dear MJ, Wolch JR: Landscapes of Despair: From Deinstitutionalization to Homelessness. Princeton, NJ, Princeton University Press, 1992

Desapriya EB, Nobutada I: Stigma of mental illness in Japan. Lancet 359:1866, 2002

Dickey B, Wagenaar H: Evaluating mental health care reform: including the clinician, client, and family perspective. J Ment Health Admin 21:313–319, 1994

Disability Rights Commission: Equal Treatment: Closing the Gap. A Formal Investigation Into Physical Health Inequalities Experienced by People With Learning Disabilities and/or Mental Health Problems. London, Disability Rights Commission, 2006

Dovidio J, Major B, Crocker J: Stigma: introduction and overview, in The Social Psychology of Stigma. Edited by Heatherton TF, Kleck RE, Hebl MR, et al. New York, Guilford, 2000, pp 1–28

Druss BG: Cardiovascular procedures in patients with mental disorders. JAMA 283:3198–3199, 2000

Dunner S, Decrey H, Burnand B, et al: Sickness certification in primary care. Sozial- und Präventivmedizin 46:389–395, 2001

Entwistle VA, Renfrew MJ, Yearley S, et al: Lay perspectives: advantages for health research. BMJ 316:463–466, 1998

Estroff SE: Making It Crazy: An Ethnography of Psychiatric Clients in an American Community. Berkeley, University of California Press, 1985

Estroff SE, Penn DL, Toporek JR: From stigma to discrimination: an analysis of community efforts to reduce the negative consequences of having a psychiatric disorder and label. Schizophr Bull 30:493–509, 2004

Evans E, Hawton K, Rodham K: In what ways are adolescents who engage in self-harm or experience thoughts of self-harm different in terms of help-seeking, communication and coping strategies? J Adolesc 28:573–587, 2005

Falk G: Stigma: How We Treat Outsiders. New York, Prometheus Books, 2001

Fallowfield L, Jenkins V: Communicating sad, bad, and difficult news in medicine. Lancet 363:312–319, 2004

Fallowfield L, Jenkins V: Current concepts of communication skills training in oncology. Recent Results Cancer Res 168:105–112, 2006

Flood C, Byford S, Henderson C, et al: Joint crisis plans for people with psychosis: economic evaluation of a randomised controlled trial. BMJ 333:729–732, 2006

Fogarty JS: Reactance theory and patient noncompliance. Soc Sci Med 45:1277–1288, 1997

Ford T, Goodman R, Meltzer H: The British Child and Adolescent Mental Health Survey 1999: the prevalence of DSM-IV disorders. J Am Acad Child Adolesc Psychiatry 42:1203–1211, 2003

Gasquet I, Chavance M, Ledoux S, et al: Psychosocial factors associated with help-seeking behavior among depressive adolescents. Eur Child Adolesc Psychiatry 6:151–159, 1997

Geller J, Zaitsoff SL, Srikameswaran S: Beyond shape and weight: exploring the relationship between nonbody determinants of self-esteem and eating disorder symptoms in adolescent females. Int J Eat Disord 32:344–351, 2002

Goto M: [Family psychoeducation in Japan]. Seishin Shinkeigaku Zasshi 105:243–247, 2003

Gould MS, Vetting D, Kleinman M, et al: Teenagers' attitudes about coping strategies and help-seeking behavior for suicidality. J Am Acad Child Adolesc Psychiatry 43:1124–1133, 2004

Gray-Little B, Hafdahl AR: Factors influencing racial comparisons of self-esteem: a quantitative review. Psychol Bull 126:26–54, 2000

Haldorsen EM, Brage S, Johannesen TS, et al: Musculoskeletal pain: concepts of disease, illness, and sickness certification in health professionals in Norway. Scand J Rheumatol 25:224–232, 1996

Hegner RE: Dispelling the myths and stigma of mental illness: the Surgeon General's report on mental health. Issue Brief Natl Health Policy Forum 754:1–7, 2000

Henderson C, Flood C, Leese M, et al: Effect of joint crisis plans on use of compulsory treatment in psychiatry: single blind randomised controlled trial. BMJ 329:136, 2004

Hensing G, Andersson L, Brage S: Increase in sickness absence with psychiatric diagnosis in Norway: a general population-based epidemiologic study of age, gender and regional distribution. BMC Med 4:19, 2006

Hinshaw SP, Cicchetti D: Stigma and mental disorder: conceptions of illness, public attitudes, personal disclosure, and social policy. Dev Psychopathol 12:555–598, 2000

Hugo CJ, Boshoff DE, Traut A, et al: Community attitudes toward and knowledge of mental illness in South Africa. Soc Psychiatry Psychiatr Epidemiol 38:715–719, 2003

Jain R, Thomasma DC, Ragas R: Down syndrome: still a social stigma. Am J Perinatol 19:99–108, 2002

Jaycox LH, Asarnow JR, Sherbourne CD, et al: Adolescent primary care patients' preferences for depression treatment. Adm Policy Ment Health 33:198–207, 2006

Jones S, Hayward P: Coping with Schizophrenia: A Guide for Patients, Families and Carers. Oxford, UK, Oneworld Publications, 2004

Jorm AF, Medway J, Christensen H, et al: Attitudes towards people with depression: effects on the public's help-seeking and outcome when experiencing common psychiatric symptoms. Aust N Z J Psychiatry 34:612–618, 2000

Kessler RC, Demler O, Frank RG, et al: Prevalence and treatment of mental disorders, 1990 to 2003. N Engl J Med 352:2515–2523, 2005

Kim Y, Berrios GE: Impact of the term schizophrenia on the culture of ideograph: the Japanese experience. Schizophr Bull 27:181–185, 2001

Kohn R, Saxena S, Levav I, et al: The treatment gap in mental health care. Bull World Health Organ 82:858–866, 2004

Lai YM, Hong CP, Chee CY: Stigma of mental illness. Singapore Med J 42:111–114, 2001

Lakoff A: Pharmaceutical Reason: Knowledge and Value in Global Psychiatry. New York, Cambridge University Press, 2006

Lancet Global Mental Health Group, Chisholm D, Flisher AJ, et al: Scale up services for mental disorders: a call for action. Lancet 370:1241–1252, 2007

Lee S, Lee MT, Chiu MY, et al: Experience of social stigma by people with schizophrenia in Hong Kong. Br J Psychiatry 186:153–157, 2005

Leese M, Johnson S, Slade M, et al: User perspective on needs and satisfaction with mental health services. PRiSM Psychosis Study, 8. Br J Psychiatry 173:409–415, 1998

Lefley HP: Family burden and family stigma in major mental illness. Am Psychol 44:556–560, 1989

Lester H, Tritter JQ, England E: Satisfaction with primary care: the perspectives of people with schizophrenia. Fam Pract 20:508–513, 2003

Lieberman JA, First MB: Renaming schizophrenia. BMJ 334:108, 2007

Link BG, Struening EL, Neese-Todd S, et al: Stigma as a barrier to recovery: the consequences of stigma for the self-esteem of people with mental illnesses. Psychiatr Serv 52:1621–1626, 2001

Littlewood R: Cultural variation in the stigmatisation of mental illness. Lancet 352:1056–1057, 1998

McClure GM: Suicide in children and adolescents in England and Wales 1970–1998. Br J Psychiatry 178:469–474, 2001

Miller CT, Downey KT: A meta-analysis of heavyweight and self-esteem. Pers Soc Psychol Rev 3:68–84, 1999

Mino Y, Yasuda N, Tsuda T, et al: Effects of a one-hour educational program on medical students' attitudes to mental illness. Psychiatry Clin Neurosci 55:501–507, 2001

Mueser KT, Gingerich S: Coping with Schizophrenia: A Guide for Families. New York, Guilford, 2005

Mueser KT, Meyer PS, Penn DL, et al: The Illness Management and Recovery program: rationale, development, and preliminary findings. Schizophr Bull 32(suppl):S32–S43, 2006

O'Toole MS, Ohlsen RI, Taylor TM, et al: Treating first episode psychosis—the service users' perspective: a focus group evaluation. J Psychiatr Ment Health Nurs 11:319–326, 2004

Okin RL, Dolnick JA, Pearsall DT: Patients' perspectives on community alternatives to hospitalization: a follow-up study. Am J Psychiatry 140:1460–1464, 1983

Oliver MI, Pearson N, Coe N, et al: Help-seeking behaviour in men and women with common mental health problems: cross-sectional study. Br J Psychiatry 186:297–301, 2005

Perlick D, Clarkin JF, Sirey J, et al: Burden experienced by care-givers of persons with bipolar affective disorder. Br J Psychiatry 175:56–62, 1999

Perlick DA, Rosenheck RA, Clarkin JF, et al: Impact of family burden and affective response on clinical outcome among patients with bipolar disorder. Psychiatr Serv 55:1029–1035, 2004

Phelan JC, Bromet EJ, Link BG: Psychiatric illness and family stigma. Schizophr Bull 24:115–126, 1998

Phelan JC, Yang LH, Cruz-Rojas R: Effects of attributing serious mental illnesses to genetic causes on orientations to treatment. Psychiatr Serv 57:382–387, 2006

Polivy J, Herman CP: Causes of eating disorders. Annu Rev Psychol 53:187–213, 2002

Potts Y, Gillies ML, Wood SF: Lack of mental well-being in 15-year-olds: an undisclosed iceberg? Fam Pract 18:95–100, 2001

Pyne JM, Bean D, Sullivan G: Characteristics of patients with schizophrenia who do not believe they are mentally ill. J Nerv Ment Dis 189:146–153, 2001

Quinn DM, Kahng SK, Crocker J: Discreditable: stigma effects of revealing a mental illness history on test performance. Pers Soc Psychol Bull 30:803–815, 2004

Repper J, Perkins R: Social Inclusion and Recovery. Edinburgh, Balliere Tindall, 2003

Rose D: Users' Voices: The Perspectives of Mental Health Service Users on Community and Hospital Care. London, The Sainsbury Centre, 2001

Rose D, Lucas J: The User and Survivor Movement in Europe, in Mental Health Policy and Practice Across Europe: The Future Direction of Mental Health Care. Edited by Knapp M, McDaid D, Mossialos E, et al. Maidenhead, Berkshire, UK, Open University Press, 2006

Rose D, Ford R, Lindley P, et al: In Our Experience: User-Focused Monitoring of Mental Health Services. London, Sainsbury Centre for Mental Health, 1998

Rose D, Fleischmann P, Tonkiss F, et al: User and carer involvement in change management in a mental health context: review of the literature. London, National Co-ordinating Centre for NHS Service Delivery and Organisation R & D (NCCSDO), 2002

Rose D, Fleischmann P, Wykes T, et al: Patients' perspectives on electroconvulsive therapy: systematic review. BMJ 326:1363, 2003

Rose D, Wykes TH, Bindman JP, et al: Information, consent and perceived coercion: patients" perspectives on electroconvulsive therapy. Br J Psychiatry 186:54–59, 2005

Rose D, Thornicroft G, Slade M: Who decides what evidence is? Developing a multiple perspectives paradigm in mental health. Acta Psychiatr Scand Suppl (429):109–114, 2006

Saldivia S, Vicente B, Kohn R, et al: Use of mental health services in Chile. Psychiatr Serv 55:71–76, 2004

Salyers MP, Godfrey JL, Mueser KT, et al: Measuring illness management outcomes: a psychometric study of clinician and consumer rating scales for illness self management and recovery. Community Ment Health J 43:459–480, 2007

Sartorius N: International perspectives of psychiatric classification. Br J Psychiatry 152 (suppl):9–14, 1988

Sartorius N, Schulze H: Reducing the Stigma of Mental Illness: A Report From a Global Programme of the World Psychiatric Association. Cambridge, UK, Cambridge University Press, 2005

Sawyer MG, Arney FM, Baghurst PA, et al: The mental health of young people in Australia: key findings from the child and adolescent component of the national survey of mental health and well-being. Aust N Z J Psychiatry 35:806–814, 2001

Saxena S, Thornicroft G, Knapp M, et al: Resources for mental health: scarcity, inequity and inefficiency. Lancet 370:878–889, 2007

Secker J, Armstrong C, Hill M: Young people's understanding of mental illness. Health Educ Res 14:729–739, 1999

Shepherd G, Murray A, Muijen M: Perspectives on schizophrenia: a survey of user, family carer and professional views regarding effective care. J Ment Health 4:403–422, 1995

Shiels C, Gabbay MB, Ford FM: Patient factors associated with duration of certified sickness absence and transition to long-term incapacity. Br J Gen Pract 54:86–91, 2004

Simon GE, Gleck M, Lucas R, et al: Prevalence and predictors of depression treatment in an international primary care study. Am J Psychiatry 161:1626–1634, 2004

Slade M, Phelan M, Thornicroft G: A comparison of needs assessed by staff and by an epidemiologically representative sample of patients with psychosis. Psychol Med 28:543–550, 1998

Slade M, Thornicroft G, Loftus L, et al: CAN: the Camberwell Assessment of Need. London, Royal College of Psychiatrists, 1999

Smart L, Wegner D: Covering up what can't be seen: concealable stigma and mental control. J Pers Soc Psychol 77:474–486, 1999

Smart L, Wegner D: The hidden costs of hidden stigma, in The Social Psychology of Stigma. Edited by Heatherton TF, Kleck RE, Hebl MR, et al. New York, Guilford, 2000, pp 220–242

Social Exclusion Unit: Mental Health and Social Exclusion: Social Exclusion Unit Report. London, Office of the Deputy Prime Minister, 2004

Steinberg BE, Shaw RJ: Bulimia as a disturbance of narcissism: self-esteem and the capacity to self-soothe. Addict Behav 22:699–710, 1997

Stoep AV, Weiss NS, Kuo ES, et al: What proportion of failure to complete secondary school in the US population is attributable to adolescent psychiatric disorder? J Behav Health Serv Res 30:119–124, 2003

Strategies for Living: Surviving User-Led Research. London, Mental Health Foundation, 2003

Struening EL, Perlick DA, Link BG, et al: Stigma as a barrier to recovery: the extent to which caregivers believe most people devalue consumers and their families. Psychiatr Serv 52:1633–1638, 2001

Stuart H, Arboleda-Flórez J: Community attitudes toward people with schizophrenia. Can J Psychiatry 46:245–252, 2001

Takizawa T: Patients and their families in Japanese mental health. New Dir Ment Health Serv (60):25–34, 1993

Thara R, Srinivasan TN: How stigmatising is schizophrenia in India? Int J Soc Psychiatry 46:135–141, 2000

Thomas J, Harden A, Oakley A, et al: Integrating qualitative research with trials in systematic reviews.BMJ 328:1010–1012, 2004

Thornicroft G: Shunned: Discrimination Against People With Mental Illness. Oxford, UK, Oxford University Press, 2006

Thornicroft G, Sartorius N, Rose D, et al: Renaming schizophrenia: the need for evidence (letter). BMJ Rapid Response, 2 February 2007

Tylee A: Depression in the community: physician and patient perspective. J Clin Psychiatry 60(suppl):12–16, 1999

Tyssen R, Røvik JO, Vaglum P, et al: Help-seeking for mental health problems among young physicians: is it the most ill that seeks help? A longitudinal and nationwide study. Soc Psychiatry Psychiatr Epidemiol 39:989–993, 2004

Wahl OF, Harman CR: Family views of stigma. Schizophr Bull 15:131–139, 1989

Wakefield JC: On winking at the facts, and losing one's Hare: value pluralism and the harmful dysfunction analysis. World Psychiatry 4:88–89, 2005

Wang PS, Aguilar-Gaxiola S, Alonso J, et al: Use of mental health services for anxiety, mood, and substance disorders in 17 countries in the WHO world mental health (WMH) surveys. Lancet 370:841–850, 2007

Wasow M: Parental perspectives on chronic schizophrenia. J Chronic Dis 36:337–343, 1983

Weiss MF: Children's attitudes toward the mentally ill: an eight-year longitudinal follow-up. Psychol Rep 74:51–56, 1994

Williams DR: Race, socioeconomic status, and health: the added effects of racism and discrimination. Ann N Y Acad Sci 896:173–188, 1999

Wittchen HU, Jacobi F: Size and burden of mental disorders in Europe: a critical review and appraisal of 27 studies. Eur Neuropsychopharmacol 15:357–376, 2005

World Health Organization: The ICD-10 Classification of Mental and Behavioural Disorders: Clinical Descriptions and Diagnostic Guidelines. Geneva, World Health Organization, 1992

World Health Organization: Mental Health Atlas 2005. Geneva, World Health Organization, 2005

Wright A, Jorm AF, Harris MG, et al: What's in a name? Is accurate recognition and labelling of mental disorders by young people associated with better help-seeking and treatment preferences? Soc Psychiatry Psychiatr Epidemiol 42:244–250, 2007

Zachrisson HD, Rodje K, Mykletun A: Utilization of health services in relation to mental health problems in adolescents: a population based survey. BMC Public Health 6:34, 2006

Zwaanswijk M, Van der Ende J, Verhaak PF, et al: Factors associated with adolescent mental health service need and utilization. J Am Acad Child Adolesc Psychiatry 42:692–700, 2003

2

PREVENTION OF MENTAL DISORDERS

*Implications for Revision of
Psychiatric Diagnosis and Classification*

Shekhar Saxena
Pratap Sharan
Michel Botbol
Deborah Hasin
Helen Herrman
Clemens Hosman
Eva Jané-Llopis
David Reiss
Shona Sturgeon

Introduction

PREVENTION OF MENTAL DISORDERS IS A PUBLIC HEALTH PRIORITY, AND THE EVIDENCE BASE TO SUPPORT PREVENTIVE EFFORTS HAS ACCRUED

About 450 million people have mental and behavioral disorders worldwide. One person in four will develop one or more of these disorders during his or her lifetime. Neuropsychiatric conditions account for 13% of total disability-adjusted life-years (DALYs) lost due to all diseases and injuries in the world, and the prevalence of these conditions is estimated to increase to 15% by the year 2020 (World Health Organization 2001b). Five of the 10 leading causes of disability and premature death globally are mental and behavioral disorders, including depression, harmful alcohol use, schizophrenia, and compulsive disorder (World Health Organization 2002). In addition to the health burden, the social and economic costs of ill mental health for societies are wide ranging, long lasting, and enormous and have been estimated at 3%–4% of gross domestic product (International Labour Organization 2000; Smit et al. 2006). Besides the health and social service costs in terms of lost employment and reduced productivity; the effect on families and caregivers, levels of crime, and public safety; and the negative impact of premature mortality, many other immeasurable costs have not been taken into account, such as lost opportunity costs to individuals and families (World Health Organization 2001b). Although evidence-based treatments for many mental and behavioral disorders have advanced greatly in the past few decades, many people with these disorders do not receive the treatments, do not benefit fully from them, or do not benefit at all. Given these limitations in access (Kohn et al. 2004) and effectiveness, prevention can be an additional method for reducing the burden (morbidity and disability as well as economic and social costs) caused by these disorders.

Although medical care can improve prognosis for some illnesses, the social and economic conditions that make people ill and in need of medical care in the first place are more important for the health of the population as a whole (Wilkinson and Marmot 2003). Genetic and individual susceptibilities to disorders are important, but the common causes of the ill health that affects populations are environmental. This is why life expectancy has improved so dramatically over recent generations; it is also why some countries have improved the health of their populations whereas others have not, and it is why health differences between different social groups have widened or narrowed as social and economic conditions have changed (Wilkinson and Marmot 2003; World Health Organization 2002). Populations living in poor socioeconomic circumstances are at increased risk for poor mental health, depression, and lower subjective well-being (European Commission 2005). Other major factors such as urbanization, war and displacement, racial discrimination, and economic instability have been linked to increased levels of psychiatric symptomatology and psychiatric morbidity (Saxena et al. 2006).

For instance, war and war-related traumas increase rates of depression, anxiety, posttraumatic stress disorder, and alcohol-related disorders through exposure both to the traumas and to the resulting poverty and social disruption. Adverse social factors can be even more detrimental when exposure to such events happens during sensitive periods. Numerous studies have provided evidence that severe adverse life events during the prenatal, neonatal, and infancy periods predispose individuals to development of stress-related psychiatric disorders, especially mood and anxiety disorders in adolescence and adulthood (Dawson et al. 2000; Heim and Nemeroff 1999; Sánchez et al. 2001). Social and environmental influences also are associated with alcohol and drug use disorders, including availability (e.g., alcohol outlet density, alcohol policy including state-level alcohol tax [Henderson et al. 2004]); religiosity; country of origin; potentially reflecting contrasting social norms (Hasin et al. 2002a, 2002b); and age-cohort-related exposure to advertising and other purposeful efforts to affect consumption. These influences appear to interact with genetic vulnerability (Spivak et al. 2007).

The approach to mental disorder prevention lies in the concept of public health. Beaglehole et al. (2004) defined *public health* as "collective (or collaborative or organized) action for sustained population-wide health improvement (and the reduction of health inequalities)." They stressed that public health efforts work best if they have a focus on whole populations; an emphasis on prevention, especially primary prevention; and a concern for underlying socioeconomic determinants of health and disease, as well as more proximal risk factors.

Two recent World Health Organization publications present evidence that mental health promotion and mental disorder prevention can be effective in leading to health, social, and economic gains (Herrman et al. 2005; World Health Organization 2004a, 2004b). Prevention strategy can be particularly cost-effective, because small effect sizes in a large number of people can lead to a greater population gain than a large effect size in a small number of people (Rose 1992). The effectiveness and efficiency of prevention strategies are likely to be high and to increase over time because simultaneous positive changes in risk and protective factors have the potential to improve multiple outcomes parameters at a given time point (e.g., symptoms such as anxiety and depression) and also to reduce the occurrence of secondary conditions (e.g., comorbid disorders). A meta-analysis of 69 programs aimed at prevention of depression or depressive symptoms showed them to be equally effective in reducing depressive symptoms, risk factors, and other psychiatric symptoms such as anxiety (Jané-Llopis et al. 2003).

DIAGNOSIS AND CLASSIFICATION INFLUENCE POLICY, PRACTICE, EDUCATION, AND RESEARCH ON PREVENTION

DSM-IV (American Psychiatric Association 1994) and ICD-10 (World Health Organization 1992) are perceived by many as giving scientific credibility to the definition of mental illness and legitimacy to the practice of psychiatry and other mental health disciplines (Regier et al. 2002). Thus, DSM-IV and ICD-10 influence policy decisions, the focus of interventions, pathways to care, and financing of services and research. The research implication is illustrated by the general tendency to give priority to treatment studies over primary prevention research addressing major causes of psychopathology.

THE STRUCTURE OF CURRENT CLASSIFICATORY SYSTEMS IS INADEQUATE FOR COMPREHENSIVE COVERAGE OF PREVENTIVE APPROACHES

Current classificatory systems have been useful to the prevention field by providing an internationally shared framework of concepts, a rule-based classification, and explicit diagnostic criteria. These systems have helped in establishing the epidemiology of disorders, in studying their long-term outcomes and burden to society, in providing comparable rubrics for the study of risk factors, and in testing the effectiveness of preventive measures. These systems do not, however, consider a range of key topics related to prevention because they focus on a relatively narrow segment of psychiatry and essentially serve clinical practice, research, and educational areas of the subject (American Psychiatric Association 2000; Spitzer 2001; World Health Organization 1992).

The perspectives of clinicians and prevention experts overlap partially but not entirely. A clinician is focused on treatment and rehabilitation of individuals or groups—that is, secondary and tertiary prevention. A prevention expert seeks to employ a broader range of health interventions that include preventive, curative, and rehabilitative strategies—that is, primary, secondary, and tertiary prevention—aimed at populations and groups at risk. Clinicians are mainly interested in the current condition of a patient and in diagnostic categories that are narrow and predict treatment response. Prevention experts are relatively more interested in risk (proximal and distal) and causative factors, developmental processes, and diagnostic categories that vary in breadth—broad to general (macro- and meso-level) interventions and narrow for some specific (micro-level) interventions—and are predictive of response to the entire range of preventive (primary, secondary, and tertiary) actions. Perhaps as a consequence of the differences in approach between a clinician and a prevention expert, classificatory systems, which have hitherto focused on clinical conditions, have mostly failed to address issues relevant to prevention adequately. For example, the new diagnoses in the appendix of DSM-IV, namely, mixed anxiety depression, premenstrual dysphoric disorders, age-related cognitive decline, and minor depressive disorder, have great relevance to prevention, yet their inclusion in official classification systems is disputed based on the argument that their boundaries with normalcy are insufficiently precise and their severity is below an appropriate (meaning clinical) threshold, thus they should not be labeled bona fide disorders.

Treatment and prevention start from different perspectives. The clinical approach focuses on an individual with an existing illness. Most evidence-based preventive trials over the past three decades focused on so-called common, or generic, protective and risk factors relevant to the promotion of mental health or on reducing risks of several mental disorders—for example, interventions for increasing self-esteem, emotional resilience, problem-solving and coping skills, prosocial and social skills, parenting behaviors, and social support systems—or on reducing social stressors and emotional vulnerability to social stressors (Jané-Llopis et al. 2003; Mrazek and Haggerty 1994; Mrazek and Hosman 2002). As far as effective preventive efforts that targeted the reduction of symptoms, disability, and disorders, the efforts typically addressed broad categories such as depression (e.g., "Jobs Project for the Unemployed," Caplan et al. 1997; "Penn Resiliency Program," Freres et al. 2002); anxiety symptoms and disorders (e.g., "Friends for Children 7–14 Years," Dadds et al. 1999); externalizing problems and substance abuse (e.g., "Children of Divorce Programs," Wolchik et al. 2000); disruptive child behavior and family relationships ("Positive Parenting Program," Sanders et al. 2002); and suicidal behavior ("Comprehensive School Program," Zenere and Lazarus 1997). Because several mental disorders have major proximal risk factors in common, subdivisions are less relevant to prevention at the macro level of intervention. When subtypes have major subtype-specific and malleable determinants, fine divisions of categories are relevant for prevention (e.g., indicated prevention [meso and micro levels of prevention]). Evidence for effectiveness of indicated prevention is available for many disorders and conditions (Ballesteros et al. 2004; Boath et al. 2005; Cipriani et al. 2005; Cororve Fingeret et al. 2006; Cuijpers et al. 2005; Elder at al. 2004; Faggiano et al. 2005; Tait and Hulse 2003).

THE GAP BETWEEN PREVENTION AND TREATMENT/ REHABILITATION IS NARROWING, MAKING NEGLECT OF PREVENTION ANACHRONISTIC

A focus on prevention in classification is becoming even more relevant as the gap between clinical and preventive fields is narrowing. Clinicians are becoming increasingly involved in treatment of prodromal (premonitory or early signs or symptoms of disorders) and subsyndromal (occurrence of fewer than the required number of signs and symptoms that are believed to characterize a particular abnormality when they occur together as a group) conditions. The response of society to ill mental health is changing, and preventive and promotive interventions are featuring more often on the stakeholders' demand list. Therefore, it is important to develop a classification that serves the range of interventions that can prevent mental disorders.

Prevention of Mental Disorders: Basic Concepts

Clarity about similarities and boundaries between the concepts of mental health and mental illness, and between prevention and promotion, respectively, is an important starting point. The World Health Organization (2001a, p. 1) defines *health* as "a state of complete physical, mental and social well-being and not merely the absence of disease or infirmity." *Positive mental health* is a state of well-being in which the individual realizes his or her own abilities, can cope with the normal stresses of life, can work productively and fruitfully, and is able to make a contribution to his or her community (World Health Organization 2007). *Ill mental health* refers to mental health problems, symptoms, and disorders, including mental health strain and symptoms related to temporary or persistent distress. *Mental disorders* are health conditions characterized by alterations in thinking, mood, or behavior (or some combination thereof) associated with persistent distress. These disorders usually cause substantial impairment in functioning.

Because mental health promotion and mental disorder prevention both deal primarily with enhancement of mental health and the influence of its antecedents, promotion and prevention are best understood as interrelated but conceptually distinct approaches. The distinction between health promotion and prevention lies in their targeted outcomes (Saxena et al. 2006). Mental health promotion aims to promote positive mental health by increasing psychological well-being, competence, and resilience and by creating supporting living conditions and environments. Mental disorder prevention has as its target the reduction of symptoms and, ultimately, of mental disorders. Public health actions of advocacy, communication, policy and legislative change, community participation, and research and evaluation—often in nonhealth sectors—are relevant to promotion and prevention. Evidence is growing for the effectiveness of these actions in several settings for promotion and prevention as well as for improved physical health and productivity. Effective interventions across the life span include support for parents of infants, school-based interventions, workplace and unemployment programs, and activity programs for older adults (Herrman et al. 2005; World Health Organization 2004a, 2004b). Other, more proximal preventive interventions focus predominantly on reducing risk factors and enhancing protective factors associated with mental disorders.

Prevention aims at reducing the incidence, prevalence, and recurrence of mental disorders; the time spent with symptoms; or the risk condition for a mental illness, preventing or delaying recurrences and also decreasing the impact of illness in the affected person, their families, and society. Mrazek and Haggerty's (1994) concept of mental disorder prevention leads to a relevant public-health framework for reducing risk factors and enhancing protective factors. The framework of preventive intervention for mental disorders is based on the classification of physical illness prevention and classic public-health distinctions between primary, secondary, and tertiary prevention. *Primary* prevention is directed toward preventing the initial occurrence of a disorder, and it includes universal, selective, and indicated preventive interventions (Table 2–1). *Secondary* prevention seeks to lower the rate of established cases of the disorder or illness in the population (prevalence) through early detection and treatment of diagnosable diseases. *Tertiary* prevention includes interventions that reduce disability, enhance rehabilitation, and prevent relapses and recurrences of the illness. However, we should emphasize that secondary and primary preventive interventions also affect (reduce or prevent) disability outcomes (Von Korff et al. 2003).

In this chapter, we provide a selective review of universal, selective, and indicated prevention in relation to diagnosis and classification of mental disorders and recommend changes that should be considered during the revision of diagnosis and classification of mental disorders. The focus is on primary prevention of mental disorders, and the supporting literature quoted mostly relates to depression and anxiety; however, that should not be construed to mean that other forms of prevention are less important or unrelated to primary prevention or that literature on other disorders does not exist. Considering that epidemiological data show up to half of lifetime psychiatric disorders, and an even larger percentage of chronic and seriously impairing disorders occur in people with a history of another disorder, we emphasize here the concept of primary prevention of secondary disorders and suicides due to mental disorders (Harkavy-Friedman 2006; Kessler and Price 1993). Connection between primary and other forms of prevention (e.g., treatment) should be kept in mind; for example, there should be no effort to create specific preventive categories that have no clear links with pathological categories, because this could be an obstacle to uniformity in classification and intervention approaches.

Addressing Prevention in the Revision of Classification

Within the spectrum of mental health intervention, prevention and promotion have become realistic and evidence-based options supported by a fast-growing body of knowledge from fields as diverse as developmental psychopathology, psychobiology, and prevention and health promotion sciences. These options bring a new challenge to a classification system: that of defining boundaries of disorders, risk conditions, and normality.

Suggestion: Prevention and articulation between prevention and care should be addressed in revisions of the classification systems. The structure of classification needs to change to address prevention, especially with regard to the following points:

- Risk and protective factors
- Prevention-relevant subthreshold conditions
- Children of mentally ill parents
- Dimensional conceptualization better suited to prevention
- Developmental and longitudinal perspectives
- Accentuation of refined subcategories and consequent comorbidity
- Multiaxial system

TABLE 2–1.   Definitions of various types of prevention and preventive interventions

	Definition
Prevention type	
Primary	Primary prevention attempts to decrease number of *new* cases of a disorder.
Secondary	Secondary prevention is directed at prevalence and seeks to lower the rate of established cases of a disorder.
Tertiary	Tertiary prevention seeks to decrease amount of disability associated with a disorder.
Intervention type	
Prevention	Prevention refers to interventions that occur before initial onset of a disorder.
Universal	Universal preventive interventions are targeted to the general public or a whole population group not identified on the basis of individual risk. The intervention is desirable for everyone (e.g., seat belts, encouragement of safe drinking, reduction of cigarette smoking, healthy eating, exercise).
Selective	Selective preventive interventions are targeted to individuals, or a subgroup of the population, whose risk of developing disorders is significantly higher than average. The risk may be imminent or may be a lifetime risk (e.g., good antenatal and perinatal care in pregnant women; health interventions in young unsupported teenage mothers; and social support for socially isolated elderly people).
Indicated	Indicated preventive interventions are targeted to high-risk individuals who are identified as having minimal but detectable signs or symptoms foreshadowing a disorder but who do not currently meet the diagnostic threshold (e.g., person with prodromal symptoms of schizophrenia when a genetic susceptibility is strongly suspected, or children exposed to disasters or violence).

RISK AND PROTECTIVE FACTORS

Data on disorder or injury outcomes alone, such as death or hospitalization, tend to focus on the need for curative or palliative services. Reliable and comparable analyses of risks to health are critical for preventing disease and injury. After obtaining improved estimates of deaths and disease burden, the World Health Organization invested in the assessment of the disease and injury burden from major risk factors (Ezzati et al. 2004; Murray et al. 2002; World Health Organization 2002). A small number of risks account for large contributions to the global loss of healthy life. Globally, an estimated 45% of mortality and 36% of disease burden were attributable to the joint effects of 19 selected risk factors (high blood pressure; smoking; high cholesterol; childhood underweight; unsafe sex; low fruit and vegetable intake; overweight and obesity; physical inactivity; alcohol use; indoor smoke from household use of solid fuels; unsafe water, sanitation, and hygiene; zinc deficiency; urban air pollution; vitamin A deficiency; iron-deficiency anemia; contaminated injections in health care settings; illicit drug use; use of ineffective methods or nonuse of contraception; and childhood sexual abuse). Furthermore, several risk factors are relatively prominent in some regions at all stages of development. The large global disease burden attributable to the selected risk factors highlights the relevance and importance of prevention policies and programs that reduce risk-factor exposure. Diagnosis and classification need to take into account this shift.

Over the past decade, researchers have made much progress in developing evidence-based strategies to reduce the risk of mental disorders (Clarke et al. 1995; Cuijpers et al. 2005; Faggiano et al. 2005; Hannan et al. 2005; Harnett and Dadds 2004; Hosman and Jané-Llopis 1999; Kowalenko et al. 2005; Mifsud and Rapee 2005; Mrazek and Haggerty 1994; O'Kearney et al. 2006; Roberts et al. 2004; Sheffield et al. 2006; Spence et al. 2005; World Health Organization 2004a, 2004b). Some examples of evidence-supported risk and protective factors with a bearing on mental health and ill health are listed in Table 2–2. As discussed later in this chapter, the current classificatory systems are structurally inadequate to support understanding of—and interventions related to—risk and protective factors.

Proximal and Distal Causes

The chain of events leading to an adverse health outcome includes both proximal and distal causes: *proximal* factors act directly, or almost directly, to cause disorder, whereas *distal* factors are farther back in the causal chain and act via a number of intermediary causes. Many risk factors can contribute to one outcome (*equifinality,* or multiple pathways to the same disorder). Equally, one risk factor can lead to many outcomes (*multifinality,* or overlapping pathways to different disorders). For example, lower economic and educational status, preterm delivery and antenatal complications, and thyroid peroxidase antibodies are all risk factors for postpartum depression (Stuart et al. 1998), whereas violence against women can lead to depression, anxiety, posttraumatic stress disorder, dissociative disorders, somatoform disorders, sexual dysfunction, and self-harm as well as comorbidities of these disorders (Fischbach and Herbert 1997).

TABLE 2–2.   Selected protective and risk factors

Risk factor	Protective factor
Social and environmental	
Access to drugs and alcohol	Empowerment
Lack of education, transport, housing	Ethnic minorities integration
Neighborhood disorganization	Positive interpersonal interactions
Peer rejection	Social participation
Poverty	Social services
Racial injustice and discrimination	Social support/community networks
Urbanization	
Violence and delinquency	
War	
Work stress or unemployment	
Individual and family	
Academic failure/scholastic demoralization	Ability to face adversity
Child abuse and neglect	Autonomy
Chronic insomnia or chronic pain	Early cognitive stimulation
Early pregnancies	Exercise
Elder abuse	Good parenting
Excessive substance use	Literacy
Exposure to aggression, violence, trauma	Positive attachment/early bonding
Family conflict or family disorganization	Problem-solving skills
Low social class	Pro-social behavior
Medical illness or organic handicaps	Self-esteem
Neurochemical imbalance	Social/conflict management skills
Parental mental illness or substance abuse	Stress management
Perinatal complications	Social support of family/friends
Personal loss, bereavement	
Poor work skills and habits	
Stressful life events	
Substance use during pregnancy	

The factors that lead to someone developing a disorder are likely to have their roots in a complex chain of environmental events that in turn was shaped by broader socioeconomic determinants. Indeed, many risks cannot be disentangled in order to be considered in isolation because they act at different levels that vary over time. As one moves farther from the direct, proximal causes of disorder, there can be a decrease in causal certainty and consistency, often accompanied by increasing complexity. Conversely, distal causes are likely to have amplifying effects; distal causes can affect many different sets of proximal causes and so have the potential to make very large differences.

Furthermore, there is a nonlinear relationship between risk factors and outcomes. Although one or two risk factors may show little prediction to poor outcome, rates of disorders increase rapidly with additional risk factors (Greenberg et al. 2001; Rutter 1979). For example, several separate environmental risk factors may impinge on a person's development (e.g., poverty, mental illness, minority status, and many others), but the most detrimental effects are caused when multiple risk factors act on a single individual (Anders 1989; Sameroff 1998; Sameroff et al. 1987). Many distal risks to health, such as socioeconomic disparity, cannot be defined appropriately at the individual level. The current classificatory systems overall are ill-equipped to either benefit from or enhance the understanding of relationships between distal causes and mental disorders.

Population-Wide Risks and High-Risk Individuals

Many risks to health are widely distributed in the population. This leads to one of the most fundamental axioms in preventive medicine: "A large number of people exposed to a small risk may generate many more cases than a small number exposed to high risk" (Rose 1992). The distribution and determinants of risks in a population have major implications for strategies of prevention. Wherever this axiom applies, a preventive strategy focusing on high-risk individuals will deal only with the margin of the problem and will not affect the large proportion of disease occurring in the large proportion of people who are at moderate risk. This approach does not work for disorders where the underlying risk factors are not continuously distributed in the population. However, for most common diseases and disorders, underlying risk factors form a continuous distribution in the population, probably because there are multiple underlying causes of vulnerability. Fortunately, the population-wide and high-risk individual approaches are complementary (Weich 1997). A key challenge is finding the right balance between population-wide and high-risk approaches.

The current classificatory systems can easily accommodate the concepts of targeted prevention interventions and relative risk (likelihood of an adverse health outcome in people exposed to a particular risk compared with those not exposed) related to individuals and specific disorders. Such approaches are effective in reducing symptoms and incidence of mental disorders such as depression (Clarke et al. 1995, 2001). Subgroups identified as at increased risk benefit the most (Gillham et al. 1995; Price et al. 1992), a finding consistent with the prevention paradox: that is, a preventive measure that brings large benefits to the community appears to offer little to each participating individual.

The existing framework of classification, with its clinical (and consequently, individual) focus, is less serviceable for considering universal preventive interventions with a focus on populations and the population burden of disorders. The need for and effectiveness of universal interventions depend on understanding the population attributable risk (the proportion of disease in a population that results from a particular risk to health). Although universal interventions, such as FRIENDS (Barrett et al. 2006) and Resourceful Adolescents Program (Shochet and Ham 2004), have proven efficacy and cost-effectiveness in unselected populations for prevention of anxiety and depression among adolescents, universal interventions can be beneficial, even for those at risk, because of lowered stigma and better socialization (Kellam et al. 1998; Reid et al. 1999). Most experts support both of these directions and see merit in programs that combine universal and targeted prevention (Conduct Problems Prevention Research Group 2000; Royal College of Psychiatrists 2002; World Health Organization 2004a, 2004b).

The fact that many risks to mental health are widely distributed in the population, with individuals differing in the *extent* of their risk rather than whether they *are* at risk, means that binary categorization into "exposed" and "unexposed" can substantially underestimate the importance of continuous risk factor–disorder relationships. This suggests a need for dimensional classification of risk factors and disorders, a theme we will pick up later.

Predisposing Factors and Precipitating Factors

There is an important distinction between predisposing factors for illness (e.g., loss of mother in childhood and genetic predisposition) and precipitating factors (e.g., stressful life events). More practical preventive opportunities arise for prevention with precipitating, rather than predisposing, factors. This has meant a shift in focus from high-risk populations to high-risk situations, partly because it is easier to identify those in high-risk situations in clinical practice than it is to access those in high-risk populations and partly because the immediate prevention payoff or return is greater in the short term, if one concentrates on those in high-risk situations, because these are more likely to be followed by illness in the short term. Those in high-risk populations may not develop illness for many years, and thus the prevention return takes longer to achieve (Royal College of Psychiatrists 2002).

Life Course Approach to Risk

Risk factors can be separated from outcomes in time, sometimes by many decades. Early material and psychosocial disadvantage may have an adverse effect on psychological and cognitive development that in turn may affect health and labor-market success later in life. Disadvantage can be accumulated across the life course. The inadequacy of the current classificatory systems for a life-course approach to prevention and disorders is discussed in a later section (World Health Organization 2002).

Generic and Specific Risk Factors

Determinants of disorders can be disorder specific or more generic factors that are common to several mental health problems and disorders. Interventions that successfully address such generic factors may generate a broad spectrum of preventive effects. There are also interrelationships between mental and physical health: for example, cardiovascular disease can lead to depression, and vice versa. Mental and physical health also can be related through common risk factors, such as poor housing leading to both poor mental and physical health (Saxena et al. 2006). Interventions that address risk and protective factors with a large impact or that are common to a range of related problems, including social and economic ones, will be most cost-effective and attractive to policy makers and other stakeholders (Saxena et al. 2006).

Monitoring of risk factors can lead to better preventive efforts; for example, multicausality offers opportunities to tailor prevention because different sets of interventions can produce the same goal, and the choice of intervention can be based on considerations of cost, availability, and preferences. Prevention need not wait until further causes are elucidated; in many cases, considerable gains can be achieved by reducing risks to health that are already known. However, to achieve this, policy makers, health insurance and other funding agencies, and health providers should be provided with knowledge of evidence-based and malleable determinants of mental health and their links to ill mental health. This effort would need synergy between the field of prevention and the development of the classification system.

Addition of an axis for risk factors in the classificatory system would be useful for more than one reason. Andreasen and Carpenter (1993) suggested that risk factors may help in identifying subtypes (of schizophrenia), which might aid in the exploration of pathophysiology and etiology. Thus, the axis on risk factors could be used as a matrix with Axis I (clinical diagnosis) to eliminate the need for some specifiers. For example, postpartum depression could be labeled as depression on Axis I, and the specifier "postpartum" would appear on the axis for risk factors. The axis for risk factors could also serve as a link between etiological understanding—the ultimate requirement of every classificatory system (Jablensky 1999; Kendell and Jablensky 2003; Spitzer 1999; Widiger and Clark 2000)—and promotive, preventive, curative, and rehabilitative interventions. Adding a risk factor axis will increase relevance of the classification systems for assessment and selection of effective interventions in each of these sectors of public mental health.

To illustrate the working of the axis, let us take an example of a patient who has made a suicide attempt (Table 2–3). Each year, about 90,000 people die from suicide, more than the total annual deaths from road traffic accidents, wars, and intentional injuries (World Health Organization 2002). Yet most countries still have no suicide prevention policy, even though evidence-based measures for sui-

---

TABLE 2–3.   Illustration of protective and risk factor axis and its utility

A patient with a suicide attempt could be diagnosed to have

> **Disorder axis:** Deliberate self-harm, psychiatric disorder (if any), physical disorder (if any)
>
> **Protective and risk factor axis:** Social/cultural/racial (e.g., social isolation)
> Psychological (e.g., impulsive aggression)
> Biological (e.g., genetic risk factors)
> Environmental (e.g., availability of gun)

A diagnosis on these lines would help in comprehensive assessment of the biopsychosocial context of the event and thus in planning intervention at the individual level. Aggregation of such information could help in a balanced exploration of etiology and directing public health interventions: for example, if surveillance of suicide attempts shows an increasing trend of use of firearms for suicide, it may call for legislation (or change in legislation) on licensing firearms. The comprehensiveness (beyond a few contextual and physical disease factors) of recording would help in choosing public health approaches that maximize use of resources.

---

cide prevention, including both population-wide and high-risk approaches, are effective and available (Mann et al. 2005).

> **Suggestion:** An axis for protective and risk factors should be added in the classificatory system, or in appendices, or a descriptive section on protective and risk factors should be included in the text.

PREVENTION-RELEVANT SUBTHRESHOLD CONDITIONS

Several general population surveys have demonstrated that minor differences in the definition of individual syndromes, such as major depression, can result in large differences in recorded prevalence, suggesting that boundaries identified by the definition do not correspond with a natural zone of rarity. Evidence from several sources now challenges the assumption of a distinct boundary between psychopathology and homeostatic responses and between normal emotions and mood disorders (Mayberg et al. 1999). Also, there is little support for the DSM-IV requirement of 2 weeks' duration, five symptoms, or clinically significant impairment in defining a distinct diagnostic category of depression. In a sample of personally interviewed female twins from a population-based registry, Kendler and Gardner (1998) reported that an increasing number and severity of depressive symptoms predicted a greater risk for future depressive episodes in the index twin and risk for major depression in the co-twin. Specifically, four or fewer symptoms, syndromes composed of symptoms involving no or minimal impairment, and episodes of less than 14 days' duration all significantly predicted both future depressive episodes in the index twin and risk of major depression in the co-twin (Kendler and Gardner 1998). Judd et al. (1996) showed that significantly more people with subsyndromal depressive symptoms or major depression reported impairment in 8 of 10 functional domains than did subjects with no disorder. Except for lower self-ratings of health status, no significant differences were found between subjects with subsyndromal symptoms and those with major depression (Judd et al. 1996). Similarly, Klein et al. (1996) reported that hypomanic traits were normally distributed and were associated with elevated lifetime rates of mood, disruptive behavior, and substance use disorders and with a broad range of indices of psychosocial dysfunction both concurrently and at 1-year follow-up. Concerns have been raised also that the DSM-IV requirements of 6 months' duration, excessive worry, and three associated symptoms exclude a substantial number of people with clinically significant anxiety from a diagnosis of generalized anxiety disorder (Ruscio et al. 2007). Hasin et al. (2006, 2007) found little support for any particular boundary for a diagnostic threshold for DSM-IV alcohol and cannabis dependence; instead, they showed that a model of alcohol dependence and cannabis dependence as continuous linear conditions fit national U.S. data best.

In DSM and ICD, the threshold is set in terms of number or duration of symptoms, or both, and it is not immediately obvious from the literature or classification why the precise threshold has been chosen (Andrews and Slade 2002). However, the emphasis on clinical and research uses for the classification systems suggests that the diagnostic thresholds reflect an emphasis on treatment over prevention (Regier et al. 2002). Altering the threshold for caseness will change the latitude for prevention and treatment within the public mental health spectrum, because the domains of treatment and prevention are separated by the definition of the term *disorder* (Figure 2–1). Drawing the definition of the threshold upward or downward has significant implications for estimates of morbidity (or hidden morbidity), burden (or hidden burden), services delivery (or denial of the same), costs of treatment and service delivery (or costs of untreated illnesses), and policy (or lack of policy) decisions. For primary prevention, it will have a bearing on targets selected for indicated, selective, and universal strategies.

A substantial literature now suggests that subthreshold conditions have considerable public health importance (Horwath et al. 1994; Pincus et al. 1999). Subthreshold depressions (e.g., mixed anxiety depression, recurrent brief depression, minor depression, subsyndromal symptomatic depression) are particularly common. Depressive symptoms in various combinations are reported to occur in up to 24% of the general adult (Horwath et al. 1994; Pincus et al. 1999; Rowe and Rapaport 2006) and 52% of the elderly (Pincus et al. 1999) populations. Subthreshold depressions are associated with substantial morbidity and dysfunction (Broadhead et al. 1990; Johnson et al. 1992; Rowe and Rapaport 2006; Wells et al. 1989) comparable to those experienced with other medical conditions (DeGruy and

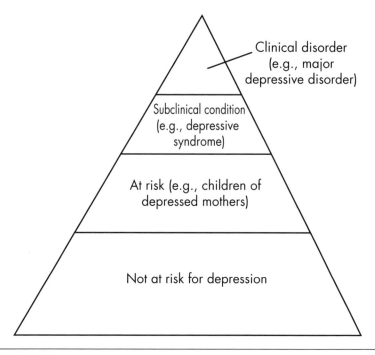

FIGURE 2–1.   Clinical iceberg.

Pincus 1996; Wells and Sherbourne et al. 1999). Subthreshold depressions account for five times as many disability days as major depressive disorders and dysthymia combined (Broadhead et al. 1990). High prevalence, high rates of comorbidity and service use, and significant impairment also can be found in individuals with subthreshold forms of anxiety disorders (Carter et al. 2001; Mendlowicz and Stein 2000) and bipolar disorders (Merikangas et al. 2007). Annual per capita cost of subthreshold anxiety was more than 60% the cost of threshold panic disorder in the Kingdom of the Netherlands (Batelaan et al. 2007). Finally, at least at the level of primary care, patients with common mental disorders and subthreshold disorders seem to have no significant difference in the level of disability.

Subthreshold depression is poorly differentiated from threshold depression. At 1-year follow-up, more than a third of the major depression group was diagnosed to have minor depressions of various types (Broadhead et al. 1990). Judd et al. (1998) found that patients with major depression had subthreshold depression for 43% of a 12-year follow-up period. Patients with subthreshold depressions and major depressive disorder have similar demographic and clinical characteristics (Sadek and Bona 2000) and medical and psychiatric comorbidity (Sherbourne et al. 1994). People with subthreshold depressions have significantly elevated rates of chronicity and suicide (Sadek and Bona 2000) and a family vulnerability for major depression (Sherbourne et al. 1994). Studies on outpatients with early insidious onset and chronic but fluctuating subthreshold manifestations falling short of full syndromal depression lend credibility to relatedness of subthreshold depression with depressive disorder. These patients have shortened rapid eye movement (REM) sleep latency, increased REM sleep percentage, redistribution of REM sleep to the first part of the night, classic diurnality, high rates of family history for mood disorders, positive response to antidepressants and sleep deprivation, and (on followup) a course marked by major affective episodes (Akiskal et al. 1997).

Subthreshold forms of mental illnesses are becoming a focus of research as quality of life and prevention of serious mental illness are recognized as important public health concerns (Rowe and Rapaport 2006). Subthreshold depression is an indicator of risk for developing threshold depression and a focus for indicated prevention. Some forms of subthreshold depression are conditions suitable for treatment and secondary prevention. In the mental health services sector, subthreshold depression has often been treated at par with mood disorders, and many patients have received antidepressants. Moreover, patients felt that they needed help for depression (Sherbourne et al. 1994). However, only a small proportion (fewer than one-third) of subjects with minor depression goes on to develop major depression (Broadhead et al. 1990; Wells et al. 1992).

Similarly, mild cognitive impairment can be regarded as a risk state for dementia. Its identification could lead to indicated prevention by controlling risk factors, such as systolic hypertension (Gauthier et al. 2006). Mild cognitive impairment is a syndrome defined as cognitive decline greater than expected for an individual's age and education level that does not interfere notably with activities of daily life. Prevalence in population-based epidemiological studies ranges from 3% to 19% in adults older than 65 years. Some people with mild cognitive impairment seem to remain stable or return to normal over time, but more than half progress to dementia within 5 years.

A recent study also suggested that subthreshold manifestations of generalized anxiety disorder are related to elevated risk of subsequent psychopathology (Ruscio et al. 2007), a finding with implications for primary prevention of secondary disorders. The challenges confronting psychiatric nosologists include developing a consensus about identification of subthreshold conditions and increasing public recognition of the impact of the entire spectrum of mental illnesses to facilitate the discovery of appropriate interventions (Rowe and Rapaport 2006)

Inclusion of subthreshold conditions in classificatory systems has been hotly debated (Kessler et al. 2004; Regier et al. 2004). The problem with lower thresholds has always been the increase in false positives, which may encourage allocation of resources to people less in need of them. Ideally, arbitrary thresholds should not govern the presumed presence of—or need for treatment for—mental disorder. In medicine, this problem is now increasingly considered, where possible, through assignment of boundaries between normal states, high-risk states, and disorders on the basis of empirical studies of risk (Vasan et al. 2002). Boundaries of illness should be addressed by empirical studies of risk or harm, and the threshold for intervention should be addressed by empirical studies of disease-related risk versus the risks and benefits of the intervention (Hyman 2003). Definition of prevention-relevant categories would encourage studies aimed at understanding disease causation (Pincus et al. 1999, 2003) and early intervention for those at risk for future morbidity, comorbidity, and mortality rather than limiting intervention to a situation in which significant morbidity has occurred. This should result in cost savings (Batelaan et al. 2007; Magruder and Calderone 2000).

Ethical dilemmas related to treatment of nondisorder conditions, social stigma, and lowered self-esteem are legitimate causes for concern when considering inclusion of subthreshold categories in classification systems. These concerns may be balanced and perhaps alleviated, however, if the subthreshold conditions are conceptualized as prevention-relevant categories. As etiological/pathogenetic data accumulate, prevention-relevant categories would be useful rubrics for future inclusion of early manifestations and risk states predictive of disorders; for example, family members of patients with Alzheimer's disease who are homozygous for Apo E ε4 alleles (Steffens and Krishnan 2003) or schizotaxia as predictive of schizophrenia (Tsuang et al. 2003).

We suggest that prevention-relevant subthreshold categories be included, as required, in various phenomenological groups of DSM-IV and ICD-10 (e.g., eating disorder, tic disorder) (First and Pincus 2002). Some members of the group felt that the concept of prodrome, rather than subsyndrome, may be a safer and wiser course, because a *prodrome* denotes "at-risk mental state," which is directly relevant to prevention, whereas *subsyndrome* conflates "at-risk mental state" with "early stage of mental illness," which may be more stigmatizing and may call for preventive as well as treatment approaches.

Suggestion: Prevention-relevant subthreshold conditions should be included, as required, in various phenomenological groups—for example, depressive disorder, eating disorder, alcohol and drug dependence—as categories or text descriptions.

CHILDREN OF MENTALLY ILL PARENTS

Children of parents with mental disorders have significantly higher rates of diagnosable mental disorders (Kim-Cohen et al. 2006; Lieb et al. 2002a, 2002b; O'Connor et al. 2003). These children also are at an elevated risk for experiencing multiple caregiving abuses and neglect (Chang et al. 2001; Dunn 1993; Goodman 1987; Nair et al. 1997). Data gathered from genetic epidemiology, linkage and association studies, high-risk investigations, and twin studies consistently suggest that many psychiatric disorders are heritable (Young et al. 2004). However, twin studies also show that genes and environment influence the process of development of psychiatric disorders. Genes interact with various types of stress in the risk for mental (e.g., major depression) (Caspi et al. 2003) and substance use disorders (e.g., alcohol) (Covault et al. 2007; Kaufman et al. 2007). Genetic testing for children who may be at risk would be a potential means of early detection of psychiatric disorders, although the information available on specific genes that may be responsible, and on their interactions with other factors, is currently insufficient to justify this on scientific grounds (Cannon 2005). Furthermore, using genetic information for early detection is replete with ethical ramifications that need very careful consideration in the public arena. The modern history in Europe, and elsewhere, of abuses in the name of eugenics is a continuing reminder of the need for caution in the way genetic and other information about risk for disorders is used.

High-risk studies have contributed significantly to the notion that prodromal features and biobehavioral anomalies can be detected in offspring of persons with mental disorders such as schizophrenia and bipolar disorder (Masi et al. 2005; Mirsky and Elliott 2005). Studies have delineated specific risk and protective factors that may be unique to these children (Brennan et al. 2003). These findings have led to trials of preventive interventions, some of which have been found to be effective in conditions such as attention-deficit/hyperactivity disorder, mood disorders, and substance use disorders (Aberson 1997; Beardslee et al. 1997, 2003; Brennan et al. 2003). A few intervention efforts have been launched for serious illnesses, such as schizophrenia and bipolar disorder, often based on the notion that shorter duration between first episode and subsequent treatment is associated with better prognosis (Birchwood et al. 1998; Christodoulou 1991; Johannessen et al. 2001). These efforts included pharmacological treatment with antipsychotics initiated during the prodromal phase or perhaps earlier (Melle et al. 2004; Woods et al. 2003). Although several early detection and intervention programs have yielded promising results, they also have generated controversy; perhaps the most major concerns involve ethical principles (Corcoran et al. 2005), such as the tension between balancing patient autonomy and provision of information necessary for informed consent, with beneficent concerns related to labeling a young person as "at risk" for psychosis. A number of questions have been raised in terms of how to best identify who is at risk and the potential stigmatization, loss of confidentiality, and insurability problems these individuals may encounter. There also are concerns about the risks of treating false-positive subjects with unnecessary medication (Verdoux and Cougnard 2003). The risks of sanctioning medication use for the prodrome of psychosis in children are significant because medication tends to be overused, and children may be more prone to side effects, including dyskinesia, as well as weight gain and diabetes (Remschmidt et al. 1996; Towbin 2006). Hence alternative strategies of both pharmacological and nonpharmacological nature need to be explored (Cornblatt 2002; Montero et al. 2001). On a more positive side, early detection may avoid treatments (e.g., antidepressants, stimulants in bipolar disorder) that may worsen the clinical course of the disorder (Soutullo et al. 2002). Research has shown that new onset of depression can be prevented in children of parents with a mental illness by identifying the children as high risk and providing a cognitive-behavioral preventive intervention (Clarke et al. 2001). Importantly, such intervention has also been shown to be cost-effective (Lynch et al. 2005).

> **Suggestion:** The classification system should list 1) early/prodromal symptoms and biobehavioral markers; 2) features of parental psychopathology; and 3) relevant risk factors associated with disorders, where there is adequate evidence.

DIMENSIONAL CONCEPTUALIZATION BETTER SUITED TO PREVENTION

Despite broad agreement that the many mental disorder categories are heterogeneous and are best described on a continuum of severity, illness definitions of the mental disorders in current classificatory systems are categorical (dichotomous). There are many advantages to categorical diagnoses, in terms of clarity, simplicity of communication, and timely treatment decisions. However, a dichotomous (categorical) diagnosis is disadvantageous for other purposes, such as etiological/associational studies and even for clinical decision making. Dimensional models have not found favor in earlier revisions of the diagnosis and classification systems but are under active discussion for many disorder categories for DSM-5, such as the substance use disorders category (Helzer et al. 2006).

Dimensional systems allow one to model the severity of a condition, not simply its presence versus absence (Clarke et al. 1995). For example, increasing severity of alcohol dependence (indicated by number of diagnostic criteria met) is associated with monotonically increasing disability levels (Hasin et al. 2007). A large body of evidence also indicates that the artificial dichotomization of continuous measures leads to substantial losses in reliability and stability (Widiger 1992). However, the relative validity of these two approaches rests on empirical considerations (Widiger and Samuel 2005). The nature of underlying distributions is important. Taxometric studies suggest that both latent categories and dimensions for various disorders are distributed. Dimensional models receive extensive support in the broad neurotic spectrum, predominating among the mood and anxiety disorders (e.g., chronic worry and posttraumatic stress) (Ruscio et al. 2001). Analyses of depression yielded mixed results but generally gave evidence of continuity rather than discontinuity (Haslam and Beck 1994; Ruscio and Ruscio 2002). However, melancholic depression appears to be better understood as a latent category, and latent categories are possible in the domains of social anxiety and inhibition. Categorical models enjoy more support in the domain of personality disorders than we might have anticipated (Haslam 2003).

Rose's (1992) model of disease prevention, which underpins much of modern epidemiology, is based on the assumption that population interventions work because exposure to many risk factors is continuously distributed. In addition, for most people, vulnerability is a result of multiple underlying causes. A small reduction in exposure to risk factors will reduce the number of people in the population with mental disorders as well as the numbers of those at high risk for disorder. The relevance of the model to mental health has been demonstrated in population studies showing that symptoms or risk factors for common mental disorders form a continuous distribution throughout the population and that the prevalence of disorder is related to the mean level of symptoms in the population (Anderson et al. 1993; Melzer et al. 2002; Whittington and Huppert 1996). Huppert and Whittington (1995) established a relationship between life expectancy and severity of mental symptoms. Therefore, interventions that reduce the mean number of psychological symptoms in a population should not only reduce the number of people with common mental disorders but also reduce premature deaths.

A dimensional model of pathology supports population intervention (Rose 1992). It also elicits help for individuals who may not quite meet diagnostic criteria for disorder but whose struggle may have serious effects on their family lives, work, and health (Huppert 2004). A dimensional approach may also help prepare for future inclusion of genetic, imaging, and biochemical elements in psychiatric diagnoses.

Suggestion: An axis should be provided for classification of agreed-upon dimensions.

An axis on dimensions, including those dimensions with relatively good literature support and consensual validity, could first be included in the appendix. For example, dependence severity (Hasin et al. 2007); the three-syndrome model of schizophrenia (deficit, nondeficit-delusional, nondeficit-disorganized) (Arndt et al. 1991; Chemerinski et al. 2006); positive affect, negative affect, and physiological hyperarousal (Watson 2005); personality (Costa and McCrae 1992); or personality disorder factors—intelligence, internalizing syndrome, externalizing syndrome (Slade 2007) could be considered for inclusion at the first step. It may also be possible, initially, to include alternative conceptualizations of dimensions for related conditions (e.g., personality and personality disorder) and agree on one set after a detailed review of its respective validity. Keeping the axis for categories and dimensions separate would be empirically accurate and would encourage research into valid models and the relationship between the two models (e.g., some disorders may be taxonic-dimensional—that is, have both categorical and dimensional aspects). This separation also would allow the flexibility of using either of the two approaches in case of need (e.g., categorical for briefing policy makers and dimensional for etiological research).

DEVELOPMENTAL AND LONGITUDINAL PERSPECTIVES

Mounting evidence in areas related to the individual and sex differences of certain disorders, continuity and change of behavior, risk and protective factors, and turning points in development suggests a need for a developmental and longitudinal perspective in classification; however, at present, classification systems take a largely cross-sectional view of disorders. Duration criteria have been included, but with a few exceptions (e.g., schizophrenia) the requirements are minimal and have only a secondary role. These criteria have served mainly to rule out alternative hypotheses about the occurrence of the disorder; for example, the relation of mood or anxiety symptoms to transient stressors (Wakefield 1999). An artificial temporal distinction also exists between disorders of childhood and adulthood. Some information is provided in DSM-IV about variation in each disorder's presentation across the life span, and some DSM-III-R (American Psychiatric Association 1987) childhood and adulthood diagnoses were collapsed into a single diagnosis to provide a more developmental perspective—for example, gender identity disorder, social phobia, and generalized anxiety disorder. Similarly, there is little emphasis on the course of disorders, again, with some exceptions. For example, the history of manic episode requires a diagnosis of a bipolar mood disorder in someone who is currently within a depressive episode, and the subtyping of mood disorders depends on the longitudinal course. This relative neglect of a longitudinal perspective is at odds with the life-course approach to study of health and illness. The life-course approach has come to dominate public health, following the recognition that risks (and their valences), as well as symptomatic expression of disorders, vary across developmental spans (Ingram and Price 2001) and that exposure to disadvantageous experiences and environments accumulate throughout life to increase the risk of illnesses (World Health Organization 2002).

The need for a developmentally informed diagnostic system is most acute for definition of psychopathology in children and adolescents. Most of the current diagnostic systems are based solely on models of adult psychopathology. Children, especially preschoolers with depressive disorders, often present with somatic complaints and aggressive behavior, and most have psychomotor agitation (Kashani et al. 1997; Ryan et al. 1987). The diagnosis may be overlooked because of the presence of these associated symptoms, suggestive of an externalizing disorder, and younger children may not be capable of experiencing or reporting the symptoms of major depression (Kovacs 1986). Similarly, children with bipolar disorder commonly have a mixed mood state, with co-occurring symptoms of depression and mania, and typically have a more malignant course than do adults with adult-onset bipolar disorders (Biederman et al. 2000, 2003, 2004; Findling et al. 2003; Geller et al. 2002; Post et al. 2004). These findings emphasize the need to have developmentally relevant criteria for diagnosis.

Other studies emphasize the need for greater attention to the life-course approach to mental disorders. Several prospective longitudinal studies of population-based samples of children and adolescents show that retrospective adult studies may seriously overestimate the age at onset of many disorders (Costello et al. 1999; Lewinsohn et al. 2000). Early use of alcohol increases the lifelong risk for alcohol and drug dependence and further problems (Grant and Dawson 1997; Lynskey et al. 2003). In addition, disorders explicitly recognized in DSM-IV as developmental conditions (e.g., attention-deficit/hyperactivity disorder [ADHD] and other syndromes such as major psychoses) may show early prodromes (Pine et al. 2002). Homotypic continuity of internalizing and externalizing disorders has been documented on follow-up of children with psychiatric conditions. An episode of depression or anxiety is a risk factor for further episodes of same general type of disorder—for example, major depression and suicide (Kovacs and Devlin 1998; Mineka et al. 1998)—and ADHD is a predictor of conduct disorder/antisocial personality disorder, substance use disorder, and bipolar disorder (Babinski et al. 1999; Biederman et al. 1998; Faraone et al. 1997). Some heterotypic associations are also apparent. High levels of anxiety in children predict increase in depression over time; however, high levels of reported depression in children did not predict increase in anxiety (Cole et al. 1998; Kolvin and Trowell 2002). Tic disorder shows longitudinal association with obsessive-compulsive disorder, with tics decreasing and obsessive symptoms increasing over time (Peterson et al. 2001; Pine et al. 2002). Interplay of biological and environmental risk factors could influence courses, both singly and across related disorders: for example, childhood sexual abuse for externalizing disorders (Brown et al. 1996; Wilsnack et al. 1997) and kindling for schizophrenia, bipolar, and other disorders (Frances and Egger 1999). Failure to take a life-course approach makes the occurrence of such comorbidity perplexing. It is important to recognize that the life-course approach extends across the life span. Studies suggest that patients with a history of alcohol dependence (who stopped drinking more than 1 year ago) have an increased risk of current major depressive disorder by a factor of four (Hasin and Grant 2002), and patients with depressive or bipolar disorder may be at increased risk for developing dementia later in life (Kessing and Anderson 2004).

There is no escaping the conclusion that common mental disorders have their onset among the young and that early intervention and prevention programs must be aimed at school-age children to avoid distortion of life trajectories (Andrews 2006). Although ICD and DSM were initially created as tools for clinicians to diagnose specific illnesses, future modifications should acknowledge the growing emphasis on prevention and early intervention in the process of developing an illness—a characteristic of all of medicine in the current era. Routine "well surveillance," along with the identification and classification of high-risk individuals, high-risk environments, and early signs and symptoms of brain disorders, represent important clinical goals that are as important for mental disorders as for cancer or diabetes. Examples abound from pediatrics and developmental medicine of early environmental modification (primary prevention) or intervention (secondary prevention/early detection) acting to reduce the likelihood of disorders later in life (Smith et al. 2000; van Spronsen et al. 2001). It is desirable that classificatory systems provide guidance on the range and limits of normal development, developmentally safe environments, and the boundary conditions that are risk markers rather than disorders while noting the caveats about the interactions and the way that the "fit" between environments and temperament and other individual factors or experience will produce different outcomes.

A life-course approach would also help in improved validity of diagnoses. Subthreshold symptoms, for example, are common during the course of disorders such as unipolar and bipolar depression (Angst 1992; Solomon et al. 1995), obsessive-compulsive disorder (Eisen and Steketee 1997), generalized anxiety disorders (Yonkers et al. 1996), panic disorder (Katschnig and Amering 1998), and substance use disorders (Stöffelmayr et al. 1994). In fact, patients may be in such a condition for long periods; as noted earlier, patients with major depression had subthreshold symptoms for 43% of the time in a 12-year follow-up study (Judd et al. 1998). Use of arbitrary thresholds for diagnosis yields a lower estimate of diagnostic stability than would a more nuanced approach to diagnosis (Widiger and Clarke 2000). Similarly, the duration cutoff for diagnosis of brief psychoses, schizophreniform disorder, and schizophrenia may lead to different diagnoses being given in different episodes when the patient may more likely have one disorder (Bertelsen 1999).

A system that provides a longitudinal framework is required to map etiology, onset, course, and remission. Two changes are proposed: 1) use of diagnostic criteria that are developmentally informed and 2) listing of relevant information on axes for clinical disorders (e.g., history of anxiety disorder), strengths/resilience factors (e.g., efficient use of problem-solving skills during a major stress in the past), and risk factors (e.g., child abuse).

Suggestion: A system that provides a longitudinal framework is required to map etiology, onset, course, and remission. Two changes are proposed: 1) use of diagnostic criteria that are developmentally informed and 2) listing of relevant developmental information on a risk and protective factor axis or in descriptive text.

ACCENTUATION OF REFINED CATEGORIES AND CONSEQUENT COMORBIDITY

Critical Reexamination of Hyperrefined Subcategories

The preoccupation with overrefined categories and subcategories has led to complex diagnostic systems that are difficult to use in the community setting. Definition of broad categories (e.g., depression [nonbipolar]) is useful from the population intervention perspective. Over the past three decades, most prevention trials have focused on so-called common, or generic, protective and risk factors as relevant for the promotion of mental health in general or for the reduction of risks for several mental disorders. These preventive efforts targeted broad categories, such as depression (Caplan et al. 1997), anxiety symptoms and disorders (Dadds et al. 1999), externalizing problems and substance abuse (Wolchik et al. 2000), or suicidal behavior (Zenere and Lazarus 1997). However, apart from utility, validity concerns also suggest caution with hyperrefined categories. Broad categories may be more valid than narrow categories in some circumstances; for example, genetic research suggests that the DSM concept of schizophrenia may be too narrow (Maziade et al. 1997; Tsuang et al. 2003). Jablensky (1999) proposed that the use of restrictive DSM-IV and ICD-10 definitions, rather than broader clinical concepts, as sampling criteria in recruiting subjects for epidemiological research carries the risk of replacing random error (due to diagnostic inconsistency) with systematic error (due to consistent exclusion of segments of the syndrome). In current classificatory systems, the division of diagnostic categories (e.g., depression) into subcategories is not based on studies of causative factors. Testing a theory regarding specific etiology does not depend on first refining a homogeneous patient cluster and then seeking the cause or causes of the patients' conditions, because etiology often is not uniquely associated with clinical phenomena; for example, exposure to disasters may lead to a number of conditions along the depressive-anxious spectrum (Caine 2003). Varying clinical presentations of depression may have major risk factors in common, independent of subtype predictors. Broad categories also have the advantage of facilitating communication with policy makers and public groups.

When subtypes have major subtype-specific and malleable determinants, finely divided categories could be relevant for indicated prevention. However, some subcategories may be redundant (e.g., single episode of depression and recurrent depression, Alzheimer's dementia with early or late onset, Alzheimer's dementia with or without behavioral disturbance) (Kopelman and Fleminger 2002; Paykel 2002). Increasing the number of refined categories will reduce the likelihood (and the cost) of identifying risk factors as well as the efficacy of primary preventive interventions because of power problems (Muñoz et al. 1995). In some circumstances, subtyping may be useful for prevention, wherein strategies are targeted at early symptoms (indicated prevention) or secondary morbidity (prevention of comorbidity) (McGorry 1992). Definition of broad categories will ideally sit alongside the existence of selected narrower categories.

Comorbidity

The increase in number of disorders has added to the problems of comorbidity; nearly one-third of people detected as cases in the general population have comorbid psychiatric problems (Wittchen 1996). The high rate of co-occurrence of substance use disorders and other psychiatric disorders is also well established (Grant et al. 2004; Jané-Llopis and Matytsina 2006; Ziedonis 2004). At least some of these comorbidities are artifacts, a function of the number of available categories. A high degree of co-occurrence is seen across a wide range of disorders (Clarke et al. 1995; Kolvin and Trowell 2002; Sher and Trull 1996; Weiss et al. 1995). Psychometric studies also show an incomplete separation of psychotic, mood, anxiety, somatoform, and substance use symptoms from other psychopathologies (Cloninger et al. 1985; Hasin et al. 2005, 2007; Sigvardsson et al. 1986). Both concurrent and successive comorbidity have been reported. The latter may take the form of same phenomena over time (homotypic continuity) or different forms of disorder over time (heterotypic continuity) (Kolvin and Trowell 2002).

Preventive interventions aimed at subthreshold categories and risk factors with broad spectrum effects would contribute to reducing both concurrent and successive comorbidity. Epidemiological data show the value of preventing successive comorbidity. Up to half of lifetime psychiatric disorders, and an even larger proportion of chronic and seriously impairing disorders, occur in people with a history of another condition (Kessler and Price 1993). As an illustration, consider the study by Verdoux et al. (2005), who found a dose-response relationship between cannabis exposure and risk of early psychosis. Because a large percentage of subjects from the general population are exposed to cannabis, even a small increase in the risk of adverse effects can have significant deleterious consequences for the health of the population. Hence, reducing exposure to cannabis may contribute to prevention of some incident cases of psychosis (Verdoux et al. 2005). In a similar vein, a study by Hasin et al. (2002c) showed that among patients with long-term, sustained remissions from substance dependence, the occurrence of an episode of major depression substantially increased the risk of subsequent relapse to substance dependence. Because leaving the "comorbid" problem unattended runs the risk of poor outcomes, authorities suggest that integrated treatment of both disorders may be more effective than separate treatments offered in parallel or in sequence (Brunette and Mueser 2006; Ziedonis 2004).

Creation of subthreshold categories has a potential to increase the rate of comorbidity (Widiger and Clark 2000). As pathogenesis of psychiatric disorders becomes better understood, however, recognition of links among disorders will enable a broadening of some categories and a reduction in the overall number of disorders and thus of artifactual comorbidity. Some clusters are already considered single disorders (e.g., panic with agoraphobia), and others may follow. Genetic and environmental risk factors may contribute to diagnostic co-occurrence (Kendler et al. 1995; Livesley et al. 1998). For example, Brown et al. (1996) showed that childhood adversity increased the risk of comorbidity between anxiety and depression, and Mineka et al. (1998) found that anxiety and depressive symptoms and disorders were due to common genetic factors that also influenced neuroticism. Krueger et al. (1998) found support for a two-factor model for explaining comorbidity: a latent internalizing factor (depression and anxiety) and a latent externalizing factor (conduct disorder, marijuana, and alcohol dependence). This study supported the position of other authors who had suggested that a general distress factor can partly explain the internalizing symptoms found across many disorders, including such disparate ones as depression, conduct disorder, and schizophrenia (Trull and Sher 1994; Watson and Clark 1994), and that an externalizing, or disinhibition, factor would similarly explain substance abuse, conduct disorder, and antisocial personality disorders (Clark 1989; Watson and Clark 1993, 1994). Continuing studies of risk and etiological factors, and acceptance of dimensional models, are likely to decrease the need for hyperrefinement of categories.

> **Suggestion:** During the revision of classifications, close attention should be paid to the number, hierarchy, and specificity of categories; broader categories should be preferred, and where feasible, categories should be combined—for example, the category of adjustment disorders could be merged with subthreshold categories in relevant phenomenological groups. The presence or absence of stressors could be coded on the risk and protective factor axis.

MULTIAXIAL SYSTEM FOR THE SUGGESTED CHANGES

Multiaxial evaluation provides a vehicle for describing different aspects of a patient's condition in order to improve our understanding of the condition and thereby to improve its management. Many multiaxial systems have been proposed, with different specific axes (Mezzich et al. 1987). Only a limited number of axes can be included in a manageable system for regular work internationally. Mezzich et al. (1987) found two broad and pervasive themes in their review of multiaxial systems: phenomenology and etiological and associated factors. The latter could accommodate subthemes such as biological, psychological, cultural, and spiritual aspects.

> **Suggestion:** A multiaxial system comprising five axes should be adopted:
>
> - Axis I: Categorical diagnoses
> - Axis II: Dimensions related to mental disorders
> - Axis III: Protective and risk factors
> - Axis IV: Function and dysfunction
> - Axis V: Quality of life

Axis I (categorical diagnoses) would comprise

- Mental disorders (including subthreshold conditions, mental retardation, personality disorders, and psychological factors that influence general medical conditions)
- Mental conditions (not amounting to disorders) requiring preventive or treatment intervention (e.g., self-harm [Z codes])

Axis II (dimensions related to mental disorders) would comprise agreed dimensions, such as

- Dependence severity (Hasin et al. 2007)
- The three-syndrome model of schizophrenia (deficit, nondeficit-delusional, nondeficit-disorganized) (Arndt et al. 1991; Chemerinski et al. 2006)
- Positive affect, negative affect, physiological hyperarousal (Watson 2005)
- Personality (Costa and McCrae 1992) or personality disorder factors (Livesley 2007)
- Intelligence, internalizing syndrome, externalizing syndrome (Slade 2007)

These dimensions would be included at the first step. This axis could also provisionally accommodate endophenotypes (i.e., quantitative traits hypothesized to underlie disease syndromes that may be reflections of genetic risk), cognitive structures, defense mechanisms, and so on, for further study.

Axis III (protective and risk factors) could include agreed risk, protective, formative, precipitating, and perpetuating factors. The axis can be subdivided into the following dimensions: biological (e.g., genetic, drug use), psychological (e.g., avoidant coping), social (e.g., social disintegration), and transcendental (e.g., spirituality, sense of coherence).

Axes IV and V are self-explanatory.

The practitioner requires a considerable amount of information about a patient to use the axes. This is to be welcomed because it places the human being at the center of the intervention exercise. It may also be a practical limitation and become a criticism of the approach. A compromise approach could keep some of the axes as optional (e.g., axis on dimensions) for use in specific settings or with specific populations.

Some Implications of Making Classification Prevention Friendly

FINANCING OF PREVENTIVE INTERVENTIONS

A combination of well-targeted treatment and prevention programs in the field of mental health, within overall public strategies, could avoid years lived with disability and deaths, reduce the stigma attached to mental disorders, increase considerably the social capital, help reduce poverty, and promote a country's development. When determining what will be financed from a given amount of resources, the overall objective should be to ensure that health interventions maximize the benefits to society. Available evidence-based prevention programs have also been found to improve positive mental health, to contribute to better physical health, and to generate social and economic benefits (Field et al. 1986; World Health Organization 2004a, 2004b). Such multiple-outcome interventions illustrate that prevention can be cost-effective because the accumulation of multiple proximal outcomes across domains of functioning can bring about more efficient strategies than collections of programs with fragmented outcomes. Even at the level of indicated prevention, prevention of comorbid disorders could lead to more efficient use of available resources (Lynch et al. 2005). Here it is important to mention that financing of prevention efforts need not always occur at the cost of treatment or rehabilitation, because an increase in resources for prevention can also be sought from other sources (e.g., public health, health promotion budgets, social welfare budgets).

The current devotion of a disproportionately small share of resources to preventive interventions should be reconsidered in a more systematic way in light of the evidence presented here. If preventive considerations are included in the classificatory system, financing for prevention may increase. Including the proposed changes in the diagnostic system will lead to identification of those who are entitled to preventive interventions and facilitate their receipt of the interventions (and might lead to changes in policy and service delivery within health care systems, which would include prevention as one of their intervention modalities). This, in turn, could save later treatment costs.

Research

Research on prevention may be facilitated if there is greater correspondence between risk factors and diagnostic categories. Such a correspondence would reveal many research challenges, for example, identification of risk groups likely to benefit from preventive strategies, nonmedical alternatives, nonspecialist providers, and the effectiveness of prevention and promotion strategies. More research on risk factors and their uses in classification will also improve understanding of the development of disorders and the potential for short-term or low-intensity treatments rather than long-term, intensive treatments. This is an important consideration in light of the large treatment gap for mental disorders worldwide (Kohn et al. 2004). The changes in the classification to include prevention will improve overall mental health practice.

Resistance From Clinicians and Consumers

Community physicians may see the changes as adding to their workload or to the difficulty in discriminating disorder from non-disorder. Overall, however, their task is likely to be simplified by the use of broad categories. For the milder forms of disorder, the emerging areas of self-management and (evidence-based) help through nonspecialist and peer providers will be relevant (Magruder and Calderone 2000).

Consumers with subthreshold conditions may not understand the need for intervention. Some subjects with subthreshold depression, however, recognized the need for help (Sherbourne et al. 1994). The use of "prevention" terminology may facilitate the quest for help in some groups with significant levels of disability.

Recommendations

The reality of society's response to the burden of mental and behavioral disorders in the population is changing. Within the spectrum of mental health interventions, prevention and promotion have become realistic and evidence-based components supported by a fast-growing body of knowledge from fields as varied as developmental psychopathology, psychobiology, and prevention and health promotion sciences. Also, mental health interventions are now offered by diverse service providers in varied settings. The classification of psychiatric disorders needs to keep pace with these changing realities.

Although a clinical approach may appear more appropriate to clinicians and clinical taxonomists, it can have only a limited impact on the mental health status of the population, because it does not tap the full spectrum of psychopathology or the full spectrum of etiological leads. In contrast, a prevention-based strategy seeks to shift the focus to the entire range of psychopathology and health, and the associated social, environmental, and risk factors, and considers the entire spectrum of interventions. The clinical and public health approaches are complementary.

For the present, we suggest the following:

1. An axis or text description for risk and protective factors should be added.
2. Prevention-relevant subthreshold/prodromal categories/descriptions should be included in various phenomenological categories—for example, depressive disorders, eating disorders, substance use disorders, and so on.
3. An axis for classification of agreed-upon dimensions should be provided.
4. Close attention should be paid to the number, hierarchy, and specificity of categories during the exercise of revising classifications. Broader categories should be preferred, and where feasible, categories should be combined.
5. A system that provides a longitudinal framework is required. Two changes are proposed: 1) use of diagnostic criteria that are developmentally informed and 2) listing of relevant information on a risk and protective factor axis or in text description.
6. Multiaxial classification comprising the following should be provided:
   - Axis I: categorical diagnoses
   - Axis II: dimensions related to mental disorders
   - Axis III: protective and risk factors
   - Axis IV: function and dysfunction
   - Axis V: quality of life

The revision of diagnosis and classification presented could have far-reaching implications in ensuring that prevention of mental disorders becomes an integral part of mental health practice. By firmly bringing the "four P's" (Predisposing [risk], Precipitating, Perpetuating, and Protective [strengths]) into the multiaxial system, it would require that mental health professionals think more seriously about, and record, developmental and current factors in the patient's environmental, social, familial, and other background when trying to understand the patient's condition. This would have the effect of alerting both mental health professionals and others concerned with funding, policy, and so on to the significance of prevention. This would also provide data that can improve research in the area. The general thrust of this initiative is, in fact, putting the "person" back into the process rather than a "label." It also fits very closely with the whole move toward community mental health, in which the patient is viewed holistically within his or her whole context, developmentally and currently. Regarding prodromal and subthreshold conditions, it would be very helpful for these conditions to be acknowledged and receive some attention, because currently not only is "prevention" not addressed in terms of policy, but also, on a humanistic level, people with these symptoms fall outside any current services.

References

Aberson BD: An intervention for improving executive functioning and social/emotional adjustment of ADHD children: three single case design studies. Doctoral dissertation, Miami Institute of Psychology of the Caribbean Centre for Advanced Studies. Diss Abstr Int 57:10–B, 6553, 1997

Akiskal HS, Judd LL, Gillin JC, et al: Subthreshold depressions: clinical and polysomnographic validation of dysthymic, residual and masked forms. J Affect Disord 45:53–63, 1997

American Psychiatric Association: Diagnostic and Statistical Manual of Mental Disorders, 3rd Edition, Revised. Washington, DC, American Psychiatric Association, 1987

American Psychiatric Association: Diagnostic and Statistical Manual of Mental Disorders, 4th Edition. Washington, DC, American Psychiatric Association, 1994

American Psychiatric Association: Diagnostic and Statistical Manual of Mental Disorders, 4th Edition, Text Revision. Washington, DC, American Psychiatric Association, 2000

Anders TF: Clinical syndromes, relationships disorders and their assessment, in Relationship Disturbances in Early Childhood. Edited by Sameroff AJ, Emde RN. New York, Basic Books, 1989, pp 125–144

Anderson J, Huppert F, Rose G: Normality, deviance and minor psychiatric morbidity in the community: a population-based approach to General Health Questionnaire data in the Health and Lifestyle Survey. Psychol Med 23:475–485, 1993

Andreasen NC, Carpenter WT Jr: Diagnosis and classification of schizophrenia. Schizophr Bull 19:199–214, 1993

Andrews G: Implications for intervention and prevention from the New Zealand and Australian mental health surveys. Aust N Z J Psychiatry 40:827–829, 2006

Andrews G, Slade T: The classification of anxiety disorders in ICD-10 and DSM-IV: a concordance analysis. Psychopathology 35:100–106, 2002

Angst J: How recurrent and predictable is depressive illness?, in Long-term Treatment of Depression. Edited by Montgomery SA, Rouillon F. New York, Wiley, 1992, pp 1–13

Arndt S, Alliger RJ, Andreasen NC: The distinction of positive and negative symptoms: the failure of a two-dimensional model. Br J Psychiatry 158:317–322, 1991

Babinski LM, Hartsough CS, Lambert NM: Childhood conduct problems, hyperactivity-impulsivity, and inattention as predictors of adult criminal activity. J Child Psychol Psychiatry 40:347–355, 1999

Ballesteros J, Duffy JC, Querejeta I, et al: Efficacy of brief interventions for hazardous drinkers in primary care: systematic review and meta-analyses. Alcohol Clin Exp Res 28:608–618, 2004

Barrett PM, Farrell J, Ollendick TH, et al: Long-term outcomes of an Australian universal prevention trial of anxiety and depression symptoms in children and youth: an evaluation of the friends program J Clin Child Adolesc Psychol 35:403–411, 2006

Batelaan N, Smit F, deGraaf R, et al: Economic costs of full-blown and subthreshold panic disorder. J Affect Disord 104:127–136, 2007

Beaglehole R, Bonita R, Horton R, et al: Public health in the new era: improving health through collective action. Lancet 363:2084–2086, 2004

Beardslee WR, Salt P, Versage EM, et al: Sustained change in parents receiving preventive interventions for families with depression. Am J Psychiatry 154:510–515, 1997

Beardslee WR, Gladstone TR, Wright EJ, et al: A family based approach to the prevention of depressive symptoms in children at risk: evidence of parental and child change. Pediatrics 112:e119–e131, 2003

Bertelsen A: Comments on the diagnosis of the schizophrenic syndrome, in Schizophrenia: WPA Series Evidence and Experience in Psychiatry, Vol 2. Edited by Maj M, Sartorius N. Chichester, UK, Wiley, 1999, pp 60–62

Biederman J, Wilens TE, Mick E, et al: Does attention-deficit hyperactivity disorder impact the developmental course of drug and alcohol abuse and dependence? Biol Psychiatry 44:269–273, 1998

Biederman J, Mick E, Spencer TJ, et al: Therapeutic dilemmas in the pharmacotherapy of bipolar depression in the young. J Child Adolesc Psychopharmacol 10:185–192, 2000

Biederman J, Mick E, Faraone SV, et al: Current concepts in the validity, diagnosis and treatment of paediatric bipolar disorder. Int J Neuropsychopharmacol 6:293–300, 2003

Biederman J, Faraone SV, Wozniak J, et al: Further evidence of unique developmental phenotypic correlates of pediatric bipolar disorder: findings from a large sample of clinically referred preadolescent children assessed over the last 7 years. J Affect Disord 82(suppl):S45–S58, 2004

Birchwood M, Todd P, Jackson C: Early intervention in psychosis: the critical period hypothesis. Br J Psychiatry Suppl 172:53–59, 1998

Boath E, Bradley E, Henshaw C: The prevention of postnatal depression: a narrative systematic review. J Psychosom Obstet Gynaecol 26:185–192, 2005

Brennan PA, Le Brocque R, Hammen C: Maternal depression, parent-child relationships, and resilient outcomes in adolescence. J Am Acad Child Adolesc Psychiatry 42:1469–1477, 2003

Broadhead WE, Blazer DG, George LK, et al: Depression, disability days, and days lost from work in a prospective epidemiologic survey. JAMA 264:2524–2528, 1990

Brown GW, Harris TO, Eales MJ: Social factors and comorbidity of depressive and anxiety disorders. Br J Psychiatry Suppl 30:50–57, 1996

Brunette MF, Mueser KT: Psychosocial interventions for the long-term management of patients with severe mental illness and co-occurring substance use disorder. J Clin Psychiatry 67(suppl):10–17, 2006

Caine ED: Determining causation in psychiatry, in Advancing DSM Dilemmas in Psychiatric Diagnosis. Edited by Phillips KA, First MB, Pincus HA. Washington, DC, American Psychiatric Association, 2003, pp 1–22

Cannon TD: The inheritance of intermediate phenotypes for schizophrenia. Curr Opin Psychiatry 18:135–140, 2005

Caplan RD, Vinokur AD, Price RH: From job loss to reemployment: field experiments in prevention-focused coping, in Primary Prevention Works. Edited by Albee GW, Gullotta TP. Thousand Oaks, CA, Sage Publications, 1997, pp 341–379

Carter RM, Wittchen HU, Pfister H, et al: One-year prevalence of subthreshold and threshold DSM-IV generalized anxiety disorder in a nationally representative sample. Depress Anxiety 13:78–88, 2001

Caspi A, Sugden K, Moffitt TE, et al: Influence of life stress on depression: moderation by a polymorphism in the 5-HTT gene. Science 301:386–389, 2003

Chang KD, Blasey C, Ketter TA, et al: Family environment of children and adolescents with bipolar parents. Bipolar Disord 3:73–78, 2001

Chemerinski E, Reichenberg I, Kilpatrick B, et al: Three dimensions of clinical symptoms in elderly patients with schizophrenia: prediction of six-year cognitive and functional status. Schizophr Res 85:12–19, 2006

Christodoulou GN: Prevention of psychopathology with early interventions. Psychother Psychosom 55:201–207, 1991

Cipriani A, Pretty H, Hawton K, et al: Lithium in the prevention of suicidal behavior and all-cause mortality in patients with mood disorders: a systematic review of randomized trials. Am J Psychiatry 162:1805–1819, 2005

Clark LA: Depressive and anxiety disorders: descriptive psychopathology and differential diagnosis, in Anxiety and Depression: Distinctive and Overlapping Features. Edited by Kendall PC, Watson D. New York, Academic Press, 1989, pp 83–129

Clarke GN, Hawkins W, Murphy M, et al: Targeted prevention of unipolar depressive disorder in an at-risk sample of high school adolescents: a randomized trial of a group cognitive intervention. J Am Acad Child Adolesc Psychiatry 34:312–321, 1995

Clarke GN, Hornbrook M, Lynch F, et al: A randomized trial of a group cognitive intervention for preventing depression in adolescent offspring of depressed parents. Arch Gen Psychiatry 58:1127–1134, 2001

Cloninger CR, Martin RL, Guze SB, et al: Diagnosis and prognosis in schizophrenia. Arch Gen Psychiatry 42:15–25, 1985

Cole DA, Peeke LG, Martin JM, et al: A longitudinal look at the relation between depression and anxiety in children and adolescents. J Consult Clin Psychol 66:451–460, 1998

Conduct Problems Prevention Research Group: Merging universal and indicated prevention programs: the Fast Track model. Conduct Problems Prevention Research Group. Addict Behav 25:913–927, 2000

Corcoran C, Malaspina D, Hercher L: Prodromal interventions for schizophrenia vulnerability: the risks of being "at risk." Schizophr Res 73:173–184, 2005

Cornblatt B: The New York high risk project to the Hillside recognition and prevention (RAP) Program. Am J Med Genet 114:956–966, 2002

Cororve Fingeret M, Warren CS, Cepeda-Benito A, et al: Eating disorder prevention research: a meta-analysis. Eat Disord 14:191–213, 2006

Costa PT Jr, McCrae RR: Normal personality assessment in clinical practice: the NEO Personality Inventory. Psychol Assess 4:5–13, 1992

Costello EJ, Erkanli A, Federman E, al: Development of psychiatric comorbidity with substance abuse in adolescents: effects of timing and sex. J Clin Child Psychol 28:298–311, 1999

Covault J, Tennen H, Armeli S, et al: Interactive effects of the serotonin transporter 5-HT-TLPR polymorphism and stressful life events on college student drinking and drug use. Biol Psychiatry 61:609–616, 2007

Cuijpers P, Van Straten A, Smit F: Preventing the incidence of new cases of mental disorders: a meta-analytic review. J Nerv Ment Dis 193:119–125, 2005

Dadds MR, Holland DE, Laurens KR, et al: Early intervention and prevention of anxiety disorders in children: results at 2-year follow-up. J Consult Clin Psychol 67:145–150, 1999

Dawson G, Ashman SB, Carver LJ: The role of early experience in shaping behavioral and brain development and its implications for social policy. Dev Psychopathol 12:695–712, 2000

DeGruy FV 3rd, Pincus HA: The DSM-IV-PC: a manual for diagnosing mental disorders in the primary care setting. J Am Board Fam Pract 9:274–281, 1996

Dunn B: Growing up with a psychotic mother: a retrospective study. Am J Orthopsychiatry 63:177–189, 1993

Eisen J, Steketee G: Course of illness in obsessive-compulsive disorder, in Review of Psychiatry, Vol 16. Edited by Dickstein JJ, Riba MB, Oldham JM. Washington, DC, American Psychiatric Press, 1997, pp 73–95

Elder RW, Shulls RA, Sleet DA, et al: Effectiveness of mass media campaigns for reducing drinking and driving and alcohol-involved crashes: a systematic review. Am J Prev Med 27:57–65, 2004

European Commission: Green Paper: Improving the Mental Health of the Population: Towards a Strategy on Mental Health for the European Union. Brussels, Belgium, European Commission, 2005

Ezzati M, Lopez AD, Rodgers A, et al: Comparative Quantification of Health Risks: The Global and Regional Burden of Disease Attributable to Selected Major Risk Factors. Geneva, World Health Organization, 2004

Faggiano F, Vigna-Taglianti FD, Version E, et al: School-based prevention for illicit drugs' use. Cochrane Database of Systematic Reviews 2005, Issue 2. Art. No.: CD003020. DOI: 10.1002/14651858.CD003020.pub2.

Faraone SV, Biederman J, Mennin D, et al: Attention-deficit hyperactivity disorder with bipolar disorder: a familial subtype? J Am Acad Child Adolesc Psychiatry 36:1378–1387, 1997

Field TM, Schanberg SM, Scafidi F, et al: Tactile/kinesthetic stimulation effects on preterm neonates. Pediatrics 77:654–658, 1986

Findling R, Calabrese J, Youngstrom E: Divalproex sodium vs. placebo in the treatment of youth at genetic high-risk for developing bipolar disorder, in Program and Abstracts of the Fifth International Conference on Bipolar Disorder; Pittsburgh, PA, June 12–14, 2003

First MB, Pincus HA: The DSM-IV Text Revision: rationale and potential impact on clinical practice. Psychiatr Serv 53:288–292, 2002

Fischbach RL, Herbert B: Domestic violence and mental health: correlates and conundrums within and across cultures. Soc Sci Med 45:1161–1176, 1997

Frances AJ, Egger HL: Wither psychiatric diagnosis. Aust N Z J Psychiatry 33:161–165, 1999

Freres DR, Gillham JE, Reivich K, et al: Preventing depressive symptoms in middle school students: the Penn Resiliency Program. Int J Emerg Ment Health 4:31–40, 2002

Gauthier S, Reisberg B, Zandig M, et al: Mild cognitive impairment. Lancet 367:1262–1270, 2006

Geller B, Craney JL, Bolhofner K, et al: Two-year prospective follow-up of children with a prepubertal and early adolescent bipolar disorder phenotype. Am J Psychiatry 159:927–933, 2002

Gillham JE, Reivich KJ, Jaycox LH, et al: Prevention of depressive symptoms in school children: two year follow-up. Psychol Sci 6:343–351, 1995

Goodman SH: Emory University Project on Children of Disturbed Parents. Schizophr Bull 13:411–423, 1987

Grant BF, Dawson DA: Age at onset of alcohol use and its association with DSM-IV alcohol abuse and dependence: results from the National Longitudinal Alcohol Epidemiologic Survey. J Subst Abuse 9:103–110, 1997

Grant BF, Stinson FS, Dawson DA, et al: Prevalence and co-occurrence of substance use disorders and independent mood and anxiety disorders: results from the National Epidemiologic Survey on Alcohol and Related Conditions. Arch Gen Psychiatry 61:807–816, 2004

Greenberg MT; Domitrovich C, Bumbarger B: The prevention of mental disorders in school-aged children: current state of the field. Prevention & Treatment 4(1), March 2001 [doi: 10.1037/1522-3736.4.1.41a]

Hannan AP, Rapee RM, Hudson JL: The prevention of depression in children: a pilot study. Behav Change 17:78–83, 2005

Harkavy-Friedman JM: Can early detection of psychosis prevent suicidal behavior? Am J Psychiatry 163:768–770, 2006

Harnett PH, Dadds MR: Training school personnel to implement a universal school-based prevention of depression program under real-world conditions. J School Psychol 42:343–357, 2004

Hasin DS, Grant BF: Major depression in 6050 former drinkers: association with past alcohol dependence. Arch Gen Psychiatry 59:794–800, 2002

Hasin DS, Aharonovich E, Liu X, et al: Alcohol and ADH2 in Israel: Ashkenazis, Sephardics, and recent Russian immigrants. Am J Psychiatry 159:1432–1434, 2002a

Hasin D, Aharonovich E, Liu X, et al: Alcohol dependence symptoms and alcohol dehydrogenase 2 polymorphism: Israeli Ashkenazis, Sephardics, and recent Russian immigrants. Alcohol Clin Exp Res 26:1315–1321, 2002b

Hasin D, Liu X, Nunes E, et al: Effects of major depression on remission and relapse of substance dependence. Arch Gen Psychiatry 59:375–380, 2002c

Hasin DS, Goodwin RD, Stinson FS, et al: Epidemiology of major depressive disorder: results from the National Epidemiologic Survey on Alcoholism and Related Conditions. Arch Gen Psychiatry 62:1097–1106, 2005

Hasin DS, Liu X, Alderson D, et al: DSM-IV alcohol dependence: a categorical or dimensional phenotype? Psychol Med 36:1695–1705, 2006

Hasin DS, Stinsoon FS, Ogburn E, et al: Prevalence, correlates, disability, and comorbidity of DSM-IV alcohol abuse and dependence in the United States: results from the National Epidemiologic Survey on Alcohol and Related Conditions. Arch Gen Psychiatry 64:830–842, 2007

Haslam N: Categorical versus dimensional models of mental disorder: the taxometric evidence. Aust N Z J Psychiatry 37:696–704, 2003

Haslam N, Beck AT: Subtyping major depression: a taxometric analysis. J Abnorm Psychol 103:686–692, 1994

Heim C, Nemeroff CB: The impact of early adverse experiences on brain systems involved in the pathophysiology of anxiety and affective disorders. Biol Psychiatry 46:1509–1522, 1999

Helzer JE, Bucholz KK, Bierut LJ, et al: Should DSM-V include dimensional diagnostic criteria for alcohol use disorders? Alcohol Clin Exp Res 30:303–310, 2006

Henderson C, Liu X, Diez Roux AV, et al: The effects of US state income inequality and alcohol policies on symptoms of depression or alcohol dependence. Soc Sci Med 58:565–575, 2004

Herrman H, Saxena S, Moodie R: Promoting Mental Health: Concepts, Emerging Evidence and Practice. Geneva, World Health Organization, 2005

Horwath E, Johnson J, Klerman GE, et al: What are the public health implications of subclinical depressive symptoms? Psychiatr Q 65:323–337, 1994

Hosman CMH, Jané-Llopis E: Effective Mental Health Promotion and Mental Disorders Prevention. Brussels, European Union for Health Promotion and Education, 1999

Huppert FA: A population approach to positive psychology: the potential for population interventions to promote well-being and prevent disorder, in Positive Psychology in Practice. Edited by Linley PA, Joseph S. New York, Wiley, 2004, pp 693–709

Huppert FA, Whittington JE: Symptoms of psychological distress predict 7-year mortality. Psychol Med 25:1073–1086, 1995

Hyman SE: Foreword, in Advancing DSM Dilemmas in Psychiatric Diagnosis. Edited by Phillips KA, First MB, Pincus HA. Washington, DC, American Psychiatric Association, 2003, pp xi–xxi

Ingram RE, Price JM: Vulnerability to Psychopathology: Risk Across the Lifespan. New York, Guilford, 2001

International Labour Organization: Mental Health in the Workplace. Geneva, International Labour Organization, 2000

Jablensky A: The nature of psychiatric classification: issues beyond ICD-10 and DSM-IV. Aust N Z J Psychiatry 33:137–144, 1999

Jané-Llopis E, Matytsina I: Mental health and alcohol, drugs and tobacco: a review of the comorbidity between mental disorders and the use of alcohol, tobacco and illicit drugs. Drug Alcohol Rev 25:515–536, 2006

Johannessen JO, McGlashan TH, Larsen TK, et al: Early detection strategies for untreated first-episode psychosis. Schizophr Res 51:39–46, 2001

Johnson J, Weissman MM, Klerman GL: Service utilization and social morbidity associated with depressive symptoms in the community. JAMA 267:1478–1483, 1992

Judd LL, Paulus MP, Wells KB, et al: Socioeconomic burden of subsyndromal depressive symptoms and major depression in a sample of the general population. Am J Psychiatry 153:1411–1417, 1996

Judd LL, Akiskal HS, Maser JD, et al: A prospective 12-year study of subsyndromal and syndromal depressive symptoms in unipolar major depressive disorders. Arch Gen Psychiatry 55:694–700, 1998

Kashani JH, Allan WD, Beck NC Jr, et al: Dysthymic disorder in clinically referred preschool children. J Am Acad Child Adolesc Psychiatry 36:1426–1433, 1997

Katschnig H, Amering M: The long-term course of panic disorder and its predictors. J Clin Psychopharmacol 18(suppl):6S–11S, 1998

Kaufman J, Yang BZ, Douglas-Palumberi H, et al: Genetic and environmental predictors of early alcohol use. Biol Psychiatry 61:1228–1234, 2007

Kellam SG, Ling X, Merisca R, et al: The effect of the level of aggression in the first grade classroom on the course and malleability of aggressive behavior into middle school. Dev Psychopathol 10:165–185, 1998

Kendell R, Jablensky A: Distinguishing between the validity and utility of psychiatric diagnoses. Am J Psychiatry 160:4–12, 2003

Kendler KS, Gardner CO Jr: Boundaries of major depression: an evaluation of DSM-IV criteria. Am J Psychiatry 155:172–177, 1998

Kendler KS, Walters EE, Neale MC, et al: The structure of the genetic and environmental risk factors for six major psychiatric disorders in women: phobia, generalized anxiety disorder, panic disorder, bulimia, major depression, and alcoholism. Arch Gen Psychiatry 52:374–383, 1995

Kessing LV, Andersen PK: Does the risk of developing dementia increase with the number of episodes in patients with depressive disorder and in patients with bipolar disorder? J Neurol Neurosurg Psychiatry 75:1662–1666, 2004

Kessler RC, Price RH: Primary prevention of secondary disorders: a proposal and agenda. Am J Community Psychol 21:607–633, 1993

Kessler RC, Merikangas KR, Berglund P, et al: For DSM-V, it's the "disorder threshold," stupid: author reply. Arch Gen Psychiatry 61:1051–1052, 2004

Kim-Cohen J, Caspi A, Rutter M, et al: The caregiving environments provided to children by depressed mothers with or without an antisocial history. Am J Psychiatry 163:1009–1018, 2006

Klein DN, Lewinsohn PM, Seeley JR: Hypomanic personality traits in a community sample of adolescents. J Affect Disord 38:135–143, 1996

Kohn R, Saxena S, Levav I, et al: The treatment gap in mental health care. Bull World Health Organ 82:858–866, 2004

Kolvin I, Trowell J: Diagnosis and classification in child and adolescent psychiatry: the case of unipolar affective disorder. Psychopathology 35:117–121, 2002

Kopelman MD, Fleminger S: Experience and perspectives on the classification of organic mental disorders. Psychopathology 35:76–81, 2002

Kovacs M: A developmental perspective on methods and measures in the assessment of depressive disorders: the clinical interview, in Depression in Young People: Developmental and Clinical Perspectives, Vol 1. Edited by Rutter M, Izard CR, Read PB. New York, Guilford, 1986, pp 435–465

Kovacs M, Devlin B: Internalizing disorders in childhood. J Child Psychol Psychiatry 39:47–63, 1998

Kowalenko N, Rapee RM, Simmons J, et al: Short-term effectiveness of a school-based early intervention program for adolescent depression. Clin Child Psychol Psychiatry 10:493–507, 2005

Krueger RF, Caspi A, Moffitt TE, et al: The structure and stability of common mental disorders (DSM-III-R): a longitudinal-epidemiological study. J Abnorm Psychol 107:216–227, 1998

Lewinsohn PM, Rohde P, Seeley JR, et al: Natural course of adolescent major depressive disorder in a community sample: predictors of recurrence in young adults. Am J Psychiatry 157:1584–1591, 2000

Lieb R, Isensee B, Hofler M, et al: Parental depression and depression in offspring: evidence for familial characteristics and subtypes? J Psychiatr Res 36:237–246, 2002a

Lieb R, Isensee B, Hofler M, et al: Parental major depression and the risk of depression and other mental disorders in offspring: a prospective-longitudinal community study. Arch Gen Psychiatry 59:365–374, 2002b

Livesley WJ: A framework for integrating dimensional and categorical classifications of personality disorder. J Pers Disord 21:199–224, 2007

Livesley WJ, Jang KL, Vernon PA: Phenotypic and genetic structure of traits delineating personality disorder. Arch Gen Psychiatry 55:941–948, 1998

Lynch FL, Hornbrook M, Clarke GN, et al: Cost-effectiveness of an intervention to prevent depression in at-risk teens. Arch Gen Psychiatry 62:1241–1248, 2005

Lynskey MT, Heath AC, Bucholz KK, et al: Escalation of drug use in early onset cannabis users vs co-twin controls. JAMA 289:427–433, 2003

Magruder KM, Calderone GE: Public health consequences of different thresholds for the diagnosis of mental disorders. Compr Psychiatry 41 (suppl):14–18, 2000

Mann JJ, Apter A, Bertolote J, et al: Suicide prevention strategies: a systematic review. JAMA 294:2064–2074, 2005

Masi G, Akiskal HS, Akiskal K: Detecting the risk for affective spectrum disorders in children of bipolar parents, in Early Detection and Management of Mental Disorders. Edited by Maj M, Lopez-Ibor JJ Jr, Sartorius N, et al. New York, Wiley, 2005, pp 163–182

Mayberg HS, Liotti M, Brannan SK, et al: Reciprocal limbic-cortical function and negative mood: converging PET findings in depression and normal sadness. Am J Psychiatry 156:675–682, 1999

Maziade M, Bissonnette L, Rouillard E, et al: 6p24–22 region and major psychoses in the eastern Quebec population. Le Groupe IREP. Am J Med Genet 74:311–318, 1997

McGorry PD: The concept of recovery and secondary prevention in psychotic disorders. Aust N Z J Psychiatry 26:3–17, 1992

Melle I, Larsen TK, Haahr U, et al: Reducing the duration of untreated first-episode psychosis: effects on clinical presentation. Arch Gen Psychiatry 61:143–150, 2004

Melzer D, Tom BD, Brugha TS, et al: Common mental disorder symptom counts in populations: are there distinct case groups above epidemiological cut-offs? Psychol Med 32:1195–1201, 2002

Mendlowicz MV, Stein MB: Quality of life in individuals with anxiety disorders. Am J Psychiatry 157:669–682, 2000

Merikangas KR, Akiskal HS, Angst J, et al: Lifetime and 12-month prevalence of bipolar spectrum disorder in the National Comorbidity Survey replication. Arch Gen Psychiatry 64:543–552, 2007

Mezzich JE, Fabrega H, Mezzich AC: On the clinical utility of multiaxial diagnosis: experience and perspectives, in Diagnosis and Classification in Psychiatry: A Critical Appraisal of DSM-III. Edited by Tischler GL. Cambridge, UK, Cambridge University Press, 1987, pp 449–463

Mifsud C, Rapee RM: Early intervention for childhood anxiety in a school setting: outcomes for an economically disadvantaged population. J Am Acad Child Adolesc Psychiatry 44:996–1004, 2005

Mineka S, Watson D, Clark LA: Comorbidity of anxiety and unipolar mood disorders. Annu Rev Psychol 49:387–412, 1998

Mirsky AF, Elliott AK: Children of persons with schizophrenia: an overview of empirical research, in Early Detection and Management of Mental Disorders. Edited by Maj M, Lopez-Ibor JJ Jr, Sartorius N, et al. New York, Wiley, 2005, pp 111–133

Montero I, Ascensio A, Hernandez I, et al: Two strategies for family intervention in schizophrenia: a randomized trial in a Mediterranean environment. Schizophr Bull 27:661–670, 2001

Mrazek P, Haggerty RJ (eds): Reducing Risks for Mental Disorder: Frontiers for Preventive Intervention Research. Washington, DC, National Academies Press, 1994

Mrazek P, Hosman CMH (eds): Toward a Strategy of Worldwide Action to Promote Mental Health and Prevent Mental and Behavioral Disorders. Alexandria, VA, World Federation for Mental Health, 2002

Muñoz RF, Ying YW, Bernal G, et al: Prevention of depression with primary care patients: a randomized controlled trial. Am J Community Psychol 23:199–222, 1995

Murray CJL, Salomon JA, Mathers CD, et al: Summary Measures of Population Health: Concepts, Ethics, Measurement, and Applications. Geneva, World Health Organization, 2002

Nair P, Black MM, Schuler M, et al: Risk factors for disruption in primary caregiving among infants of substance abusing women. Child Abuse Negl 21:1039–1051, 1997

O'Connor TG, Heron J, Golding J, et al: Maternal antenatal anxiety and behavioural/emotional problems in children: a test of a programming hypothesis. J Child Psychol Psychiatry 44:1025–1036, 2003

O'Kearney R, Gibson M, Christensen H, et al: Effects of a cognitive-behavioural internet program on depression, vulnerability to depression and stigma in adolescent males: a school-based controlled trial. Cogn Behav Ther 35:43–54, 2006

Paykel ES: Mood disorders: review of current diagnostic systems. Psychopathology 35:94–99, 2002

Peterson BS, Pine DS, Cohen P, et al: Prospective, longitudinal study of tic, obsessive-compulsive, and attention deficit/hyperactivity disorders in an epidemiological sample. J Am Acad Child Adolesc Psychiatry 40:685–695, 2001

Pincus HA, Davis WW, McQueen LE: "Subthreshold" mental disorders: a review and synthesis of studies on minor depression and other "brand names." Br J Psychiatry 174:288–296, 1999

Pincus HA, McQueen LE, Ellison L: Subthreshold mental disorders: nosological and research recommendations, in Advancing DSM: Dilemmas in Psychiatric Diagnosis. Edited by Phillips KA, First MB, Pincus HA. Washington, DC, American Psychiatric Association, 2003, pp 129–144

Pine DS, Alegría M, Cook EH Jr, et al: Advances in developmental science and DSM-V, in A Research Agenda for DSM-V. Edited by Kupfer DJ, First MB, Regier DA. Washington, DC, American Psychiatric Association, 2002, pp 85–122

Post RM, Chang KD, Findling RL, et al: Prepubertal bipolar I disorder and bipolar disorder NOS are separable from ADHD. J Clin Psychiatry 65:898–902, 2004

Price RH, Van Ryn M, Vinokur AD: Impact of a preventive job search intervention on the likelihood of depression among the unemployed. J Health Soc Behav 33:158–167, 1992

Regier DA, Narrow WE, First MB, et al: The APA classification of mental disorders: future perspectives. Psychopathology 35:166–170, 2002

Regier DA, Narrow WE, Rae DS: For DSM-V, it's the "disorder threshold," stupid. Arch Gen Psychiatry 61:1051, 2004

Reid JB, Eddy JM, Fetrow RA, et al: Description and immediate impacts of a preventive intervention for conduct problems. Am J Community Psychol 27:483–517, 1999

Remschmidt H, Schulz E, Herpertz-Dahlmann B: Schizophrenia psychoses in childhood and adolescence. Disease Management 6:100–112, 1996

Roberts C, Kane R, Bishop B, et al: The prevention of depressive symptoms in rural school children: a follow-up study. International Journal of Mental Health Promotion 6:4–16, 2004

Rose G: The Strategy of Preventive Medicine. Oxford, UK, Oxford University Press, 1992

Rowe SK, Rapaport MH: Classification and treatment of sub-threshold depression. Curr Opin Psychiatry 19:9–13, 2006

Royal College of Psychiatrists: Prevention in Psychiatry: Report of the Public Policy Committee Working Party. London, Royal College of Psychiatrists, 2002

Ruscio AM, Ruscio J: The latent structure of analogue depression: should the Beck Depression Inventory be used to classify groups? Psychol Assess 14:135–145, 2002

Ruscio AM, Borkovec TD, Ruscio J: A taxometric investigation of the latent structure of worry. J Abnorm Psychol 110:413–422, 2001

Ruscio AM, Chiu WT, Roy-Byrne P, et al: Broadening the definition of generalized anxiety disorder: effects on prevalence and associations with other disorders in the National Comorbidity Survey Replication. J Anxiety Disord 21:662–676, 2007

Rutter M: Protective factors in children's responses to stress and disadvantage, in Primary Prevention of Psychopathology, Vol 3: Social Competence in Children. Edited by Kent MW, Rolf J. Hanover, NH, University Press of New England, 1979, pp 49–74

Ryan ND, Puig-Antich J, Ambrosini P, et al: The clinical picture of major depression in children and adolescents. Arch Gen Psychiatry 44:854–861, 1987

Sadek N, Bona J: Subsyndromal symptomatic depression: a new concept. Depress Anxiety 12:30–39, 2000

Sameroff AJ: Environmental risk factors in infancy. Pediatrics 102(suppl):1287–1292, 1998

Sameroff A, Seifer R, Zax M, et al: Early indicators of developmental risk: Rochester Longitudinal Study. Schizophr Bull 13:383–394, 1987

Sánchez MM, Ladd CO, Plotsky PM: Early adverse experience as a developmental risk factor for later psychopathology: evidence from rodent and primate models. Dev Psychopathol 13:419–449, 2001

Sanders MR, Turner KM, Markie-Dadds C: The development and dissemination of the Triple P-Positive Parenting Program: a multilevel, evidence-based system of parenting and family support. Prev Sci 3:173–189, 2002

Saxena S, Jané-Llopis E, Hosman C: Prevention of mental and behavioural disorders: implications for policy and practice. World Psychiatry 5:5–14, 2006

Sheffield JK, Spence SH, Rapee RM, et al: Evaluation of universal, indicated, and combined cognitive-behavioral approaches to the prevention of depression among adolescents. J Consult Clin Psychol 74:66–79, 2006

Sher KJ, Trull TJ: Methodological issues in psychopathology research. Annu Rev Psychol 47:371–400, 1996

Sherbourne CD, Wells KB, Hays RD, et al: Subthreshold depression and depressive disorder: clinical characteristics of general medical and mental health specialty outpatients. Am J Psychiatry 151:1777–1784, 1994

Shochet IM, Ham D: Universal school-based approaches to preventing adolescent depression: past findings and future directions of the Resourceful Adolescent Program. International Journal of Mental Health Promotion 6:17–25, 2004

Sigvardsson S, Bohman M, von Knorring AL, et al: Symptom patterns and causes of somatization in men, I: differentiation of two discrete disorders. Genet Epidemiol 3:153–169, 1986

Slade T: The descriptive epidemiology of internalizing and externalizing psychiatric dimensions. Soc Psychiatry Psychiatr Epidemiol 42:554–560, 2007

Smit F, Cuijpers P, Oostenbrink J, et al: Costs of nine common mental disorders: implications for curative and preventive psychiatry. J Ment Health Policy Econ 9:193–200, 2006

Smith ML, Saltzman J, Klim P, et al: Neuropsychological function in mild hyperphenylalaninemia. Am J Ment Retard 105:69–80, 2000

Solomon DA, Keitner GI, Miller IW, et al: Course of illness and maintenance treatments for patients with bipolar disorder. J Clin Psychiatry 56:5–13, 1995

Soutullo CA, DelBello MP, Ochsner JE, et al: Severity of bipolarity in hospitalized manic adolescents with history of stimulant or antidepressant treatment. J Affect Disord 70:323–327, 2002

Spence SH, Sheffield JK, Donovan CL: Long-term outcome of a school-based, universal approach to prevention of depression in adolescents. J Consult Clin Psychol 73:160–167, 2005

Spitzer RL: Harmful dysfunction and the DSM definition of mental disorder. J Abnorm Psychol 108:430–432, 1999

Spitzer RL: Values and assumptions in the development of DSM-III and DSM-III-R: an insider's perspective and a belated response to Sadler, Hulgus, and Agich's "On values in recent American psychiatric classification." J Nerv Ment Dis 189:351–359, 2001

Spivak B, Frisch A, Maman Z, et al: Effect of ADH1B genotype on alcohol consumption in young Israeli Jews. Alcohol Clin Exp Res 31:1297–1301, 2007

Steffens DC, Krishnan KRR: Laboratory testing and neuroimaging: implications for psychiatric diagnosis and practice, in Advancing DSM: Dilemmas in Psychiatric Diagnosis. Edited by Phillips KA, First MB, Pincus HA. Washington, DC, American Psychiatric Association, 2003, pp 85–103

Stöffelmayr BE, Mavis BE, Kasim RM: The longitudinal stability of the Addiction Severity Index. J Subst Abuse Treat 11:373–378, 1994

Stuart S, O'Hara MW, Blehar MC: Mental disorders associated with childbearing: report of the Biennial Meeting of the Marcé Society. Psychopharmacol Bull 34:333–338, 1998

Tait RJ, Hulse GK: A systematic review of the effectiveness of brief interventions with substance using adolescents by type of drug. Drug Alcohol Rev 22:337–346, 2003

Towbin KE: Gaining: pediatric patients and use of atypical antipsychotics. Am J Psychiatry 163:2034–2036, 2006

Trull TJ, Sher KJ: Relationship between the five-factor model of personality and Axis I disorders in a nonclinical sample. J Abnorm Psychol 103:350–360, 1994

Tsuang MT, Stone WS, Tarbox, BA: Insights from the neuroscience for the concept of schizotaxia and the diagnosis of schizophrenia, in Advancing DSM: Dilemmas in Psychiatric Diagnosis. Edited by Phillips KA, First MB, Pincus HA. Washington, DC, American Psychiatric Association, 2003, pp 105–127

van Spronsen FJ, van Rijn, Bekhof J, et al: Phenylketonuria: tyrosine supplementation in phenylalanine-restricted diets. Am J Clin Nutr 73:153–157, 2001

Vasan RS, Beiser A, Seshadri S, et al: Residual lifetime risk for developing hypertension in middle-aged women and men: the Framingham Heart Study. JAMA 287:1003–1010, 2002

Verdoux H, Cougnard A: The early detection and treatment controversy in schizophrenia research. Curr Opin Psychiatry 16:175–179, 2003

Verdoux H, Tournier M, Cougnard A: Impact of substance use on the onset and course of early psychosis. Schizophr Res 79:69–75, 2005

Von Korff M, Katon W, Rutter C, et al: Effect on disability outcomes of a depression relapse prevention program. Psychosom Med 65:938–943, 2003

Wakefield JC: Evolutionary versus prototype analyses of the concept of disorder. J Abnorm Psychol 108:374–399, 1999

Watson D: Rethinking the mood and anxiety disorders: a quantitative hierarchical model for DSM-V. J Abnorm Psychol 114:522–536, 2005

Watson D, Clark LA: Behavioral disinhibition versus constraint: a dispositional perspective, in Handbook of Mental Control. Edited by Wegner DM, Pennebaker JW. New York, Prentice Hall, 1993, pp 506–527

Watson D, Clark LA (eds): Special issue on personality and psychopathology. J Abnorm Psychol 103:1–158, 1994

Weich S: Prevention of the common mental disorders: a public health perspective. Psychol Med 27:757–764, 1997

Weiss MG, Raguram R, Channabasavanna SM: Cultural dimensions of psychiatric diagnosis: a comparison of DSM-III-R and illness explanatory models in south India. Br J Psychiatry 166:353–359, 1995

Wells KB, Sherbourne CD: Functioning and utility for current health of patients with depression or chronic medical conditions in managed, primary care practices. Arch Gen Psychiatry 56:897–904, 1999

Wells KB, Stewart A, Hays RD, et al: The functioning and well-being of depressed patients: results from the Medical Outcomes Study. JAMA 262:914–919, 1989

Wells KB, Burnam MA, Rogers W, et al: The course of depression in adult outpatients: results from the Medical Outcomes Study. Arch Gen Psychiatry 49:788–794, 1992

Whittington JE, Huppert FA: Changes in the prevalence of psychiatric disorder in a community are related to changes in the mean level of psychiatric symptoms. Psychol Med 26:1253–1260, 1996

Widiger TA: Categorical versus dimensional classification: implications from and for research. J Pers Disord 6:287–300, 1992

Widiger TA, Clark LA: Toward DSM-V and the classification of psychopathology. Psychol Bull 126:946–963, 2000

Widiger TA, Samuel DB: Diagnostic categories or dimensions? A question for the Diagnostic and Statistical Manual of Mental Disorders—Fifth Edition. J Abnorm Psychol 114:494–504, 2005

Wilkinson R, Marmot M (eds): Social Determinants of Health: The Solid Facts, 2nd Edition. Copenhagen, Denmark, World Health Organization Regional Office for Europe, 2003. Available at: http://www.euro.who.int/document/e81384.pdf. Accessed September 23, 2009.

Wilsnack SC, Vogeltanz ND, Klassen AD, et al: Childhood sexual abuse and women's substance abuse: national survey findings. J Stud Alcohol 58:264–271, 1997

Wittchen HU: What is comorbidity: fact or artefact? Br J Psychiatry Suppl (30):7–8, 1996

Wolchik SA, West SG, Sandler IN, et al: An experimental evaluation of theory-based mother and mother-child programs for children of divorce. J Consult Clin Psychol 68:843–856, 2000

Woods SW, Breier A, Zipursky RB, et al: Randomized trial of olanzapine versus placebo in the symptomatic acute treatment of the schizophrenic prodrome. Biol Psychiatry 54:453–464, 2003

World Health Organization: The ICD-10 Classification of Mental and Behavioural Disorders: Clinical Descriptions and Diagnostic Guidelines. Geneva, World Health Organization, 1992

World Health Organization: WHO Document: Fact Sheet No 220, November 2001. Geneva, World Health Organization, 2001a

World Health Organization: The World Health Report 2001—Mental Health: New Understanding, New Hope. Geneva, World Health Organization, 2001b. Available at: http://www.who.int/whr/2001/en/. Accessed September 23, 2009.

World Health Organization: The World Health Report 2002—Reducing Risks, Promoting Healthy Life. Geneva, World Health Organization, 2002. Available at: http://www.who.int/whr/2002/en/. Accessed September 23, 2009.

World Health Organization: Prevention of Mental Disorders: Effective Interventions and Policy Options: Summary Report. Geneva, World Health Organization, 2004a. Available at: http://www.who.int/mental_health/evidence/en/prevention_of_mental_disorders_sr.pdf. Accessed September 23, 2009.

World Health Organization: Promoting Mental Health: Concepts, Emerging Evidence, Practice: A Summary Report. Geneva, World Health Organization, 2004b. Available at: http://www.who.int/mental_health/evidence/en/promoting_mhh.pdf. Accessed September 23, 2009.

World Health Organization: The World Health Report 2007—A Safer Future: Global Public Health Security in the 21st Century. Geneva, World Health Organization, 2007

Yonkers KA, Warshaw MG, Massion AO, et al: Phenomenology and course of generalized anxiety disorder. Br J Psychiatry 168:308–313, 1996

Young RM, Lawford BR, Nutting A, et al: Advances in molecular genetics and the prevention and treatment of substance misuse: implications of association studies of the A1 allele of the D2 dopamine receptor gene. Addict Behav 29:1275–1294, 2004

Zenere FJ 3rd, Lazarus PJ: The decline of youth suicidal behavior in an urban, multicultural public school system following the introduction of a suicide prevention and intervention program. Suicide Life Threat Behav 27:387–403, 1997

Ziedonis DM: Integrated treatment of co-occurring mental illness and addiction: clinical intervention, program, and system perspectives. CNS Spectr 9:892–904, 925, 2004

3

CAPTURING COMPLEXITY

*The Case for a New Classification System for
Mental Disorders in Primary Care*

Linda Gask
Christopher Dowrick
Sandra Fortes
David A. Katerndahl
Oye Gureje
Michael S. Klinkman
Bruce Arroll
Khalid Saeed
Frank deGruy III

This chapter was prepared by the Primary Care Conference Expert Group for the Conference on Public Health Aspects of Diagnosis and Classification in September 2007. The specific remit of the group was to consider adaptation of new diagnosis and classification systems in primary care; implementation of these systems in primary care settings; and training issues in relation to primary care (in liaison with Group D).

In the first section of this chapter, we present the primary care context, which differs considerably from the specialist mental health setting. Understanding this difference is essential if we are to fully explore the issues surrounding the use of diagnostic systems in the primary care setting. We describe the varying international forms of primary care. We show how problems are often presented in undifferentiated forms, with consequent difficulties in distinguishing between distress and mental disorder and with a complex relationship between psychological, mental, and social problems and their temporal variations. We explain how diagnosis in primary care often carries different meanings from diagnosis in specialist settings.

In the second section, we consider the validity of existing diagnostic systems for application in primary care. We discuss evidence for comorbidity between depression, anxiety, medically unexplained symptoms, and other related disorders and argue that this is more likely to be related to diagnostic confusion than to the coexistence of discrete conditions. We explain the substantial prevalence of subthreshold disorders in primary care and argue that current classification systems do not adequately address the importance of these disorders. We consider problems with cross-cultural application of current classification systems. We then consider the relative merits of categorical and hierarchical classification systems and provide evidence that severity and impairment should be considered separately.

In the third section, we summarize previous mental health classification systems devised or modified for primary care settings, including the primary health care version of ICD-10 (ICD-10-PHC; World Health Organization 1996) and the primary care version of DSM-IV (DSM-IV-PC; American Psychiatric Association 1995). We explain that their focus on diagnosis may be too restrictive and that, to date, attempts to introduce them into routine practice have met with limited success.

In the fourth section, we describe—and explain the uses and limitations of—tools developed for use in primary care, including interview schedules, screening instruments, severity measures, and measures of impairment and disability.

In conclusion, we argue that existing classification systems are unsatisfactory for primary care because they fail to adequately capture the clinical complexity of psychological disorders as manifest in primary care settings. We propose a classification system for primary care that is characterized by simplicity; addresses not only diagnosis but also severity, chronicity, and disability; is linked both to routine data gathering and to training; and facilitates communication between primary and specialist care.

We emphasize the importance of evidence throughout this chapter and employ the following classification of evidence, with reference by Roman numeral in the text:

- Type I: supported by large studies conducted among representative (primary care) samples in different cultures and different socioeconomic groups
- Type II: large studies conducted among (or replicated in) representative (primary care) samples in more than one country
- Type III: at least one large (and/or high-quality) study conducted in primary care
- Type IV: qualitative study

- Type V: expert opinion, including the opinions of international institutions, service users, and carers
- Type VI: clinical or anecdotal reports or experience

We specifically devised this system to classify evidence from epidemiological and descriptive studies rather than treatment studies, which is the purpose for which such systems have usually been devised.

The Context of Primary Care: What Is the Clinical Significance and Utility of Mental Health Diagnosis in Primary Care?

WHAT IS PRIMARY CARE?

Primary care has been defined by the Institute of Medicine (1996, p. 1) in the United States as the "provision of integrated, accessible health care services by clinicians who are accountable for addressing a large majority of personal health needs, developing a sustained partnership with patients, and practicing in the context of the family and community." In many countries, such care is provided by a range of different professionals and paraprofessionals, including doctors, nurses, medical assistants, health visitors, social workers, and lay workers, and there is a considerable overlap between *primary care* and *general medical* settings.

Primary care systems can be further categorized according to whether they

- Act as gatekeepers to specialist services (as in the United Kingdom and Northern Ireland), whether they provide free-market services in parallel to specialist services, or whether they function in a blended system containing both free-market and gatekeeper functionality (as in the United States);
- Are free to patients at the point of care delivery;
- Are led by doctors or nonmedical personnel; and
- Provide continuity of care, and the degree to which they do so, from fixed-list systems to systems in which very little continuity of care is the norm.

Primary care teams also can represent the level within health systems where health promotion and disease prevention can be organized, together with community interventions, as in the Family Health Program in the Federative Republic of Brazil (Ministério da Saúde 1998). This type of primary care system is one of four types of primary care interventions cited by the Pan American Health Organization (PAHO) document "Renovação da Atenção Primária em Saúde nas Américas, Documento de Posicionamento da Organização Pan-Americana da Saúde/OMS, Agosto 2005," (originally in English) (Type V), which include

- Selective and specific interventions, such as immunization or oral rehydration, especially directed to the poorest populations all over the world;
- Primary care, as in Europe and North America, which is the entrance for the health system and the locus for continuous care for most of the population, usually based on family doctors or general practitioners;
- The Alma-Ata Primary Care model, which considers primary care not only as the first level of assistance but also as the place for coordination of all intersectoral interventions needed to deal with and overcome a broader group of health problems determinants, including community interventions that go from dealing with garbage to improving self-esteem; and
- Primary care as a human rights and health promotion approach, a more ideological and philosophical perspective.

The average duration of a primary care consultation varies considerably throughout the world, from less than 5 minutes in some countries in the developing world, where more than 100 people may be seen in one clinic session, to 20 minutes or even longer, in parts of Northern Europe and North America. Two points are probably worth noting here: 1) in some developing countries, the Federal Republic of Nigeria being an example, the notion of "primary care," to both the lay public and policy makers, carries an implicit assumption that the provision of such care does not involve medical doctors; and 2) the diversity of the nature of primary care may have implications for how patients present their problems. For example, there is evidence that "somatizers" are fewer in settings in which a more personalized type of care is common than in those where it is less common (Type I) (Gureje 2004).

UNDIFFERENTIATED PROBLEMS ARE MORE COMMON IN PRIMARY CARE

Patients in primary care settings are much less likely to present with clearly identifiable diagnostic syndromes. People present to primary care workers with a wide variety of symptoms, concerns, worries, and problems. These are not only *undifferentiated* (Type VI), as originally described by Balint (1957), but also, at least at first presentation, *unrehearsed* by prior discussion with doctors versed in the *agenda and language of diagnosis*. When people present to specialist professionals, they will either 1) be seeking that professional by choice because they consider that the problem is within the clinical domain of that professional (where there is no gatekeeping by primary care), or 2) have had a negotiation about the likely cause of their symptoms and possible diagnosis by the signposting primary care professional (where gatekeeping by primary care exists). The critical point to understand is that primary care clinicians will often encounter unfiltered and unrecognized symptoms that may or may not be identifiable as mental health syndromes, whereas specialty mental health clinicians will encounter filtered symptoms that are recognized and understood as representative of a mental health problem.

DISTRESS VERSUS DISORDER IN PRIMARY CARE

It is important to understand the difference between *distress* and *disorder*. Distress can be present in patients for many reasons other than the presence of a mental health disorder, and patients with threshold disorders may not display any distress. Many primary care patients are clearly distressed but do not show other symptoms of mental illness (Type III) (Katerndahl et al. 2005), yet primary care physicians often recognize this distress and manage these patients differently from those without distress. These physicians do so without guidance from most existing nosological systems, which—with one or two exceptions discussed later in this chapter—do not account for "distress." In our view, neither the DSM nor the ICD classification system reflects the richness and complexity of mental health in the primary care settings. The adverse consequences of the confusion between these two constructs can be seen in the misidentification of distressed patients as "depressed" by casefinding instruments, such as the Center for Epidemiologic Studies Depression Scale or Hamilton Rating Scale for Depression, when they are used in primary care (Santor and Coyne 2001a, 2001b) (Type III).

We consider the merits and shortcomings of the adaptations that have been made specifically for primary care in a later section of this chapter (see "Classification Systems Developed or Modified for Primary Care").

THE COMPLEX RELATIONSHIP BETWEEN PHYSICAL, MENTAL, AND SOCIAL PROBLEMS

Primary care patients frequently present with a mixture of psychological, physical, and social problems. Mental health problems occur more frequently in people with common chronic physical illness, such as diabetes, arthritis, and heart disease, and their comorbid mental health problems may not be recognized because attention is focused on their physical illnesses. The primary care context of life events and medical comorbidity plays an important role in how primary care patients experience and cope with their mental health symptoms (Type I) (Kisely and Simon 2005). In turn, those symptoms reciprocally affect subjective perceptions of health and objective measures of disease outcomes (Type I) (Sherbourne et al. 1996; Sinclair et al. 2001). One of the most important aspects of a classification of mental disorders for primary care should be to enable primary care workers to accurately record core elements of the context of care, such as life events, undifferentiated symptoms, and patient perceptions, goals, and preferences for care; this will, in turn, allow clinicians to more effectively help patients with "mixed" physical, mental, and social suffering. The traditional biomedical model that still dominates the training pattern of health professionals makes it difficult for them to deal with these patients because there is often not a specific problem that can be solved.

Therefore, classification of mental disorders in primary care should contribute to the organization of a therapeutic strategy that links different interventions: medication, psychotherapy, and social support interventions such as groups, family therapy, or community work. This is particularly necessary where primary care interventions incorporate the Alma-Ata model (see earlier description in subsection titled "What Is Primary Care?")—which specifically incorporates social interventions—as is the case in Latin America. This model is also applicable internationally across many different systems of "primary care."

PSYCHIATRIC "CASENESS" IN INDIVIDUALS WITH TRANSIENT, RECURRENT, OR CHRONIC SYMPTOMS

Even when primary care patients meet diagnostic criteria for specific disorders, their symptoms often fluctuate over time and their "caseness" may be transient. Of patients with at least one disorder, 20% recover within 3 months (Type III) (Berti Ceroni et al. 1992). Nosological diagnoses have been reported to last less than 4 weeks 30% of the time and less than 6 months 65% of the time (Type III) (Lamberts and Hofmans-Okkes 1993). We lack good research on the long-term validity and prognosis of "threshold" mental health diagnoses in primary care patient samples. Community-based epidemiological studies have confirmed that many patients have recurrent or chronic depression (Gask 2005; Judd et al. 1998; Kessler et al. 2005) (Type III), but the relative risk of recurrence or chronicity in depressed primary care patients and the level of disability associated with this risk are not clear (Type III) (Van Weel-Baumgarten et al. 1998; Vuorilehto et al. 2005).

The fluctuating nature of symptoms has made it difficult to assess performance of primary care workers in recognizing and treating mental health problems. Recognition of the potential long-term effect of such problems on health and function has led to aggressive case finding and treatment efforts in primary care settings in order to prevent disability. Although primary care workers have frequently been criticized for their lack of skill in recognizing threshold mental disorders, recognition in primary care is itself a complex phenomenon related, in part, to the transience of symptoms. Researchers have found higher rates of detection (and treatment) for patients with more severe symptoms and higher levels of disability (Type III) (Dowrick and Buchan 1995; Mental Health and General Practice Investigation [MaGPIe] Research Group 2004), and some evidence indicates that short-term outcomes for "detected" and "undetected" depressed primary care patients are no different (Coyne et al. 1997) (Type III).

PRAGMATIC SOLUTIONS

Diagnosis is less precise (and less frequent) in primary care than in specialty care. Family doctors are more likely to think in terms of *problems* than diagnoses and are more likely to make a diagnosis of depression if they believe they can manage and treat it: that is, diagnosis tends to follow management decisions, not precede them (Type III) (Dowrick et al. 2000). In the United States, primary care clinicians are often trained to separate patients by level of severity of symptoms and to carry out full mental health diagnostic assessment only for patients with significant and/or persistent symptoms (Klinkman and Valenstein 1997) (Type V).

Diagnoses are essentially value-based moral decisions. Fulford (2001) has argued that all mental illness concepts are derived from negatively evaluated experiences. This is a particularly relevant issue in primary care: family doctors and patients may see making and accepting a mental health diagnosis as a social and moral decision. Depressed women may seek and accept help (i.e., medication) for the sake of others, when they feel they are not adequately fulfilling their social roles. Doctors may offer diagnosis and treatment to show that they are taking their patients' suffering seriously, despite considering that the patients' problems are primarily social in origin (Type IV) (Maxwell 2005).

The stigma traditionally associated with mental disorders is reinforced by these conceptions and makes it more difficult for doctors to help people who do not consider that these professionals could offer support for emotional complaints. Such problems are usually understood as a sign of character weakness, spiritual phenomenon, or a consequence of social suffering that is to be accepted as part of life (Gask et al. 2003) (Type IV).

Limitations in Validity of Existing Diagnostic Systems for Application in Primary Care

There are a number of ways in which existing diagnostic systems may have limited validity when applied in primary care settings. We specifically consider the following problems:

- Comorbidity: real or apparent?
- Subthreshold disorders
- Cross-cultural application of systems
- The basis for current classification systems
- Categorical and hierarchical classification systems
- Severity and impairment

COMORBIDITY

In primary care, overlapping psychopathology may exist along a spectrum of anxiety, depression, somatization, and substance misuse. This coexistence may be cross-sectional, in that all these symptoms appear together at the same time, or it may be longitudinal, in the sense that one set of symptoms is followed closely in time by another (Katerndahl 2005).

Much of the evidence regarding comorbidity was assembled during the 1990s in the World Health Organization Collaborative Study of Psychological Problems in General Health Care (Type I) (Üstün and Sartorius 1995), conducted in 15 centers in Asia, Africa, Europe, and the Americas. Consecutive primary care attendees between the age of majority (typically 18 years) and 65 years were screened (N= 25,916), and stratified random samples were interviewed (n = 5,438). The study found that "well-defined" psychological problems (according to ICD-10 [World Health Organization 1992]) are frequent in general health care settings (median 24% of attendees), and among the most common problems were depression, anxiety, alcohol misuse, somatoform disorders, and neurasthenia.

The most common co-occurrence was depression and anxiety (Type I) (Sartorius et al. 1996). A number of substudies considered other aspects of comorbidity:

- Across all 15 centers, 22% of primary care patients reported persistent pain, but there was wide variation in prevalence rates across centers (range, 5.5%–33%). Relative to patients without persistent pain, those with pain were more likely to have an anxiety or a depressive disorder (adjusted odds ratio [OR], 4.14; 95% confidence interval [CI], 3.52–4.86) (Type I) (Gureje et al. 1998).
- ICD-10-defined somatization disorder was relatively uncommon in most primary care settings, but a less restrictive "abridged" form (four current symptoms in males and six in females) was more common. Of particular note, somatizing patients were at elevated risk for self-reported disease burden, negative perceptions of their health, and comorbid depression and generalized anxiety disorder (GAD; Type I) (Gureje et al. 1997a).
- Although hypochondriasis is frequently described as a chronic condition, distinct from anxiety and depressive disorders, some 45% of those patients who met criteria for hypochondrias at 12-month follow-up also met criteria for a DSM-IV (American Psychiatric Association 1994) anxiety or depressive disorder (Type I) (Simon et al. 2001).
- Cases of depression were found to have an increased rate of developing a new episode of unexplained fatigue at follow-up, with an adjusted odds ratio of 4.15 (95% CI, 2.64–6.54). Similarly, cases of unexplained fatigue were found to have an odds ratio of 2.75 (95% CI, 1.32–5.78). Further adjustment for subthreshold symptoms at baseline weakened the reported associations, especially

between fatigue and the development of a new episode of depression, but these remained significant (Type I) (Skapinakis et al. 2004).

- Analysis of data from 1,617 adult primary care attendees with at least three symptoms of anxiety, depression, and/or somatization but no formal ICD-10 disorders provided support for the existence of a mixed anxiety-depression category crossing the boundaries of current anxiety and depression disorders (Type I) (Piccinelli et al. 1999).

Medically unexplained symptoms pose a particular problem in this regard, and we will return later to the shortcomings of current diagnostic systems with respect to these problems in primary care settings. Considerable empirical evidence now suggests that persistent medically unexplained symptoms frequently coexist with mood or anxiety disorders in primary care settings (Type III) (Garcia-Campayo et al. 1998; Kessler et al. 1996; Kirmayer and Robbins 1991; Toft et al. 2005). In the study by Toft et al. (2005) in the Kingdom of Denmark, comorbidity was highest for anxiety disorders, with 89% having another diagnosis, but was lowest for somatoform disorders, with 39%. The stability of somatizing symptoms and somatization disorders among primary care patients is a problem in itself, because most of the symptoms (61%) will not be recalled as a health problem 1 year later (Type I) (Simon and Gureje 1999). Other researchers have concluded that hypochondriasis is difficult to distinguish from severe depressive syndromes in the primary care setting (Type III) (Escobar et al. 1998).

In a vast majority of patients presenting with symptomatology of conversion/dissociative disorders, there is an available history suggestive of depression antedating the development of these symptoms. In a study in Pakistan of 100 patients with conversion disorder diagnosed on the basis of DSM-IV criteria, overall comorbidity of anxiety and depression symptoms was 95%, and only 5% of the patients were without any comorbid anxiety or depressive symptoms (Type III) (Khan et al. 2005).

Substance misuse also may commonly be comorbid with anxiety and depression. A recent study from the MaGPIe group in New Zealand revealed that more than one-third of people attending their general practitioner had a diagnosable mental disorder during the previous 12 months. The most common disorders identified by accepted and well-validated psychological instruments were anxiety disorders, depression, and substance use disorders, and there was high comorbidity of these three groups, with the experience of mixed pictures as common as disorders occurring alone (Type III) (MaGPIe Research Group 2003).

However, there is not universal agreement in the literature about comorbidity with chronic fatigue. Hickie and his colleagues (1999) in Australia examined longitudinal patterns of comorbidity between prolonged fatigue and other forms of psychological distress in primary care and found that the risk of developing prolonged fatigue was not increased in patients who initially had psychological distress (OR, 1.4; 95% CI, 0.2–3.6); neither was the risk of developing psychological distress increased in patients who initially had prolonged fatigue (OR, 1.4; 95% CI, 0.6–3.4) (Type III).

Do all these findings constitute evidence of true comorbidity (i.e., coexistence of two—or often more—discrete disorders) or, rather, an overlap between—and therefore confusion of—diagnostic categories? We consider the latter far more likely.

SUBTHRESHOLD DISORDERS

Subthreshold conditions (i.e., not meeting full diagnostic criteria for mental disorders in DSM-IV or ICD-10) are prevalent and associated with significant costs and disability. Pincus et al. (1999) have shown how varying conceptualizations have been applied to define these conditions. Further research is needed to apply methodological and intellectual rigor to investigation of such conditions and to systematically consider them in a broader clinical and nosological context.

The substantial degree of associated disability and clinical reality of subthreshold disorders in primary care settings is clear from existing research. Considerable attention was paid to the presence of subthreshold disorders in the World Health Organization study (Piccinelli et al. 1999). Some 9% of patients had a "subthreshold condition" (see Table 3–1) that did not meet diagnostic criteria but involved clinically significant symptoms and functional impairment (Type I) (Piccinelli et al. 1999). In the Italian subsample (Type III) (Rucci et al. 2003), the impact of subthreshold disorders on health perception, disability in daily activities, and psychological distress was analyzed by using multiple regression models. The overall prevalence of subthreshold disorders exceeded that of ICD-10 disorders. Subjects with subthreshold disorders reported levels of psychological distress, disability in daily activities, and perceived health comparable to those of patients with full-fledged ICD-10 disorders. When Rucci and colleagues analyzed the associated health characteristics of individual subthreshold disorders, they found that each subthreshold disorder was characterized by poorer health perception, after adjusting for comorbidity with defined disorders and physical illness, age, and gender. Disability in daily activities was increased in individuals with subthreshold depression and agoraphobia. They concluded that "because of the prevalence and associated characteristics of subthreshold disorders, primary-care physicians should attach adequate importance to the patient's perceived poor health, distress and inability to fulfill daily tasks. The clinical relevance of subthreshold disorders has also potential implications for ongoing revisions of classification systems" (Rucci et al. 2003, p. 171).

In a very different setting—the Nigerian subsample (Type III) (Gureje 2002)—caseness on either the General Health Questionnaire (25% of the sample, using a

TABLE 3–1. CIDI-PHC subthreshold mental disorders

Subthreshold disorder	Symptoms
I) Depression	Any of three symptoms of ICD-10 criterion B (depressed mood, loss of interest or pleasure, decreased energy, or increased fatigability) plus three or more symptoms of ICD-10 criterion C (loss of confidence or self-esteem, guilt or self-reproach feelings, suicidal behavior or death thoughts, impaired concentration, agitation or retardation, sleep disturbances, change in appetite and weight)
II) Generalized anxiety	Three or more anxiety symptoms of 1-month duration among the ICD-10 symptom criteria for generalized anxiety disorder, including apprehension, motor tension, and autonomic overactivity
III) Agoraphobia	Marked fear or avoidance of specific situations, such as crowds, public places, traveling alone, or being away from home; two symptoms of anxiety in the feared situation had to co-occur at least on one occasion
IV) Hypochondriasis	Strong belief in the presence of a serious physical disease persisting for 6 months or longer, in spite of a doctor's reassurance that there is no physical cause for the symptoms
V) Panic	Up to three spells in the previous month, with at least four panic symptoms
VI) Somatization	More than three somatization symptoms occurring in at least two of the four domains defined by genitourinary, cardiovascular, pain, and gastrointestinal symptoms

Note. The CIDI-PHC (Primary Health Care version of the Composite International Diagnostic Interview) was used to identify these subthreshold mental disorders, as defined at a consensus meeting of World Health Organization experts (Type V)—in addition to formal mental disorders.

cutoff of 5 or more) or ICD-10 (10% of the sample) was associated with poor self-rated overall health, interviewer-rated occupational disability, and more disability days in the previous month. However, at 12-month follow-up, caseness on the General Health Questionnaire but not categorical ICD-10 diagnostic status at baseline was associated with disability, poor health perception, and high health service utilization.

Other studies in primary care settings in the United States and Australia have confirmed these findings. In the Australian National Survey of Mental Health and Well-Being, considerable disability was found to be associated with symptom levels indicating distress but not reaching levels for formal diagnosis of anxiety or depression (Type III) (Korten and Henderson 2000). In a sample of 1,001 primary care patients in a large health maintenance organization (HMO) in the United States (Type III) (Olfson et al. 1996), subthreshold symptoms were as, or more, common than their respective Axis I disorders for panic (10.5% vs. 4.8%), depression (9.1% vs. 7.3%), anxiety (6.6% vs. 3.7%), obsessive-compulsive (5.8% vs. 1.4%), and alcohol (5.3% vs. 5.2%) and other drug (3.7% vs. 2.4%) cases. Patients with each of the subthreshold symptoms had significantly higher Sheehan Disability Scale scores (greater impairment) than did patients with no psychiatric symptoms. Many patients (22.6%– 53.4%) with subthreshold symptoms also met the full criteria for other Axis I disorders. After adjusting for the confounding effects of other Axis I disorders, other subthreshold symptoms, age, sex, race, marital status, and perceived physical health status, only depressive symptoms, major depressive disorder, and (to a lesser extent) panic symptoms were significantly correlated with the impairment measures. Specific diagnostic categories also proved to be problematic.

Somatization disorder was relatively uncommon in most primary care settings in the World Health Organization international sample (Type I) (Gureje et al. 1997a), but a less restrictive form of the condition was more common. This less restrictive form was not only comorbid with other disorders but also independently associated with disability. This is a finding that is well known to most primary care physicians but is a relative surprise for psychiatric epidemiologists.

The appropriateness of the current definition of *hypochondriasis* to primary care is also questionable. Although ICD-10-defined hypochondriasis was rare in primary care settings, a less restrictive form of hypochondriasis that does not require the criterion of refusal to accept medical reassurance was more common and was not different from the full syndrome in terms of comorbidity with other disorders and associated disability (Type I) (Gureje et al. 1997b).

GAD was very common in the World Health Organization international study, but using the ICD-10 definition of GAD—in which 6 months is the minimum duration and at least four associated symptoms are required for diagnosis—results in a substantial proportion of psychosocially disabled subjects characterized by anxiety, tension, and worry that do not meet the diagnostic criteria for caseness (Type I) (Maier et al. 2000).

The specific validity and utility of DSM-IV *somatoform disorder* was explored by determination of the prevalence of DSM-IV somatoform and nonsomatoform disorders in HMO patients with medically unexplained symptoms diagnosed by chart review (Type III) (Smith et al. 2005). Patients with full or abridged DSM-

IV somatoform diagnoses were labeled "DSM somatoform-positive," whereas patients without them were labeled "DSM somatoform-negative." Correlates of this DSM somatoform-negative status were female gender ($P=0.007$), less severe mental ($P=0.007$) and physical dysfunction ($P=0.004$), a decreased proportion of medically unexplained symptoms ($P<0.10$), and less psychiatric comorbidity ($P<0.10$) (c-statistic, 0.77). The authors concluded that depression and anxiety characterized patients with medically unexplained symptoms better than did somatoform disorders. They suggested radically revising the somatoform disorders for DSM-5 by incorporating a new, very large group of now-overlooked DSM somatoform-negative patients (bearing some similarity to those meeting criteria for the "abridged" syndrome in the World Health Organization study), who were typically women with less severe dysfunction.

This brief discussion of subthreshold conditions and unexplained symptoms highlights our need for improved symptom-level classification in primary care to better categorize people with physical symptoms for which doctors cannot find an organic explanation. DSM-IV criteria have much more limited validity or utility for patients seen in primary care settings than for those seen by specialist mental health workers. The scientific validity of a classification system in which the residual category (undifferentiated somatoform disorder) is far more common than the main subtype (somatization disorder) (Type I) (Janca et al. 1999) is questionable. A new classification system may result from the recent considerable growth in research into medically unexplained symptoms (Rosendal et al. 2005); this work should be expanded upon to help develop a symptom-level classification.

CROSS-CULTURAL APPLICATION OF SYSTEMS

The DSM-IV-TR (American Psychiatric Association 2000) and ICD-10 classifications in current use are direct descendants of clinical and research diagnostic classifications developed in the United States and Western Europe. As such, the classifications are based on a Western conceptual framework of mental health and mental illness, and it is highly likely that some of their diagnostic categories will have limited validity in other parts of the world. It is also highly likely that some conditions important in other non-Western cultures will have limited or inaccurate representation in DSM or ICD (Type V) (Mezzich et al. 1999). This issue may be even more relevant in cross-cultural primary care settings, because, as we have seen earlier in this chapter, this is the setting in which unfiltered symptoms present to health care workers.

Support for this view comes from research that has documented the following shortcomings:

- Some formal diagnoses may lack concept validity in certain settings (Patel and Mann 1997).

- Some "culture-bound" diagnostic labels may not fit with formal diagnostic criteria yet apparently serve a useful purpose in terms of describing a group with clinically significant levels of disturbance and disability (Type III) (Chang et al. 2005).
- Severity thresholds for clinically significant diagnoses may differ between cultures.

In the World Health Organization study of cross-national differences in depression (Type I) (Simon et al. 2002), although large cross-national variations in depression prevalence were found, the syndrome defined by DSM-IV showed a remarkably similar form at centers with low, medium, or high prevalence rates. Therefore, the authors concluded that apparent differences in depression could not be attributed to "category fallacy" (Kleinman 1977) while acknowledging that no analysis of symptom patterns could definitively establish the clinical validity of the DSM depression syndrome. However, when the authors used the effect of depression on disability to compare diagnostic thresholds, they found evidence that the same diagnostic criteria identified differing levels of depression severity.

In this large cross-national study, centers with higher prevalence of depressive symptoms generally had higher prevalence rates for the full range of psychological and somatic symptoms that were assessed (Type I) (Simon et al. 1996). The authors commented that prevalence differences are often attributed to stigmatization of psychological distress in some cultures, but there was no evidence that patients at low-prevalence centers tended to deny psychological distress and report somatic symptoms. This finding is echoed in other reports that challenge commonly held stereotypes about low reporting of psychological symptoms in South Asian populations (Type II) (Bhui et al. 2004; Patel et al. 1998).

Elevated rates of medically unexplained physical symptoms may have been observed in Latin American primary care populations, but this does not appear to be associated with strongly held beliefs about the presence of physical illness, because most of these patients recognize an emotional or at least a psychosocial origin for their symptoms, and these physical symptoms are usually associated with psychological symptoms. This also happens in other parts of the world and seems to be related to a non-Cartesian cultural model of understanding body-mind relationship (Type VI) (Okasha and Okasha 1999; Patel 2000; Patel et al. 1998). It is also important to note that some differences hitherto attributed to "culture" may indeed reflect the form and nature of the doctor-patient interaction, which may be largely dictated by the system of health service operating in the country (Institute of Medicine 1996).

PROBLEMS WITH THE BASIS FOR CURRENT CLASSIFICATION SYSTEMS

Current classification systems are generally based on research and experience in psychiatric settings. If patients with mental illness who are seen in these settings differ significantly from those seen in primary care settings, then the classification system on which that experience is based may not reflect mental illness as seen in primary care. There is mounting evidence that there are indeed important differences between patients seen in primary care and those seen in specialty mental health settings. Mentally ill patients in primary care are less distressed, less likely to have a discernible mental disorder, and less impaired than their psychiatric cohorts (Coyne and Schwenk 1997; Goldberg and Huxley 1992; Zinbarg et al. 1994).

For patients with mental illness to be seen and studied in psychiatric settings, they must present to their primary care physician, be recognized as mentally ill, be referred to the mental health sector, and keep their appointments. Although fewer than 50% of those with a mental disorder are recognized as such by their primary care physician, those who are recognized tend to be more disabled, with greater symptom severity (Type I). Once recognized, patients are more likely to be referred to the mental health sector if they are hallucinating or suicidal (Type II) (Saraceno et al. 1995) and are more likely to keep their psychiatric (Coyne et al. 1997) appointments if they have had prior mental health concerns and lack unexplained physical symptoms (Type III) (Olfson 1991). All of these filters lead to marked differences between primary care and psychiatric populations. Thus, out of 100 primary care patients with mental illness, only 3 patients are seen in a mental health setting. This distortion compromises the primary care validity of classification systems based on patients seen in mental health settings.

CATEGORICAL AND HIERARCHICAL CLASSIFICATION SYSTEMS

The advantage of dimensional measures over categorical systems of classification has been extensively debated in the literature, particularly for neurotic disorders, personality disorder, and common mental disorders (Goldberg 2000).

Categorical representation of important clinical phenomena can misrepresent dimensional qualities (Nease and Aikens 2003), and it has been more than two decades since Goldberg and colleagues (1987) demonstrated that two highly correlated symptom dimensions of anxiety and depression could be shown, by latent-trait analysis, to underlie the common psychiatric disorders in primary care. More recently, Slade and Andrews (2005) suggested that depression—as measured in the Australian National Survey of Mental Health and Well-Being, a large epidemiological survey—is best conceptualized, measured, and classified as a continuously distributed syndrome rather than as a discrete diagnostic entity (Type III).

Application of particular hierarchical rules also may have implications for management in primary care. The diagnosis of adjustment disorder is undermined by mechanistic application of current DSM-IV-TR diagnostic criteria; major depressive episode can be diagnosed when five or more depressive symptoms have been present for longer than 2 weeks, irrespective of the close temporal relationship between an identifiable stressor and symptoms (Type V) (Casey et al. 2001). If these classificatory rules are applied, the diagnosis of adjustment disorder is therefore systematically removed from clinical consideration. This is not just a semantic issue. Because adjustment disorders are more likely than depression to be considered self-limiting conditions and therefore not in need of medical intervention, ignoring or abolishing them may also have profound clinical implications. If a patient is diagnosed with an adjustment disorder, it may be reasonable to assume that the patient can deal with this him- or herself, relying on personal coping styles and problem-solving mechanisms or enlisting the help of his or her usual networks of social support. On the other hand, if the patient is diagnosed with a depressive disorder, the doctor may feel obliged to offer him or her a formal course of treatment.

SEVERITY AND IMPAIRMENT

There has been a working assumption that increasing severity of disorders is directly associated with increasing disability (Patel et al. 1998) and hence with worse outcomes. However, there are two problems with this assumption. The first, as we have already noted, is that it tends to play down the considerable levels of impairment experienced by people with subthreshold disorders. The second is that severity and impairment may not, after all, be directly associated but rather may form separate but overlapping domains. Research by Foley et al. (2003) on the Virginia Twin Registry found that although the risk factors for major depression and associated functional impairment were substantially correlated, they were not identical. The most parsimonious model suggests that more than a quarter of the variance in associated functional impairment was a result of factors unrelated to risk for major depression (Type III).

This is potentially important in primary care. Family doctors are probably better at assessing impairment than at making formal psychiatric diagnoses. If impairment is indeed a discrete problem from diagnosis, then awareness of, and emphasis on, this difference may well play to the strengths of primary care.

It seems evident that current definitions of mental health disorders do not take advantage of the capacity of primary care to assemble symptom-level data over time. A classification that incorporates this element could greatly enhance the utility of diagnosis for primary care workers.

Classification Systems Developed or Modified for Primary Care

EARLY LITERATURE

During the 1980s, there was increasing recognition of a need for an appropriate, relatively simple, and flexible classification or list of problems presenting in primary care. It was recognized that neither ICD nor the International Classification of Health Problems in Primary Care could be consistently applied by general practitioners. A multidimensional formulation was mooted, incorporating notions of severity and duration, as well category, on the dimensions of psychological illness, social stresses and supports, personality, and physical illness (Type V) (Jenkins et al. 1988). Some steps were taken toward development of a triaxial classification system of health problems containing a psychological problem list and a social problem list (Type I) (Clare et al. 1992).

During the same period, David Goldberg (1992) proposed a simpler approach to classification informed by research in primary care and based on the patient's need for intervention. He characterized these as 1) disorders requiring recognition and discussion (the largest group), 2) patients requiring social support and social intervention, and 3) disorders that require skilled intervention. Skills required for this group include the "ability to assess the severity of depressive illness and so make a rational decision about antidepressants…and the ability to assess an anxious patient. The best management of anxiety disorders will depend upon the skills of the doctor…; however, the most important skills required are those in fact needed for all groups mentioned so far, and those are counseling skills" (Goldberg 1992, p. 192). This pragmatic approach, incorporating advice on management, informed the development of ICD-10-PHC.

ADAPTED CLASSIFICATIONS FOR PRIMARY CARE: DSM-IV-PC AND ICD-10-PHC

Both DSM-IV and ICD-10 have been adapted for primary care. However, the extent to which these systems have been adopted in *routine* primary care data collection and monitoring across the world is unclear, although ICD-10-PHC has been widely disseminated. Translation between the systems (and the International Classification of Primary Care [ICPC]) is possible but complex, and clinical comparability of the same diagnosis in different systems is limited by the characteristics of the different systems (Lamberts et al. 1998).

DSM-IV-PC

The primary care version of DSM-IV was introduced in 1995 and contains several symptom-based clinical algorithms designed to guide the primary care physician through the diagnostic process (American Psychiatric Association 1995).

Some limitations are evident (Pingitore and Sansone 1998). Although the multiaxial nature of DSM-IV encompasses a variety of biopsychosocial parameters, the multiaxial schema is not emphasized in DSM-IV-PC, particularly with respect to impairment or disability. It is a large and complex volume that requires some level of familiarity before it can be used. The complexity of the diagnostic schemes, and the amount of time needed to reach a diagnosis, have been cited as conspicuous limitations.

Other general concerns with DSM-IV-PC include the need to 1) validate its diagnostic criteria in the primary care setting (Brody 1996), 2) refine comorbidity and multiaxial assessment (deGruy and Pincus 1996), and 3) reevaluate the relegation of subthreshold disorders to the diffuse category of "not otherwise specified" (Pincus et al. 1995). Additional concerns include the viability of primary care reimbursement for visits related to psychiatric care and the need to connect diagnoses with specific treatments (deGruy and Pincus 1996).

ICD-10-PHC

The primary health care version of ICD-10 for mental and behavioral disorders was first published in 1995 (Üstün et al. 1995) and was finalized after a series of field trials in different countries across the world (Type I) (Jenkins et al. 2002). It is now the most widely used system in primary care settings, although it has a range of uses and can be used as much for education and training as for data collection and coding. The ICD-10-PHC classification bears a rough correspondence to ICD-10 categories; is user friendly, based on the different types of management that various conditions require; and includes detailed advice about the sort of psychological help shown to be effective. It also provides information about each disorder that should be given to a patient and his or her family. Advice is given about drug treatments, where these are indicated, as well as features that require specialist referral. The system consists of 25 conditions (see Table 3–2) that are common in primary care settings, but each country is encouraged to adapt the system to its own needs.

This classification was field tested in 30 different centers in 19 countries, with published evidence available from two large studies (Type II) (Busnello et al. 1999; Goldberg et al. 1995). In the United Kingdom study, a total of 478 general practitioners completed all stages of the study. Nearly all participating general practitioners found the classification "very useful" or "useful." Each category was also rated, and most received high ratings; those that were criticized were amended by the group at a later meeting.

Simultaneous ratings of patients by two general practitioners were obtained for 1,691 patients, and the concurrent reliability was found to be satisfactory (κ, 0.68; in the Brazilian study, a κ of 0.79 was achieved). Concurrent validity was assessed by comparing diagnoses made by general practitioners with those made by independent raters using a semistructured interview, and this also produced a high value (κ, 0.93). However, validity ratings for individual diagnoses were quite variable: high values were obtained for psychotic disorders, mental retardation, tobacco use disorder, and enuresis, but very low values were seen for sleep problems, conduct disorder, dementia, and alcohol use. Other diagnoses were intermediate. Many suggestions made both by the participating general practitioners and by ex-

TABLE 3–2. The 25 disorders included in the primary health care version of ICD-10 (ICD-10-PHC), with full ICD-10 codes

Disorder	Code
Addictive disorders	
1 Alcohol use disorder	F10
2 Drug use disorder	F11
3 Tobacco use disorder	F17.1
Common mental disorders	
4 Depression	F32
5 Phobic disorders	F40
6 Panic disorders	F41.0
7 Generalised anxiety	F41.1
8 Mixed anxiety depression	F41.2
9 Adjustment disorder	F43
10 Dissociative disorder (conversion hysteria)	F44
11 Unexplained somatic complaints	F45
12 Neurasthenia	F48.0
13 Eating disorders	F50
14 Sleep problems	F51
15 Sexual disorders	F52
16 Bereavement	Z63
Organic disorders	
17 Dementia	F00
18 Delirium	F05
Psychotic disorders	
19 Chronic psychotic disorders	F20
20 Acute psychotic disorders	F23
21 Bipolar disorders	F3
Disorders of childhood	
22 Mental retardation	F70
23 Hyperkinetic (attention-deficit) disorder	F90
24 Conduct disorder	F91
25 Enuresis	F98.0

Note. For multipurpose health workers, a simpler version is available that consists of six categories: 1) cognitive disorders, 2) alcohol and drug use disorder, 3) psychotic disorders, 4) depression, 5) anxiety disorders, and 6) unexplained somatic complaints.

pert reviewers in each country were incorporated into modifications to the system. Each country is free to use those categories found most useful by the health professionals in that country.

In the United Kingdom, the classification has been modified further since the original publication, and the whole system has been reissued twice with a number of additional features, including information leaflets for patients and information about voluntary agencies (World Health Organization 2004) (www.mentalneurologicalprimarycare.org).

ICD-10-PHC is simple and easy to use and links diagnosis to treatment. However, it does not address issues of measurement of severity, associated disability or chronicity, or the accompanying social problems manifest in primary care settings. It is also important to note that simply disseminating guidelines developed from ICD-10-PHC did not improve outcomes in a British primary care study (Type III) (Upton et al. 1999).

INTERNATIONAL CLASSIFICATION OF PRIMARY CARE

The ICPC, first published in 1987 under the auspices of the World Organization of Family Doctors, represents a departure from the two classifications described previously. ICPC was designed to capture and code three essential elements of each clinical encounter: the patient's *reason for the encounter,* the clinician's *diagnosis,* and the (diagnostic and therapeutic) *interventions,* all organized in an *episode of care* data structure that links the initial to all subsequent encounters for the same clinical problem. This approach permits coding of 95% or more of primary care visits and enables calculation of prior and posterior probabilities for important diseases (Type V) (Okkes et al. 2002a). Published experience with ICPC has confirmed the validity of its key elements (Types I and II) (Lamberts 1989; Lamberts and Schade 1988; Okkes et al. 2001, 2002a), and worldwide experience with ICPC has confirmed its utility in creating and analyzing episodes of care for several common primary care problems (Type III) (Britt et al. 1994; Leduc et al. 1995).

ICPC (see Table 3–3) is not an exhaustive classification scheme; rather, it aims at hierarchically ordering the primary care domain in order to better understand its content. It was designed either to serve as a stand-alone classification or to be mapped to ICD, as necessary, for billing or statistical purposes. The full conversion structure between ICPC and ICD has identified areas in which ICPC offers more granularities (symptom and complaint codes) as well as areas in which ICD is far more granular (most diagnostic codes, including mental health codes). ICPC-2, released in 1998 in paper and in 2000 in electronic format, has been designed from the start to be incorporated into electronic health record software with a conversion map to ICD-10 (Okkes et al. 2002a, 2002b; World Organization of Family Doctors International Classification Committee 1998). In this use, the underlying data structure of ICPC provides the "backbone" to enable the proper organization and retrieval of clinical data. This approach has been tested in the Kingdom of the Netherlands and the Republic of Malta, where an ICPC-ICD-10 thesaurus has been embedded in the TransHis software used by dozens of Dutch and Maltese general practitioners to code diagnoses in both ICPC and ICD terms (Britt et al. 1994; Lamberts and Schade 1988; Soler 2000). More recently, teams in Australia, the Kingdom of Belgium, Canada, and the United States have created electronic health records using the combination of ICPC plus clinical terminology or ICD mapping (Bernstein et al. 1997; Nease and Green 2003) (plus World Organization of Family Doctors Classification Committee reports). One good example of the conceptual differences between ICD and ICPC can be seen in the classification of unexplained somatic complaints. ICD-10 includes rubrics F45.3–F45.9, describing limited syndromes attributed to somatization (and thus susceptible to errors in attribution); in ICPC, these symptoms are not assumed to be caused by a mental disorder and are coded simply as individual symptoms. In primary care, the high prevalence of undifferentiated symptoms described by patients raises questions about the validity of the causal attributions embedded in the ICD-10 terms. Although a considerable amount of work has been done to reconcile the conceptual differences between ICPC and ICD/DSM (Type V) (Lamberts et al. 1998), more work is clearly needed.

Although the limited diagnostic specificity available in ICPC is problematic, ICPC offers a major advantage in its more complete capture of the context of mental health problems. The episode structure of ICPC automatically accommodates mental health and biomedical comorbidity by simply noting all active problems at a point in time or over a specified time interval. The inclusion of symptoms as reasons for encounter at the beginning of a longitudinal data stream enables investigation of the relation between somatic symptoms and mental health disorders at a level of resolution not possible when using other classifications. The routine coding of social problems provides detail about the social context in which mental health problems occur that is not available anywhere else. Pilot studies to embed severity of illness and disability coding into ICPC have been completed (Type II) (Parkerson et al. 1996), but these have not yet been formally integrated into the classification.

Tools Developed for Primary Care

Four types of tools promoted for use in primary care are briefly reviewed here because they are used as *aids to diagnosis* in the primary care setting: interview schedules designed for primary care, screening tools, and tools for assessment of severity and disability.

TABLE 3–3.   International Classification of Primary Care, 2nd Edition (ICPC-2): diagnostic terms in Chapter P (psychosocial)

Term	Title
P01	Feeling anxious/nervous/tense
P02	Acute stress reaction
P03	Feeling depressed
P04	Feeling/behaving irritable/angry
P05	Senility, feeling/behaving old
P06	Sleep disturbance
P07	Sexual desire reduced
P08	Sexual fulfillment reduced
P09	Sexual preference concern
P10	Stammering, stuttering, tics
P11	Eating problems in children
P12	Bedwetting, enuresis
P13	Encopresis/bowel training problem
P15	Chronic alcohol abuse
P16	Acute alcohol abuse
P17	Tobacco abuse
P18	Medication abuse
P19	Drug abuse
P20	Memory disturbance
P22	Child behaviour symptom/complaint
P23	Adolescent behaviour symptom/complaint
P24	Specific learning problem
P25	Phase-of-life problems in adults
P27	Fear of mental disorder
P28	Limited function/disability psychosocial
P29	Psychological symptom/complaint, other
P70	Dementia
P71	Organic psychosis, other
P72	Schizophrenia
P73	Affective psychosis
P74	Anxiety disorder/anxiety state
P75	Somatisation disorder
P76	Depressive disorder
P77	Suicide/suicide attempt
P78	Neurasthenia, surmenage
P79	Phobia, compulsive disorder

TABLE 3–3. International Classification of Primary Care, 2nd Edition (ICPC-2): diagnostic terms in Chapter P (psychosocial) *(continued)*

Term	Title
P80	Personality disorder
P81	Hyperkinetic disorder
P82	Posttraumatic stress disorder
P85	Mental retardation
P86	Anorexia nervosa, bulimia
P98	Psychosis not otherwise specified, other
P99	Psychological disorders, other

INTERVIEW SCHEDULES

Interview schedules have been used primarily for research purposes. The exception is the Primary Care Evaluation of Mental Disorders, which has been widely used across the world and generates DSM-IV diagnoses (Spitzer et al. 1994). However, to what extent such a formal schedule might be adopted into routine primary care consultations, particularly in developing countries, remains unclear. It could add more difficulties to the establishment of a good doctor-patient relationship and restrict even more the approach to personal and social problems associated with the development of mental disorder, which is essential to proper management of mental health problems, especially in primary care.

SCREENING TOOLS

Screening instruments also have been widely used in research. The best known is the General Health Questionnaire (Goldberg and Williams 1998), which is available in four versions (12-, 28-, 30-, 60-item) and translated into numerous languages. The General Health Questionnaire is nonspecific and does not provide specific diagnoses, unlike the Hospital Anxiety and Depression Scale (Zigmond and Snaith 1983); the self-completion measures derived from the Primary Care Evaluation of Mental Disorders; the original comprehensive Patient Health Questionnaire (Spitzer et al. 1999); the depression-specific Patient Health Questionnaire-9 (Kroenke et al. 2001); the GAD-7 for anxiety (Spitzer et al. 2006); and the Patient Health Questionnaire-15 for severity of somatic symptoms (Kroenke et al. 2002).

However, although a variety of other tools have been developed for screening, there is considerable disagreement in the literature about whether screening is of benefit in improving psychosocial outcomes of people with psychiatric disorder who are managed in nonpsychiatric settings (Agency for Healthcare Research and Quality 2009; Gilbody et al. 2001). A brief screening tool consisting of only two written screening questions, plus the addition of a question inquiring if help is needed, that can be completed in the waiting room (or asked directly) and handed to the primary care worker has recently shown promising results in terms of diagnostic validity (Arroll et al. 2005). However, as some studies in Brazil have found, self-answered questionnaires in underdeveloped countries usually have to be read by an interviewer, even for research finalities, because a significant proportion of patients attending primary care units are semi-illiterate (Type III) (Mari and Williams 1985).

MEASURING SEVERITY

Screening questionnaires also can be used to measure severity of symptoms. The Patient Health Questionnaire has been widely used for this purpose in depression. Other tools include the Inventory to Diagnose Depression (Zimmerman et al. 1986), the Primary Care Screener for Affective Disorder (Rogers et al. 2002), and the 21-item Major Depressive Disorder subscale of the Psychiatric Diagnostic Screening Questionnaire (Zimmerman and Mattia 2001). All perform as well as the Beck Depression Inventory (Rogers et al. 2005), although most of these have not been validated for use in countries outside the United States or in languages other than English. Measurement of severity in primary care is being introduced in the United Kingdom through the next Quality Outcomes Framework, which will enable assessment of severity to be directly linked to treatment guidelines for depression that are recommended by the National Institute for Clinical Excellence (2004).

MEASURING IMPAIRMENT AND DISABILITY

Disability in relation to depression has commonly been measured using the Sheehan Disability Scale (Sheehan 1983), a three-item self-report scale measuring the severity of disability in the domains of work, family life/home responsibilities, and social/leisure activities. Each of these three domains is scored on a 10-point Likert scale, where a score of 0 is "not at all impaired," 5 is "moderately impaired," and 10 is "very severely impaired." The score provides a measure of total functional disability (range 0–30). This scale has been shown to have adequate internal reliability (α-coefficients and factor analyses) and construct/criterion-related validity (Leon et al. 1992).

The Social Functioning Questionnaire, an eight-item self-report scale (score range 0–24), was developed from the Social Functioning Schedule, a semistructured interview that has been used primarily with nonpsychotic patients and has good test-retest and interrater reliability as well as construct validity. The Social Functioning Questionnaire was developed to meet the need for a quick assessment of perceived social function (Tyrer et al. 2005).

Recent research attention has focused on the World Health Organization Disability Assessment Schedule, a brief instrument that is available in a variety of versions for rating by observer, self, or caregiver (for details of schedules, see www.who.int/icidh/whodas/index.html). This measure is derived from the International Classification of Functioning and Disability model of functioning and disability and has good internal consistency and convergent validity in the primary care setting (Chwastiak and Von Korff 2003).

Conclusions and Recommendations

SUMMARY CONCLUSIONS

Existing classification systems are unsatisfactory for primary care.

- Most systems have been *adapted for,* rather than *developed in,* primary care settings; the exception is ICPC.
- In general, the systems do not capture the complexity of psychological disorder as it manifests in primary care settings, with associated physical illness and social problems.
- Specifically, the systems do not address, in a satisfactory way, the problems of comorbidity, subthreshold disorders, cross-cultural applications, or the differences between severity and impairment/disability.

A classification system for primary care should

- Be characterized by simplicity.
- Address diagnosis, severity, and chronicity.
- Be linked to disability assessment.
- Be linked to routine data gathering, including gathering information on outcomes.
- Be linked to training.
- Facilitate communication between primary and specialist care.

LIMITATIONS OF THIS CHAPTER

The definition of primary care used in this chapter is different from the World Health Organization definition, which includes a variety of elements in addition to the provision of health care to people who come forward with a health problem. In this chapter, we deal predominantly with curative aspects of primary health care services. We do not propose a classification of mental health problems for public health purposes: such a classification would undoubtedly be useful.

Most of the evidence presented here comes from English-speaking sources. We recognize the limitations that this may impose; for example, in relating our findings and conclusions to the situation in Eastern Europe and francophone countries. We consider that evidence regarding both primary care–related psychiatric classifications and primary care mental health service delivery is relatively sparse in these parts of the world, in part because academic expertise in the field of primary care mental health is less well developed. We recommend that steps be taken, through the World Health Organization and other organizations, to address this relative deficiency.

RECOMMENDATIONS

- Measurement of *severity of symptoms* is essential in primary care settings. A solution to the problems with categorical-based systems in primary care would be to combine aspects of the categorical approach with the dimensional approach (measurement of severity of symptoms) (Nease et al. 2002).
- Impairment should be recognized as discrete from diagnosis or severity. A tailored mental health *disability* classification needs to be linked directly to the classification system. In the current system, many people with subthreshold disorders have significant levels of disability.
- We welcome the development, in ICPC, of a classification of *social problems* in primary care and recommend that this classification be reviewed and revised so it can be used to support clinical data exchange between primary medical care and social care.
- Rather than reconceptualizing the categorical system of diagnosis to include subthreshold disorders and distress, we recommend that categorical diagnoses should be more stringent and precise so that they become rarer—but more significant—events in primary care. This would reduce unnecessary medicalization (Dowrick 2004) and enhance focus on those most in need of care.

Example of Classification System

On this basis we suggest that a classification system for use in primary care would include the following key dimensions:

1. Diagnostic framework, composed of ICPC-2 codes for patients' reasons for encounter and general practitioner's diagnosis (recognizing that these may often be the same if using Codes P01 to P29)
2. Severity, using reliable self-rated measure (e.g., Patient Health Questionnaire-9 for depression)
3. Chronicity (We are not aware of reliable measures, but this may require questions about how long the patient has experienced symptoms or problems and checking of case notes.)
4. Disability, using reliable self-rated measure such as the Social Functioning Questionnaire
5. Social problems (e.g., using ICPC-2 Z codes)

These dimensions cover the range of information likely to be readily available or accessible during a routine primary care encounter. They build on the existing knowledge and skills of primary care health professionals and make sense within the current parameters of primary care. The dimensions provide both doctor and patient with sufficient information to make an accurate assessment of the patient's problems.

The dimensions also provide a much stronger basis than currently exists for considering whether and how to intervene. Rather than relying exclusively on categorical diagnoses, the assessment of chronicity, severity, disability, and social problems offers primary care clinicians (and health policy makers) crucial additional information, enabling better targeting of medical, psychological, and social interventions.

This process also, importantly, provides the patient with an opportunity to play a substantial role in both assessment and management. In assessment, reasons for encounter and evidence of severity and disability may be more reliably provided by the patient than by the physician. This multidimensional approach to assessment also intrinsically leads toward a multidimensional approach to management, offering the patient greater choice: not only about whether he or she wishes for help for the mental health problems at the moment (Arroll et al. 2005) but also about whether the focus of such help should be on symptom reduction, greater functional ability, or the resolution of social difficulties.

For a classification system to be widely adopted, it needs to be simple, grounded in primary care research and reality, locally adapted for specific populations and countries, easily used as a teaching tool, and readily adaptable for purposes of data collection. We are aware that this will have *training implications,* and it will be necessary to produce a multilingual training package—in tandem with the classification system—as well as a specific implementation strategy aimed at diffusion within, and adoption by, primary care systems to a greater degree than has been the case in the past.

The collective experiences of the World Health Organization (in developing and testing ICD-10-PHC) and the World Organization of Family Doctors (in developing and testing ICPC) provide a strong platform on which we can build a new classification.

References

Agency for Healthcare Research and Quality: U.S. Preventive Services Task Force (USPSTF). Available at: http://www.ahrq.gov/clinic/uspstfix.htm. Accessed October 6, 2009.

American Psychiatric Association: Diagnostic and Statistical Manual of Mental Disorders, 4th Edition. Washington, DC, American Psychiatric Association, 1994

American Psychiatric Association: Diagnostic and Statistical Manual of Mental Disorders, 4th Edition, Primary Care Version. Washington, DC, American Psychiatric Association, 1995

Arroll B, Goodyear-Smith F, Kerse N, et al: Effect of the addition of a "help" question to two screening questions on specificity for diagnosis of depression in general practice: diagnostic validity study. BMJ 331:884, 2005

Balint M: The Doctor, His Patient and the Illness. London, Pitman, 1957

Bernstein RM, Hollingworth GR, Viner G, et al: Reliability issues in coding encounters in primary care using an ICPC/ICD-10 based controlled clinical terminology. Proc AMIA Annu Fall Symp 843, 1997

Berti Ceroni G, Berti Ceroni F, Bivi R, et al: DSM-III mental disorders in general medical sector: a follow-up and incidence study over a two-year period. Soc Psychiatry Psychiatr Epidemiol 27:234–241, 1992

Bhui K, Bhugra D, Goldberg D, et al: Assessing the prevalence of depression in Punjabi and English primary care attenders: the role of culture, physical illness and somatic symptoms. Transcult Psychiatry 41:307–322, 2004

Britt H, Bridges-Webb C, Sayer GP, et al: The diagnostic difficulties of abdominal pain. Aust Fam Physician 23:375–377, 380–381, 1994

Brody DS: The DSM-IV-PC: toward improving management of mental disorders in primary care. J Am Board Fam Pract 9:300–302, 1996

Busnello ED, Tannous L, Gigante L, et al: Diagnostic reliability of mental disorders of the International Classification of Diseases in primary care. Rev Saúde Pública 33:487–494, 1999

Casey P, Dowrick C, Wilkinson G: Adjustment disorders: fault line in the psychiatric glossary. Br J Psychiatry 179:479–481, 2001

Chang DF, Myers HF, Yeung A, et al: Shenjing shuaruo and the DSM-IV: diagnosis, distress, and disability in a Chinese primary care setting. Transcult Psychiatry 42:204–218, 2005

Chwastiak LA, Von Korff M: Disability in depression and back pain: evaluation of the World Health Organization Disability Assessment Schedule (WHO DAS II) in a primary care setting. J Clin Epidemiol 56:507–514, 2003

Clare A, Gulbinat W, Sartorius N: A triaxial classification of health problems presenting in primary health care: a World Health Organization multicentre study. Soc Psychiatry Psychiatr Epidemiol 27:108–116, 1992

Coyne JC, Schwenk TL: Relationship of distress to mood disturbance in primary care and psychiatric populations. J Consult Clin Psychol 65:161–168, 1997

Coyne JC, Klinkman MS, Gallo SM, et al: Short-term outcomes of detected and undetected depressed primary care patients and depressed psychiatric patients. Gen Hosp Psychiatry 19:333–343, 1997

deGruy FV 3d, Pincus H: The DSM-IV-PC: a manual for diagnosing mental disorders in the primary care setting. J Am Board Fam Pract 9:274–281, 1996

Dowrick C: Beyond Depression: A New Approach to Understanding and Management. Oxford, UK, Oxford University Press, 2004

Dowrick C, Buchan I: Twelve month outcome of depression in general practice: does detection or disclosure make a difference? BMJ 311:1274–1276, 1995

Dowrick C, Gask L, Perry R, et al: Do general practitioners' attitudes towards depression predict their clinical behaviour? Psychol Med 30:413–419, 2000

Escobar JL, Gara M, Waitzkin H, et al: DSM-IV hypochondriasis in primary care. Gen Hosp Psychiatry 20:155–159, 1998

Foley D, Neale MC, Gardner CO, et al: Major depression and associated impairment: same or different genetic and environmental risk factors? Am J Psychiatry 160:2128–2133, 2003

Fulford KW: "What is (mental) disease?": an open letter to Christopher Boorse. J Med Ethics 27:80–85, 2001

Garcia-Campayo J, Lobo A, Pérez-Echeverría MJ, et al: Three forms of somatisation presenting in primary care settings in Spain. J Nerv Ment Dis 186:554–560, 1998

Gask L: Is depression a chronic illness? For the motion. Chronic Illn 1:101–106, 2005

Gask L, Rogers A, Oliver D, et al: Qualitative study of patients' perceptions of the quality of care for depression in general practice. Br J Gen Pract 53:278–283, 2003

Gilbody SM, House AO, Sheldon TA: Routinely administered questionnaires for depression and anxiety: systematic review. BMJ 322:406–409, 2001

Goldberg D: A classification of psychological distress for use in primary care settings. Soc Sci Med 35:189–193, 1992

Goldberg D: Plato versus Aristotle: categorical and dimensional models for common mental disorders. Compr Psychiatry 41 (suppl):8–13, 2000

Goldberg D, Huxley P: Common Mental Disorders: A Bio-Social Model. London, Tavistock, 1992

Goldberg D, Williams P: A User's Guide to the General Health Questionnaire. Windsor, UK, NFER-Nelson, 1988

Goldberg DP, Bridges K, Duncan-Jones P, et al: Dimensions of neuroses seen in primary-care settings. Psychol Med 17:461–470, 1987

Goldberg D, Sharp D, Nanayakkara K: The field trial of the mental disorders section of ICD-10 designed for primary care (ICD10-PHC) in England. Fam Pract 12:466–473, 1995

Gureje O: Psychological disorders and symptoms in primary care: association with disability and service use after 12 months. Soc Psychiatry Psychiatr Epidemiol 37:220–224, 2002

Gureje O: What can we learn from a cross-national study of somatic distress? J Psychosom Res 56:409–412, 2004

Gureje O, Simon GE, Üstün TB, et al: Somatization in cross-cultural perspective: a World Health Organization study in primary care. Am J Psychiatry 154:989–995, 1997a

Gureje O, Üstün TB, Simon GE, et al: The syndrome of hypochondriasis: a cross-national study in primary care. Psychol Med 27:1001–1010, 1997b

Gureje O, Von Korff M, Simon GE, et al: Persistent pain and well-being: a World Health Organization Study in Primary Care. JAMA 280:147–151, 1998

Hickie I, Koschera A, Hadzi-Pavlovic D, et al: The temporal stability and co-morbidity of prolonged fatigue: a longitudinal study in primary care. Psychol Med 29:855–861, 1999

Institute of Medicine of the National Academies: Primary Care: America's Health in a New Era. Washington, DC, Institute of Medicine, 1996. Available at: http://www.iom.edu/CMS/3809/27706.aspx. Accessed October 6, 2009.

Janca A, Tacchini G, Isaac M: WHO International study of somatoform disorders: an overview of methods and preliminary results, in Somatoform Disorders: A Worldwide Perspective, Tokyo. Edited by Ono Y, Janca A, Asai M, et al. Tokyo, Japan, Springer, 1999, pp 125–131

Jenkins R, Smeeton N, Shepherd M: Classification of mental disorder in primary care. Psychol Med Monogr Suppl 12:1–59, 1988

Jenkins R, Goldberg D, Kiima D, et al: Classification in primary care: experience with current diagnostic systems. Psychopathology 35:127–131, 2002

Judd LL, Akiskal HS, Maser JD, et al: A prospective 12-year study of subsyndromal and syndromal depressive symptoms in unipolar major depressive disorders. Arch Gen Psychiatry 55:694–700, 1998

Katerndahl D: Variations on a theme: the spectrum of anxiety disorders and problems with DSM classification in primary care settings, in New Research on the Psychology of Fear. Edited by Gower PL. Hauppauge, NY, Nova, 2005, pp 121–221

Katerndahl DA, Larme AC, Palmer RF, et al: Reflections on DSM classification and its utility in primary care: case studies in "mental disorders. J Clin Psychiatry 7:91–99, 2005

Kessler RC, Nelson CB, McGonagle KA, et al: Comorbidity of DSM-III-R major depressive disorder in the general population: results from the US National Comorbidity Survey. Br J Psychiatry Suppl 168:17–30, 1996

Kessler RC, Berglund P, Demler O, et al: Lifetime prevalence and age-of-onset distributions of DSM-IV disorders in the National Comorbidity Survey Replication. Arch Gen Psychiatry 62:593–602, 2005

Khan MN, Ahmad S, Arshad N, et al: Anxiety and depressive symptoms in patients with conversion disorder. J Coll Physicians Surg Pak 15:489–492, 2005

Kirmayer LJ, Robbins JM: Three forms of somatization in primary care: prevalence, co-occurrence and socio-demographic characteristics. J Nerv Ment Dis 179:647–655, 1991

Kisely S, Simon G: An international study of the effect of physical ill health on psychiatric recovery in primary care. Psychosom Med 67:116–122, 2005

Kleinman A: Depression, somatization and the "new cross-cultural psychiatry." Soc Sci Med 11:3–10, 1977

Klinkman MS, Valenstein M: A general approach to psychiatric problems in the primary care setting, in Primary Care Psychiatry. Edited by Knesper D, Riba M, Schwenk T. Philadelphia, PA, WB Saunders, 1997, pp 3–8

Korten A, Henderson S: The Australian National Survey of Mental Health and Well-Being: common psychological symptoms and disablement. Br J Psychiatry 177:325–330, 2000

Kroenke K, Spitzer RL, Williams JB: The PHQ-9: validity of a brief depression severity measure. J Gen Intern Med 16:606–613, 2001

Kroenke K, Spitzer RL, Williams JB: The PHQ-15: validity of a new measure for evaluating the severity of somatic symptoms. Psychosom Med 64:258–266, 2002

Lamberts H: The use of the International Classification of Primary Care as an episode-oriented database, in Medinfo 89 (World Conference on Medical Informatics//Medinfo). Edited by Barber B, Cao D, Qin D, et al. Amsterdam, The Netherlands, Elsevier, 1989, pp 835–839

Lamberts H, Hofmans-Okkes IM: Classification of psychological and social problems in general practice. Huisarts Wet 36 (suppl):5–13, 1993

Lamberts H, Schade E: Surveillance systems from primary care data: from a prevalence-oriented to an episode-oriented epidemiology, in Surveillance in Health and Disease. Edited by Eylenbosch WJ, Noah ND. Oxford, UK, Oxford University Press, 1988, pp 75–89

Lamberts H, Magruder K, Kathol RG, et al: The classification of mental disorders in primary care: a guide through a difficult terrain. Int J Psychiatry Med 28:159–176, 1998

Leduc Y, Cauchon M, Emond JG, et al: [Utilization of computerized classification system of primary care: three years of experience]. Can Fam Physician 41:1338–1345, 1995

Leon AC, Shear MK, Portera L, et al: Assessing impairment in patients with panic disorder: the Sheehan Disability Scale. Soc Psychiatry Psychiatr Epidemiol 27:78–82, 1992

Maier W, Gänsicke M, Freyberger HJ, et al: Generalised anxiety disorder (ICD-10) in primary care from a cross-cultural perspective: a valid diagnostic entity? Acta Psychiatr Scand 101:29–36, 2000

Mari JJ, Williams P: A comparison of the validity of two psychiatric screening questionnaires (GHQ-12 and SRQ-20) in Brazil using Relative Operating Characteristic (ROC) analysis. Psychol Med 15:651–659, 1985

Maxwell M: Women's and doctors' accounts of their experiences of depression in primary care: the influence of social and moral reasoning on patients' and doctors' decisions. Chronic Illn 1:61–71, 2005

Mental Health and General Practice Investigation (MaGPIe) Research Group: The nature and prevalence of psychological problems in New Zealand primary healthcare: a report on Mental Health and General Practice Investigation (MaGPIe). N Z Med J 116:U379, 2003. http://www.nzma.org.nz/journal/116–1171/379/. Accessed October 6, 2009.

Mental Health and General Practice Investigation (MaGPIe) Research Group: General practitioner recognition of mental illness in the absence of a "gold standard." Aust N Z J Psychiatry 38:789–794, 2004

Mezzich JE, Kirmayer LJ, Kleinman A, et al: The place of culture in DSM-IV. J Nerv Ment Dis 187:457–464, 1999

Ministério da Saúde: Manual para organização da Atenção Básica no sistema Único de Saúde. Saúde, Brasil, Ministério da Saúde, 1998

National Institute for Clinical Excellence: Depression: the treatment and management of depression in adults. 2009. Available at: http://publications.nice.org.uk/depression-cg90. Accessed February 1, 2012.

Nease DE Jr, Aikens JE: DSM depression and anxiety criteria and severity of symptoms in primary care: cross sectional study. BMJ 327:1030–1031, 2003

Nease DE Jr, Green LA: ClinfoTracker: a generalizable prompting tool for primary care. J Am Board Fam Pract 16:115–123, 2003

Nease DE Jr, Klinkman MA, Volk RJ: Improved detection of depression in primary care through severity evaluation. J Fam Pract 51:1065–1070, 2002

Okasha A, Okasha T: Somatoform disorders: an Arab perspective, in Somatoform Disorders: A Worldwide Perspective. Edited by Ono Y, Janca A, Asai M, et al. Tokyo, Japan, Springer, 1999, pp 38–46

Okkes IM, Groen A, Oskam SK, et al: Advantages of long observation in episode-oriented electronic patient records in family practice. Methods Inf Med 40:229–235, 2001

Okkes IM, Becker HW, Bernstein RM, et al: The March 2002 update of the electronic version of ICPC-2: a step forward to the use of ICD-10 as a nomenclature and a terminology for ICPC-2. Fam Pract 19:543–546, 2002a

Okkes IM, Oskam SK, Lamberts H: The probability of specific diagnoses for patients presenting with common symptoms to Dutch family physicians. J Fam Pract 51:31–36, 2002b

Olfson M: Primary care patients who refuse specialized mental health services. Arch Intern Med 151:129–132, 1991

Olfson M, Jenkins R, Goldberg D, et al: Subthreshold psychiatric symptoms in a primary care group practice. Arch Gen Psychiatry 53:880–886, 1996

Parkerson GR Jr, Bridges-Webb C, Gervas J, et al: Classification of severity of health problems in family/general practice: an international field trial. Fam Pract 13:303–309, 1996

Patel V: The need for treatment evidence for common mental disorders in developing countries. Psychol Med 30:743–746, 2000

Patel V, Mann A: Etic and emic criteria for non-psychotic mental disorder: a study of the CISR and care provider assessment in Harare. Soc Psychiatry Psychiatr Epidemiol 32:84–89, 1997

Patel V, Pereira J, Mann AH: Somatic and psychological models of common mental disorder in primary care in India. Psychol Med 28:135–143, 1998

Piccinelli M, Rucci P, Üstün B, et al: Typologies of anxiety, depression and somatization symptoms among primary care attenders with no formal mental disorder. Psychol Med 29:677–688, 1999

Pincus HA, Vettorello NE, McQueen LE, et al: Bridging the gap between psychiatry and primary care: the DSM-IV-PC. Psychosomatics 36:328–335, 1995

Pincus HA, Davis WW, McQueen LE: "Subthreshold" mental disorders: a review and synthesis of studies on minor depression and other "brand names." Br J Psychiatry 174:288–296, 1999

Pingitore D, Sansone RA: Using DSM-IV primary care version: a guide to psychiatric diagnosis in primary care. Am Fam Physician 58:1347–1352, 1998

Rogers WH, Wilson IB, Bungay KM, et al: Assessing the performance of a new depression screener for primary care (PC-SAD). J Clin Epidemiol 55:164–175, 2002

Rogers WH, Adler DA, Bungay KM, et al: Depression screening instruments made good severity measures in a cross-sectional analysis. J Clin Epidemiol 58:370–377, 2005

Rosendal M, Fink P, Bro F, et al: Somatization, heartsink patients, or functional somatic symptoms? Towards a clinical useful classification in primary health care. Scand J Prim Health Care 23:3–10, 2005

Rucci P, Gherardi S, Tansella M, et al: Subthreshold psychiatric disorders in primary care: prevalence and associated characteristics. J Affect Disord 76:171–181, 2003

Santor DA, Coyne JC: Evaluating the continuity of symptomatology between depressed and nondepressed individuals. J Abnorm Psychol 110:216–225, 2001a

Santor DA, Coyne JC: Examining symptom expression as a function of symptom severity: item performance on the Hamilton Rating Scale for Depression. Psychol Assess 13:127–139, 2001b

Saraceno B, Terzian E, Barquero FM, et al: Mental health care in the primary health care setting: a collaborative study in six countries of Central America. Health Policy Plan 10:133–143, 1995

Sartorius N, Üstün TB, Lecrubier Y, et al: Depression comorbid with anxiety: results from the WHO study on psychological disorders in primary health care. Br J Psychiatry Suppl 30:38–43, 1996

Sheehan DV: The Anxiety Disease. New York, Scribner, 1983

Sherbourne CD, Wells KB, Meredith LS, et al: Comorbid anxiety disorder and the functioning and well-being of chronically ill patients of general medical providers. Arch Gen Psychiatry 53:889–895, 1996

Simon G, Gureje O: Stability of somatization disorder and somatization symptoms among primary care patients. Arch Gen Psychiatry 56:90–95, 1999

Simon G, Gater R, Kisely S, et al: Somatic symptoms of distress: an international primary care study. Psychosom Med 58:481–488, 1996

Simon GE, Gureje O, Fullerton C: Course of hypochondriasis in an international primary care study. Gen Hosp Psychiatry 23:51–55, 2001

Simon GE, Goldberg DP, Von Korff M, et al: Understanding cross-national differences in depression prevalence. Psychol Med 32:585–594, 2002

Sinclair PA, Lyness JM, King DA, et al: Depression and self-reported functional status in older primary care patients. Am J Psychiatry 158:416–419, 2001

Skapinakis P, Lewis G, Mavreas V: Temporal relations between unexplained fatigue and depression: longitudinal data from an international study in primary care. Psychosom Med 66:330–335, 2004

Slade T, Andrews G: Latent structure of depression in a community sample: a taxometric analysis. Psychol Med 35:489–497, 2005

Smith RC, Gardiner JC, Lyles JS, et al: Exploration of DSM-IV criteria in primary care patients with medically unexplained symptoms. Psychosom Med 67:123–129, 2005

Soler JK: Transhis: The Maltese Experience With ICPC-2. it-Tabib tal-Familja, June 19–22, 2000

Spitzer RL, Williams JB, Kroenke K, et al: Utility of a new procedure for diagnosing mental disorders in primary care: the PRIME-MD 1000 study. JAMA 272:1749–1756, 1994

Spitzer RL, Kroenke K, Williams JB: Validation and utility of a self-report version of PRIME-MD: the PHQ primary care study. Primary Care Evaluation of Mental Disorders. Patient Health Questionnaire. JAMA 282:1737–1744, 1999

Spitzer RL, Kroenke K, Williams JB, et al: A brief measure for assessing generalized anxiety disorder: the GAD-7. Arch Intern Med 166:1092–1097, 2006

Toft T, Fink P, Oernboel E, et al: Mental disorders in primary care: prevalence and comorbidity among disorders: results from the functional illness in primary care (FIP) study. Psychol Med 35:1175–1184, 2005

Tyrer P, Nur U, Crawford M, et al: The Social Functioning Questionnaire: a rapid and robust measure of perceived functioning. Int J Soc Psychiatry 51:265–275, 2005

Upton MW, Evans M, Goldberg DP, et al: Evaluation of ICD-10 PHC mental health guidelines in detecting and managing depression within primary care. Br J Psychiatry 175:476–482, 1999

Üstün TB, Sartorius N: Mental Illness in General Health Care. Chichester, UK, Wiley, 1995

Üstün TB, Goldberg D, Cooper J, et al: New classification for mental disorders with management guidelines for use in primary care: ICD-10 PHC chapter five. Br J Gen Pract 45:211–215, 1995

Van Weel-Baumgarten E, van den Bosch W, van den Hoogen H, et al: Ten year follow-up of depression after diagnosis in general practice. Br J Gen Pract 48:1643–1646, 1998

Vuorilehto M, Melartin T, Isometsa E: Depressive disorders in primary care: recurrent, chronic, and comorbid. Psychol Med 35:673–682, 2005

World Health Organization: The ICD-10 Classification of Mental and Behavioural Disorders: Clinical Descriptions and Diagnostic Guidelines. Geneva, World Health Organization, 1992

World Health Organization: Diagnostic and Management Guidelines for Mental Disorders in Primary Care: ICD-10 Chapter V Primary Care Version. Göttingen, Germany, Hogrefe, 1996

World Health Organization: WHO Guide to Mental and Neurological Health in Primary Care, 2nd Edition. London, Royal Society of Medicine Press, 2004. Available at: http://www.mentalneurologicalprimarycare.org/. Accessed October 7, 2009.

World Organization of Family Doctors International Classification Committee: International Classification of Primary Care, Second Edition [ICPC-2]. Oxford, UK, Oxford University Press, 1998

Zigmond AS, Snaith RP: The hospital anxiety and depression scale. Acta Psychiatr Scand 67:361–370, 1983

Zimmerman M, Mattia JI: A self-report scale to help make psychiatric diagnoses: the Psychiatric Diagnostic Screening Questionnaire. Arch Gen Psychiatry 58:787–794, 2001

Zimmerman M, Coryell W, Wilson S, et al: Evaluation of symptoms of major depressive disorder: self-report vs. clinician ratings. J Nerv Ment Dis 174:150–153, 1986

Zinbarg RE, Barlow DH, Liebowitz M, et al: The DSM-IV field trial for mixed anxiety-depression. Am J Psychiatry 151:1153–1162, 1994

4

USE OF DIAGNOSIS IN FORENSIC PSYCHIATRY

Julio Arboleda-Flórez
Paul S. Appelbaum
Richard J. Bonnie
Norbert Konrad
Svetlana V. Polubinskaya
Genevra Richardson
Carlos Téllez
Liu Xiehe

Mental illness is expressed through behavioral manifestations that reflect cognitive, emotional, and volitional aspects and functions of the personality, which are the very functions that the law considers essential to assess to adjudicate guilt, label the accused a criminal, and proffer a sentence (Arboleda-Flórez and Deynaka 1999). This might explain why such a large number of mental patients end up in difficulties with the law, where they pose major challenges for diagnosis, legal adjudication, and management. Obligations to deal with these issues have traditionally fallen on forensic psychiatrists, who are often asked to provide evaluations of the mental state and competence of individuals involved in legal actions. This involvement could be either in *criminal law,* in relation to the possibility that an accused has a mental condition, or in *civil law,* in relation, for example, to the possibility that a person has entered into some contractual agreement while not entirely *compos mentis.* In any of these situations, forensic psychiatrists follow heuristic rules to arrive at a classification of symptoms that at times conforms to diagnostic entities in the general body of psychiatry but that often relates more to the legal exigencies of the case and to a need to accommodate clinical findings to determinations in law.

In this chapter, we review the elements and processes of forensic psychiatry and apply them to questions concerning the role of diagnosis in making legal decisions.

Definition of Forensic Psychiatry

Forensic psychiatry is a subspecialty of psychiatry, commonly defined as "the branch of psychiatry that deals with issues arising in the interface between psychiatry and the law" (Gutheil 2004). Although short and simple, this definition fails to emphasize that a good portion of the work in forensic psychiatry is to help mentally ill persons, who are in trouble with the law, to navigate three different, interrelated systems: mental health, justice, and corrections. Thus, the simple definition can be modified to encompass the specific problems of managing the mentally ill offender: "Forensic psychiatry is the branch of psychiatry that deals with issues arising in the interface between psychiatry and the law, and with the flow of mentally disordered offenders along a continuum of social systems" (Arboleda-Flórez 2006).

Areas of Focus in Forensic Psychiatry

The primary foci of forensic psychiatrists, as their work pertains to diagnostic issues, fall into three areas. The first focus involves matters at the interface between psychiatry and criminal law. The professional activities of many forensic psychiatrists center on assessment of defendants for court proceedings or, once defendants are found guilty, on treatment for them in either a highly specialized maximum-security forensic hospital or a prison. As a second focus, most forensic psychiatrists also deal with problems at the interface between psychiatry and civil law, for example, when evaluations of competence to enter into contracts are requested or when an assessment for damages caused by third parties is required. Finally, forensic psychiatrists also become involved in development and application of mental health legislation; however, we do not explore these activities in this chapter.

CRIMINAL LAW

Traditional legal doctrine and contemporary public policy both recognize that a population exists in which mental disorder and criminal behavior converge (Monahan and Steadman 1983), and in many jurisdictions, mental health legislation makes dangerousness—or a potential to cause grievous bodily harm to self or others—the main criterion for civil commitment (Appelbaum 1994; Arboleda-Flórez and Copithorne 1998). In most countries, mental health legislation and criminal codes assume that a relation exists between mental states and criminal offending and that this relation may be determinative in the outcome of a commitment hearing or criminal trial. Two matters arise out of a possible association between mental illness and criminality: one relates to the level of convergence between the two sets of phenomena and the other to the legal procedures that begin from the moment a person is charged with a criminal offense.

With regard to the level of convergence, a study of the relation between *crime* and *psychopathology* has to start by questioning whether the relation is causal—that is, whether the symptoms associated with mental disorders directly induce a propensity to commit crimes. At another level of discourse, it is important to differentiate clinical pathology from criminal behavior. For example, not all sexual behaviors, aberrant as they may be, and not every act of violence can be attributed to a mental disorder, and even when they can be, many offenders may not be amenable to psychiatric intervention, as is often the case with serious psychopathic offenders.

The behavioral manifestations of some mental disorders are *ipso facto* criminal offenses, so that the "patient" is a criminal because the expressed symptoms are criminal acts (e.g., some paraphilias, pyromania, and kleptomania). The convergence in these cases is one-to-one; it is absolute. In some other disorders, the convergence is not one-to-one, because the symptoms could be expressed without necessarily breaking the law, such as in psychopathic personality, antisocial personality and borderline personality disorders, pathological gambling, and other impulse-control disorders. Not all symptoms of these conditions can be categorized as crimes, and sometimes the crimes, when they occur, are not directly related to the symptoms. For example, an alcoholic person could get quite intoxicated without causing any crimes if he or she just falls asleep, but acute intoxication is a major risk factor for violence. Similarly, persons with drug dependencies could indulge their dependencies without breaking any law, but occasionally, their addictions may lead to income-generating crimes to finance the addictions. On the other hand, mere possession of drugs of abuse, including alcohol, is illegal in many countries.

The level of convergence is less straightforward among some other mental conditions. For example, although persons with schizophrenia may commit serious violent crimes (McKay and Wright 1984; Taylor 1993), and persons with major depression may display violent behavior toward others (Goodwin and Jamison 1990), this typically happens sporadically, not every time they become seriously ill. Moreover, most persons with schizophrenia or major depression never commit a criminal offense (Arboleda-Flórez 2009).

The second matter relates to legal procedures that ensue once a person is charged with a criminal offense. On entering into the legal system, three major areas are the most common objects of consideration: fitness to stand trial, insanity criteria, and dangerousness determinations.

Fitness to stand trial is a legal requirement found in countries that follow the Anglo-Saxon common law system; it pertains to the mental condition of an accused at the time of trial. In the Anglo-Saxon system, persons who are mentally ill at the time of trial cannot be tried; the trial stops until the person improves or regains his or her sanity. To this end, the person may be remanded to a forensic facility, and it is expected that, once improvement has taken place, the person will be returned to court for the trial to continue. The question for the system is how to maximize, through appropriate treatment, the competence of the accused so that the trial can proceed. The question for forensic evaluators at the facility often revolves around how to predict restorability of competence, which should be based on an adequate response to treatment (Pinals 2006). As in many other forensic functions, diagnostically, the issue is not whether the person has a particular mental condition but whether current symptoms would preclude continuation of the trial.

Most continental European and Latin American countries, as well as those colonized by the French Republic or the Portuguese Republic in Africa and the Far East, follow a Napoleonic (also known as inquisitorial) system of law, in which mental illness at time of trial is no bar to continuation of the trial but bears heavily on a finding of imputability. However, over the past decade, some countries have modified their legal systems in this respect. Although the legal construct of fitness to stand trial does not exist as such, in practice, a judge could order hospitalization and treatment of a defendant affected by a mental condition. The trial is then effectively postponed until the defendant gets better. For example, in the Republic of Chile, paragraph 10 of the Criminal Code *(Código Procesal Penal)* stipulates that if the judge doubts the capacity of a person to exercise his or her rights, the judge should adopt whatever measures are required to improve the person's capacity, including suspending the proceedings. In practice, if the person already has a history of incapacity, the judge moves directly to order a psychiatric evaluation (usually by the official Medico-Legal Service attached to the Department of Justice) and stops the proceedings until the service submits a medicolegal report. Disregarding this legal operation on the capacity of the accused to proceed to trial may lead to an annulment of the proceedings. Obviously, this legal operation is independent of an evaluation of imputability (Pffefer 2001).

Ingrained in most legal systems is the concept that offenders who are mentally capable at the time of trial, but who were mentally ill at the time the offense was committed, are dealt with differently in terms of the level of criminal responsibility and type of disposition. This constitutes the second function of forensic psychiatry in criminal law and it pertains to an ascription of the level of criminal responsibility in the Anglo-Saxon system, or a decision on imputability in the inquisitorial system and the old Soviet system of law. *Criminal responsibility* relates to issues of free will, and its determination is in the hands of the judge or jury; *imputability* is a function of the association between the agent (cause) and the result (effect), and its determination is, to a large extent, in the hands of the expert.

Although overlapping, the concepts of criminal responsibility and imputability are not entirely the same. The role of the forensic psychiatrist in criminal responsibility cases is, in part, to determine whether the accused was mentally ill at the time of the crime, but this is only a threshold determination on which eligibility to be found not criminally responsible is based. A decision on criminal responsibility hinges not on the presence of a mental condition *per se* but rather on the degree to which such condition is deemed to have affected the capacity of the individual to know that the act was wrong, to appreciate the ramifications of the act, or to control his or her behavior so as to prevent commission of the act (with the precise criteria varying across jurisdictions). Such incapacity creates a condition in which the accused either was not able to exercise free will (i.e., had volitional impairment) or substantially misconstrued the nature of his or her behavior and its consequences. A finding of not criminally responsible, although implying that the person committed the act *(actus reus),* nonetheless absolves him or her in the eyes of society for not having a guilty mind *(mens rea);* such a finding precludes criminal sanctions. Criminal responsibility is a social construct and cannot be measured scientifically; only the judge or jury can decide what level to ascribe to the accused. On the other hand, imputability refers to the fact that the accused (agent) cannot be punished (result) on account of a mental condition. The concept derives from Roman law, in which *"demens, furiosus et mentecaptus,"* as well as children younger than 7 years, were considered incapable of having committed a crime. If the person could not have committed the crime, then he or she could not be imputed with it in law. *Causality* (as caused by a mental incapacity) is, therefore, a basic element of imputability, a situation that leads to much controversy in countries where the inquisitorial system is in use regarding whether it should be attributed only by the judge or be a determination at the hand of the psychiatrist (Ribé and Martí Tusquets 2002).

In summary, insanity criteria pertain to legal tests used to decide whether the effect of mental illness on competence to know, understand, or appreciate the nature of a crime or to be able to avoid committing a crime could be used to declare an offender "not criminally responsible because of a mental condition," "not guilty by reasons of insanity," "nonimputable," or any other wording used in different countries. As in issues of fitness to stand trial, the basic mental element of an insanity defense is not the presence of a mental condition, whatever the diagnosis—although diagnosis may be required as a threshold determination—but the presence of symptoms that cause the person to be incapable of comprehending or conforming to the expectations of the law. Furthermore, it is not the forensic psychiatrist who makes those determinations, but the judge, the jury, or the tribunal.

Following a finding of legal insanity, the task for forensic psychiatrists is to gauge the level of systems interface in relation to different types of receiving and treating institutions. Hospitals for the criminally insane, mental hospitals for civilly committed patients, and penitentiary hospitals for mentally ill inmates, as well as hospital wings in local jails, are all part of the mental health system, and their interdependency has to be acknowledged for purposes of system integration and budgeting (Konrad 2002).

Another function of forensic psychiatrists in criminal proceedings is the determination of whether a particular offender is "dangerous." Declaring an offender "dangerous" usually demands a high level of expertise on the part of forensic experts, who are expected to provide courts with technical and scientific information on risk assessment and prediction of future violence. Dangerousness determinations rely heavily on the evaluee's history of violent behavior. Many clinicians believe that when such behavior has been escalating, and when the most recent offense is a continuation of the same pattern, the risk is particularly acute. In these applications, it is the focus on violent behavior and the likelihood that it will continue that is important, not the specific diagnosis of a mental condition; although, again, the diagnosis of some mental disorder may be a requirement for entry into the system. As an aside, however, it should be noted that in the United Kingdom of Great Britain and Northern Ireland, a criminal court may make a hospital disposal after a conviction for a criminal offense (excluding murder), provided the required mental disorder is present to the required degree, even if there is no causal connection between the disorder and the offense. Indeed, the onset of the disorder can postdate the offense. Also, there is no need to prove dangerousness; harm to self can be sufficient.

CIVIL LAW

The United Nations Declaration on Human Rights, paragraph 6, stipulates that "Everyone has the right to recognition everywhere as a person before the law." However, having inherent legal rights is not the same as having legal capacity to act, because this capacity may be compromised among persons who have mental disorders. Given the importance of exercising one's rights, any abrogation of that power generally requires a judicial decision. Hence, in most instances (medical treatment settings sometimes constituting an exception), a medical decision that a person has lost capacity is given effect only by a legal determination of incompetence.

Needs for forensic assessments in civil law arise out of multiple situations, which range from examinations to specify the effect of emotional injuries on a third party involved in a motor vehicle accident to evaluations of guardianship, capacity to write a will, or ability to enter into contracts; assessments of testamentary capacity; psychological autopsies in cases of suicide or sudden death; evaluations of fitness to work; and, of late, in many countries, evaluations to determine access to benefits from disability insurance. In most of these situations, the issue at hand is a determination of capacity to perform some function, including autonomous decision making by the impaired person. A determination of *incapacity* (a medical function) that could lead to a finding of *incompetence* (a legal decision) legitimizes restriction of that person's decision-making powers. The severity of these consequences imposes on clinicians an ethical duty to base their decisions on the best available clinical evidence.

Ordinarily, there is a presumption of capacity—that is, a person is assumed to be competent to make decisions unless proven otherwise (Weisstub 1994). Decision-making capacity requires the abilities to understand, appreciate, and reason about the relevant information and to make an informed choice and communicate it. In the absence of a "metacognoscope," clinicians rely on clinical judgment and assessment instruments (Chiswick 2005). However, the presence of a major mental or physical condition does not, in and of itself, produce incapacity, either in general or for specific functions. Even in the presence of a condition that may affect capacity, a person may still be competent to carry out some functions, not only because capacity fluctuates from time to time but also because competence is not an all-or-none concept and is tied to the specific decision or function to be accomplished. For example, a stroke may render a person incapacitated to drive a motor vehicle and therefore incompetent to drive, but the person could still have the capacity to enter into contracts or to manage personal financial affairs. With time and proper rehabilitation, the person might be able to regain capacity to drive. Given that incapacity is often time limited, findings of incompetence should be reviewed at appropriate intervals. Although the subjects of capacity evaluations should be informed of the purpose of the assessment, consent is not typically required for an evaluation to be completed. It is often advisable to use a screening test of capacity and to do a full assessment only if the person fails the screening test. This will reduce the burden on both the subject of the assessment and the evaluator, if the screening test is passed. As is the case in criminal law, in civil law, what is important is not just a diagnosis—which here may not even be required as a threshold determination—but the incapacity to execute some functions as a result of the symptoms of the mental condition.

The Practice of Forensic Psychiatry

Forensic evaluations proceed in two phases: investigation of the evaluee's mental state and preparation of a psychiatric legal report. Forensic psychiatrists begin with review of all materials and documents relating to the case and then proceed to examination of the person—often with the aid of assessment instruments to assist in determining diagnosis, level of functioning, and recommendations for disposition based on the incapacities (a medical finding)—as a basis for legal determinations of incompetence in criminal or in civil law.

EVALUEE'S MENTAL STATE

Quality of the Evaluator

In application of this medicolegal method, it is expected that the forensic psychiatric expert will be aware of the importance of the expert role, the need for rigorous preparation, the necessity of methodical exploration of alternative conclusions, and the need to anticipate the challenges of court appearances. In addition, experts should also strive to embody the following qualities:

- Objectivity in interpreting material evidence
- Impartiality in elucidating truth, without the goal of defending any of the parties in conflict
- Veracity, regardless of social, political, or legal consequences
- Knowledge and skills in clinical evaluation and application of the findings to the legal question
- Common sense and parsimonious application of Occam's razor
- Keen critical abilities to avoid assuming extreme positions or premature closure of alternative explanations or believing in the infallibility of one's clinical findings
- Excellent grounding in biological, medical, and social sciences
- Good understanding of legal concepts and terminology
- Grounding in, and clear understanding of, the ethical conflicts in forensic psychiatry

Ignorance of relevant medical or legal facts, inability to remain neutral, dishonesty, and blindness to the ethical quagmires of medicolegal work are incompatible with the role of an expert.

Quality of the Tools of Evaluation

Diagnostic difficulties in forensic psychiatry include the risk of observer bias and the possibility of secondary gain for the evaluee. Hence, forensic psychiatrists need to verify their conclusions, whenever possible, via information from third parties—including witnesses, family, and friends—who can relate the behavior of the defendant or litigant, the psychiatric history, and the person's mental state at the time in question. Effort should be made to obtain school, military, and hospital records as well as records from family physicians, court dockets, criminal sheets, and any other documents that could shed light on the development and the presence of symptoms and the evaluee's veracity. Similarly, in a quest for objectivity in the diagnostic formulation, clinical aids to diagnosis, such as electroencephalograms, diagnostic imaging, laboratory tests, and psychological tests are often indicated. The more the expert bases his or her conclusions on objective information, the better grounded are likely to be the diagnosis and conclusions.

PREPARATION OF THE PSYCHIATRIC LEGAL REPORT

The quality of the expert and the forensic examination should be reflected in the preparation of the medico-legal report; the expert's signature at the end testifies to the care taken by the expert in the examination of the facts as well as to his or her knowledge, reasoning abilities, impartiality, and commitment to excellence. These reports follow a typical format, including a detailed list of data used to form an opinion, personal and family history of the evaluee, an in-depth review of the legal case and particulars of the crime or the allegations, a description of all findings at examination and from medical or psychological tests and records, the formulation of a diagnosis, and an assessment of the effect of the person's symptoms on the capacity or function at issue. One of the most important parts of the report is the analysis of the case and the concatenation of all the facts into a cohesive and integrative formulation, the premises of which sustain the final diagnostic and capacity findings and recommendations.

Diagnosis in Forensic Psychiatry

Difficulties in defining caseness and in measurement of symptoms are major concerns in forensic psychiatry, where, as mentioned earlier, diagnosis per se is not as important a consideration as is the presence of symptoms, their severity, and their effects on capacity or behavior. Thus, assessment of symptoms is paramount, requiring careful evaluation of their presence, severity, and duration, taking into account problems of recall bias, malingering, and observer bias.

DIAGNOSTICS AND CLASSIFICATIONS

Descriptive psychopathology and the diagnostic systems it has spawned developed in a unique sociopolitical context (French and German in the mid- to late nineteenth century) and present certain challenges to contemporary forensic psychiatry. Diagnostic systems may act as a procrustean bed that limits the full use of psychiatric understandings of personality dynamics and criminal psychopathology in legal contexts. In other words, just because a diagnosis can be assigned to a defendant does not mean that the meaning of the act is evident.

The strictures of diagnostic classifications do not fit well with the need for the courts to comprehend the roots of behaviors in both civil and criminal contexts. Although presentation of dynamic information is not intrinsically incompatible with modern diagnostic formulations, courts tend to look to the seeming certainty of a diagnostic label and to undervalue additional information that can shed light on how a disorder has affected the person whose behavior is being assessed. The result can be a disservice to persons involved in legal proceedings, with a failure to recognize the wide variations in consequences for thought and behavior of most mental disorders.

An additional issue for forensic psychiatry relates to the tendency in DSM-IV (American Psychiatric Association 1994) and other diagnostic systems to expand the scope of subjective experiences and behaviors that are considered to represent disorders as opposed to expectable consequences of common life events or adaptations to life situations. Among the defense bar, the judiciary, and the public, the sense often exists that any disorder can be used to exculpate criminal behavior. The caveat in DSM that the categories in the manual may not be applicable to legal determinations has not entirely solved the problem. Attorneys still seek to push forensic psychiatrists to place defendants and persons involved in civil legal actions into diagnostic procrustean beds. They use the "bible of psychiatry," as some attorneys have labeled DSM, as a ramrod to prevent the introduction of more parsimonious explanations of symptoms and diagnostic formulations that encompass the totality of human experience.

LEGAL AND PSYCHIATRIC APPROACHES TO DIAGNOSIS

In the interface with the legal process, diagnostic formulations may conflict with legal categories. Legal definitions and concepts do not move as fast as changes in scientific knowledge and often seek different goals. Hence, in practically every legal system and country, legal terminology may be misguided, outmoded, and even archaic from a psychiatric perspective (Sepúlveda 2007); definitions of mental disorder may not be the same in psychiatry and in law, and legal criteria for diagnosis may be at variance with accepted psychiatric criteria. Important legal determinations that have the potential to severely affect the lives of individuals, such as determinations of *dangerousness*, require the input of forensic psychiatry, but dangerousness is a sociolegal concept, not a psychiatric diagnosis. In these cases, the diagnosis is not as relevant as the history of violent behavior. *Psychopathy* is a common diagnosis in law, but it is not included in diagnostic systems such as DSM, and some penal systems allow for a diagnosis of *temporary insanity* that includes a disparate array of psychiatric entities from febrile or metabolic deliria to twilight epileptic states, pathological intoxication, sleepwalking, automatism, drug-induced psychosis, and so on.

Other legal definitions of pathological mental states that do not have a clear corresponding equivalent in psychiatric classifications include a *state of passion* beyond the normal expression of emotions and independent of mental pathology. In most penal codes, such a state, if not considered a complete excuse leading to exoneration, is at least a major element to consider at sentencing. If proven or inferred, such a "legal diagnosis" may be used to reduce the severity of the offense charged (i.e., from first-degree murder to manslaughter) or, at sentencing, to reduce the severity of the punishment. Pathological panic, as in *homosexual panic,* is a legal construct to denote the state of a person who, fearful of a homosexual advance, panics and kills the other person. In this condition, the panic and subsequent crime depend on the provoking agent and the reactivity of the offender, which is a manifestation of the person's sexual and psychosocial development and moral attitudes. In other words, pathological panic is a subjective experience independent of any diagnosis.

The use of "syndrome defenses" or clusters of thinly related symptoms to produce the impression of an identifiable legally relevant diagnostic entity is unique to forensic settings and is not related at all to standard psychiatric diagnostic entities. *Pathological lying* is almost an entirely forensic diagnosis, and the ever-present possibility that a person under assessment might be simulating or malingering places the examiner on alert to the point that *malingering* is the diagnosis to be ruled out at practically every step in forensic psychiatry. Other diagnoses, such as *gambling, fire setting,* and *kleptomania,* may meet opposition in some legal systems so that, for example, in German-speaking countries, forensic psychiatrists may be reluctant to use these diagnoses as single entities but rather will use them as part of some other diagnosis. Finally, even within a country, some diagnoses may be differently defined because of their utility to a particular area of law. For example, although *personality disorders* or *paraphilias* can be seen as mental disorders in civil law, in German countries, they may not be so-defined for purposes of criminal law unless other diagnostic categories are present (such as in *addictive disorders*). The issue at hand in this regard is the propensity of courts to depend on diagnostic labels to conclude that effective treatment is available. Thus, as is happening now in many countries, untreatable criminals are flocking into mental institutions to be "treated" while treatable regular mental patients are piling up in prisons to be "managed."

UTILITY OF DIAGNOSIS

Seldom do forensic psychiatrists base important decisions and recommendations about criminal responsibility, emotional harms, or competence on a specific diagnosis, although some diagnosis may be required as a threshold consideration. Rather, these psychiatrists rely on the assessment of the mental state of a person at the time a crime was committed or on current functional abilities. In fact, in most penal codes and countries, a specific diagnosis should be irrelevant in criminal law because the presence of legal insanity is a decision vested in the judge or jury, not the psychiatrist. *Mental disorder* is sometimes defined circuitously to mean "any disorder or disability of the mind" or simply, "disease of the mind." By the same token, a patient may be defined as "a person who has, or appears to have, a mental disorder," "demented," "enajenado" (alienated), "loco" or "crazy," or somewhat more elegantly, as "somebody deprived of the use of reason or the ability to exercise judgment."

A diagnosis, however, may be considered as a basis for disposition for treatment and the type of institution to which a particular offender may be sent. In many countries, for example, there exist special institutions or hospitals for the intellectually disabled as well as high-security prison hospitals for the management and treatment of severe paraphilias (especially rapists) and severe personality disorders (especially psychopathic individuals). Yet even for this purpose, terms such as *mental illness* (as opposed to *schizophrenia, mood disorder, anxiety disorder,* etc.), *sexual deviation* (as opposed to a specific paraphilia), *psychopathy* (which often encompasses antisocial personality disorder), and *mental impairment* or *severe mental impairment* (as opposed to *intellectual disability* with a specific determinant and level of intellectual functioning) often provide a better shorthand communication tool in courts of law than does a diagnostic psychiatric term.

NEGATIVE EFFECTS OF FORENSIC DIAGNOSIS

In a different vein, the use of diagnostic entities—whether originating in psychiatry or in law—may be damaging in forensic settings. Labels "freeze-frame" the accused as possessing a set of categories unacceptable in law; they may pigeonhole the offender into categories of risk to the point that the ethics of it could be called into question (Grover 2005). Diagnoses such as "dangerous and severe personality disorder" (Glen 2005), "psychopathy," "alcoholism," or "drug addiction" go beyond a label because they encapsulate the whole of a personality into a frame devoid of individuality, recognition of which is vital to emotional integrity and personal identification. A label of "dangerous sexual offender" immediately means, in some countries, an indeterminate sentence and a label of "pedophile," with the connotation that the person has a criminal history of molesting children; this may be tantamount to a sentence of death in a loosely guarded penitentiary system.

DIAGNOSTIC SYSTEMS AND THEIR RELATION TO THE LAW

Given that the legal process generally focuses on mental states and functional impairments, rather than on diagnoses per se, it may be appropriate to ask whether the construction of diagnostic systems ought, at all, to take into account the needs of the legal system. In fact, sensitivity to how diagnostic systems such as DSM can be used in the courts may help to avoid unanticipated and undesirable consequences. Two such considerations can be identified.

First, diagnostic criteria or descriptions that suggest a link between a diagnosis and reduced functional capacity may be of great interest in the legal process. Attorneys and experts may rely on such descriptions to assert that the presence of a diagnostic entity necessarily implies impaired capacity. Because it is rarely the case that a diagnosis and functional impairment map on each other perfectly, drafters of diagnostic manuals should be sensitive to the ways in which descriptions of such relationships can be misused. When at all possible, descriptions of impairments associated with a disorder should acknowledge variation in the degree of impairment across affected populations and indicate the lack of a precise correspondence between diagnosis and degree of impairment.

Second, diagnostic criteria or descriptions that characterize a disorder as resulting in, or associated with, an inability to control behavior can be used, sometimes misleadingly, to argue that a person was unable to control his or her actions because of having received a given diagnosis. This is a particular issue with impulse-control disorders and addictions. For example, someone with a diagnosis of pathological gambling may argue that he was unable to refrain from illegal gambling because of his disorder, or a person with a diagnosis of drug dependence may similarly contend that her illegal behavior in obtaining and possessing substances of abuse was compelled by her disorder. Although it may be the case that being predisposed to, or being diagnosed with, an impulse-control disorder or addiction may make it more difficult for a person to control related behaviors, it is almost never the case that the predisposition or diagnosis precludes such control. Indeed, treatment of many impulse-control disorders and addictions is often based on the assumption that the affected person can take control of his or her behavior. Assertions to the contrary should be avoided as diagnostic systems are being developed.

Forensic psychiatry should not prescribe which concept of mental disorder or mental illness is adequate from a legal point of view. This is a normative question, but better validity and reliability of psychiatric diagnosis can improve discussion with lawyers. Empirical matters of science are for psychiatrists to decide, but sociopolitical and legal questions are for lawmakers to resolve. On the other hand, in the transfer of concepts between psychiatry and the law, comparative transcultural research could be helpful in clarifying the use of diagnostic entities in different legal systems.

Public Health Considerations in Forensic Psychiatry

Three major areas of import in forensic psychiatry could have major effects on the health of the general population: 1) mass violence, 2) relation between mental illness and violence, and 3) prevalence of violence, mental conditions, and infections in prison settings.

MASS VIOLENCE

War and massive terror have major effects on the mental health of civilians, especially in cases of asymmetrical wars carried out via indiscriminate terrorist attacks on the population. Mental health casualties will likely increase if weapons of mass destruction—bioterrorism, nuclear weapons, or gases—are ever used in future conflicts (Arboleda-Flórez 2007). Sadly, common victims in war situations and terrorist actions, such as children, are the most vulnerable members of the population (Levav 2006). Apart from being victims of attacks, children are also often enrolled as combatants, thus compounding their vulnerabilities.

In their capacity as clinicians, psychiatrists have a major role to play by providing diagnostic and treatment services to combatants and noncombatants in need of medical services—especially children affected by emotional conditions after exposure to war traumas (World Health Organization 2005)—as well as by advocating against the use of children as combatants. Similarly, psychiatrists should mobilize resources and become civilly active by advocating a culture of life and peace to protect the mental health of the populations affected.

MENTAL ILLNESS AND VIOLENCE

An association between mental illness and violence, hence criminality, has implications for public health because of the effect of violence on public mental health. Although a relation of causality between mental illness and violence has been proposed, because of an increased relative risk (Stueve and Link 1997), this type of relation has not yet been proven. However, given space constraints, rather than entering into this controversy, suffice it to say here that for purposes of public health, the measure to be concerned about is not the *relative* risk but the *attributable* risk, because despite a high relative risk, violence due to mental illness is not that frequent once all other causes of violence in society are taken into account. This risk has been estimated at about 3% and when substance abuse and alcoholism are included, at about 10% (Stuart and Arboleda-Flórez 2001). Other estimates place the risk at 4.3% (Swanson et al. 1997) or as low as 1% (Wessely 1993).

A basic rule of causality, however, should cast a sobering caveat about all estimates purporting to show a relation between mental illness and violence. Frequently, when a mental condition is suspected in relation to a crime, the unstated assumption is that the basic rule of temporality to infer causality has been met—that is, that the condition *preceded* the crime and hence may have actually *caused* the crime. In reality, it could have been that the mental condition that was present much earlier in life was not a factor in the current crime or that the mental condition developed after the crime had been committed.

VIOLENCE, MENTAL CONDITIONS, AND INFECTIONS IN PRISON SETTINGS

Finally, the matter of the high prevalence of violence, mental conditions, and infections in prisons is the subject matter of correctional psychiatry proper. *Correctional psychiatry* refers to all matters of psychiatric practice in the corrections system (Travin 1994). More amply, however, *correctional psychiatry* is the branch of forensic psychiatry that studies the incidence, prevalence, determinants, and management of mental disorders in prisons; the response of correctional systems to the mentally ill offender; and the relation between criminality and mental illness.

Jails (remand centers) are not only "the most important of all our institutions of imprisonment" (Steadman et al. 1986) but also the mental health asylums of our times because of the number, diversity, and complexity of cases among the mentally ill persons they serve (Konrad 2002). Jails also seem to have assumed the burden of treatment for substance abuse and alcoholism. Jails and prisons also harbor an inordinate number of persons affected with serious infections, especially hepatitis and AIDS. Infections in jails and prison settings are major public health threats, especially if prisons do not have the medical treatment systems required for their proper management. Infections in prisons are closely related to the high prevalence of mental illness in prisons, which in itself is a matter of major concern.

Reluctantly, prisons have accepted the mentally ill ever since the invention of prisons more than 200 years ago. Despite multiple government commissions and voluminous parliamentary reports in many countries, and the introduction of several alternatives to care, the problem of the mentally ill in prisons persists and appears to be getting worse. As indicated, in many cities the large number of mental patients in local jails has made the jail a practical extension of the general mental health services. The trans-institutionalization of mentally ill persons from hospitals to prisons has been documented in a plethora of studies that have also estimated their numbers at different points in the justice-correctional system (Brink et al. 2001). Penrose (1939) postulated a theory whereby lack of an adequate number of mental-hospital beds would be expected to create pressures in alternative prison systems. In the present-day systems of community psychiatry, nonexistent community alternatives are blamed for driving mental patients into committing "survival crimes" (Estroff et al. 1998). Looked at from this angle, it may be that the association between criminality and mental illness flows not from a causal relation but is only the result of inadequate health systems. However, studies do show that the high frequency of persons with mental conditions in prison is more than a lack of adequate systems; instead, it involves an association between mental illness, violence, and criminality.

Some studies have pointed toward a putative association. For example, Yarvis (1990) found in a series of 100 murderers that 29% had a diagnosis of "psychosis," of which 21% had schizophrenia and 8% had affective disorders. In addition, 35% had a diagnosis of substance abuse. Among alcoholic persons, prevalence rates for depression, suicide attempts, and violent behavior are much higher than those found among nonalcoholic persons (Swanson et al. 1990). Psychopathy is strongly associated with a high risk for criminal and violent behavior (Hare and Hart 1993). Other factors that seem to mediate an interaction between mental illness and crime include gender, age, socioeconomic status, previous criminality, and previous forensic psychiatric involvement.

Some studies seem to support the proposition that there is more than a correlation between mental illness and criminality, whether by itself or in association with other factors. A 30-year follow-up of a birth cohort in Sweden found a relation between crime and mental disorder and between crime and intellectual deficiency, with mental disorder being 2.5 times more likely to have been registered for a criminal offense and 4 times more likely to have been registered for a violent offense (Hodgins 1993). In addition, a review of computerized records in a prison showed that 13.8% of inmates without a psychiatric history or history of substance abuse had a history of recent or remote violence compared with 17% of inmates with a history of either (Toch and Adams 1989).

Like any other prisoners, mentally ill persons in prisons are vulnerable to the large pool of infections in these institutions, but mental disabilities compound the vulnerability of these individuals. Prisons are true breeding grounds for massive in-festations that can be transmitted to the population at large, especially prison systems that have a rapid turnaround of inmates (such as jails or remand centers) because, in these systems, there is no time to screen, treat, or make arrangements for community follow-up. Other prison systems simply do not have proper medical facilities for diagnosis and treatment. Apart from the high prevalence of HIV/AIDS and hepatitis (Calzavara et al. 2007; Canadian HIV/AIDS Legal Network 2007), drug-resistant *Staphylococcus* infections (Lovgren 2006) and infections with many other highly lethal pathogens thrive in the closed environments of prisons or among persons frequenting needle-exchange programs.

Finally, violence in prison occurs both against others and, frequently, against the self. Within the content of a hypernomic environment (Holley and Arboleda-Flórez 1988), suicide in jails and prisons among both prisoners and guards can be considered a major public health issue (Goss et al. 2002; World Health Organization 2000). More people die by suicide than for any other reason in prison and, given that most suicides occur within the first days of detention in jails or remand centers, special precautions and screening methods are highly recommended (Stuart 2003). To make this matter more important for public health purposes, a significant proportion of prisoners commit suicide shortly after their release from prisons (Jones et al. 2002).

Recommendations

There are three channels by which to explain the high prevalence of mental illness in prison systems. First, the high prevalence could simply be in line with the high prevalence of mental conditions among criminals, in general, at the time they committed the offense that brought them to court; so in these cases, offenders come to prison already mentally ill. Second, persons who have had a mental illness in the past could decompensate and have a relapse while in prison; persons in this group come in well but break down as part of natural expected relapses of mental conditions. Finally, persons who had never before had a mental problem may break down in prisons, by virtue of genetic or family backgrounds that manifest for the first time or simply because of stress and the harsh nature of the prison environment.

To facilitate treatment and management of mental conditions in prison systems and improve research protocols that depend heavily on adequate diagnostic systems, forensic practitioners and researchers should strive to identify groups of risk factors for mental and physical pathology. For example, substance misuse, previous suicidal behavior, and single-cell accommodation have been considered risk factors for suicide (Fazel and Lubbe 2005) in prisons. In addition, the judicious application of research findings for risk factors for violence could go a long way toward minimizing the probabilities of violence among the mentally ill in the community.

Prevention strategies could be implemented among persons who, although having a history of mental illness, are well on arrival or among those who had never had a mental condition. For those who are ill on arrival, correctional systems should have protocols for their management and treatment. From the start, and to follow a principle of equivalence, treatment options in prison should not be of lesser quality than similar services in the community (United Nations 1977) and should both address the immediate mental health needs of the inmate and, in communication with mental health systems in the community, develop adequate postrelease plans. Similarly, because of the high levels of comorbidities, there should be protocols that are all inclusive of health issues both physical and mental. Consent to treatment and other ethical safeguards pertaining to psychiatric treatment and research (Arboleda-Flórez, in press) should be the same in prison as those that apply in the community, and regulatory bodies for treatment and research watchdogs should exercise their authority in overseeing that these regulations apply behind the prison walls as well (Konrad et al. 2007).

Despite the comments in this chapter about the relative utility of diagnostics in forensic psychiatry, these comments apply almost exclusively to forensic psychiatry proper, not to correctional psychiatry. Even in forensic psychiatry, diagnostics are essential for purposes of statistical tabulations in forensic hospitals and administrative and financial operations and research. Use of diagnostics in prison medicine, including correctional psychiatry, is essential. The high frequency of mental conditions in prisons makes it mandatory to apply rigorous diagnostic systems so that patient-inmates can be properly triaged in order to use the finite health resources in any prison system in the best way possible. In addition, comorbidities between mental conditions, addictions, and physical conditions—especially infections—make it obligatory to apply standard and well-developed diagnostic systems.

These systems should not be telegraphic shorthand one-liners for communications but elaborate algorithms that could capture the totality of the personality. From the point of view of labels, diagnosticians should be trained into teasing out the few "forensic specific" diagnostic labels and into learning how to apply whole-person lifelong diagnostics that could be relevant and meaningful to a court of law. Ideally, diagnosticians should also be trained and be able to apply functional algorithms and levels of disabilities (World Health Organization 2001) for courts of law to make considered and enlightened decisions on persons with incapacities and disabilities.

An overreliance on diagnostic labels alone may lead to therapeutic nihilism and the closing of potential therapeutic alternatives in forensic settings. Exclusiveness on a diagnostic focus will preclude seeing the person behind the diagnosis in his or her humanity and with all his or her potentialities.

Conclusions

The process and ritual of diagnosis are essential components of medical practice, a shorthand communication system in clinical work and in research, and an obligatory tool for health care services research, besides forming the basis for statistical models to gauge delivery of services and financing. In forensic psychiatry, however, diagnosis is not the most important and relevant factor. In criminal proceedings, forensic psychiatrists make decisions about capacity to know and to appreciate the requisites of the law and to conduct one's behavior according to those requisites, based on the mental state of the person at the time an offense was committed or at the moment of trial. Similarly, in civil law, the capacity to make decisions and competently to carry out the functions at issue is what is important. These decisions must be conveyed to a court of law in a comprehensive formulation that encompasses the whole of the personality and the dynamics at the time of the event, matters that could hardly be accomplished with the telegraphic, clipped language of diagnostic systems. However, there are considerations regarding the use of diagnostic criteria and descriptions in the courts that should be taken into account as diagnostic systems are developed and revised; in prison systems and special hospitals, diagnostic processes follow the same routines and practices as in other hospitals in health care systems.

References

American Psychiatric Association: Diagnostic and Statistical Manual of Mental Disorders, 4th Edition. Washington, DC, American Psychiatric Association, 1994

Appelbaum P: Almost a Revolution. New York, Oxford University Press, 1994

Arboleda-Flórez J: Forensic psychiatry: contemporary scope, challenges and controversies. World Psychiatry 5:87–91, 2006

Arboleda-Flórez J: Mass violence and public health: a view from forensic psychiatry. Int Rev Psychiatry 19:211–220, 2007

Arboleda-Flórez J: Mental patients in prisons. World Psychiatry 8:187–189, 2009

Arboleda-Flórez J: Ethics in research. Bridges (in press)

Arboleda-Flórez J, Copithorne M: Mental Health Law and Practice: A Guide to the Alberta Mental Health Act and Related Canadian Legislation. Toronto, Ontario, Canada, Carswell, 1998

Arboleda-Flórez J, Deynaka C: Forensic Psychiatric Evidence. Toronto, Ontario, Canada, Butterworths, 1999

Brink JH, Doherty D, Boer A: Mental disorder in federal offenders: a Canadian prevalence study. Int J Law Psychiatry 24:339–356, 2001

Calzavara L, Ramuscak N, Burchell AN, et al: Prevalence of HIV and hepatitis C virus infections among inmates of Ontario remand facilities. CMAJ 177:257–261, 2007

Canadian HIV/AIDS Legal Network: Hard Time: Promoting HIV and Hepatitis C Prevention Programming for Prisoners in Canada. Toronto, Ontario, Canada, PASAN, 2007

Chiswick D: Test of capacity has little practical benefit. BMJ 331:1469–1470, 2005

Estroff SE, Swanson JW, Lachicotte WS, et al: Risk reconsidered: targets of violence in the social networks of people with serious psychiatric disorders. Soc Psychiatry Psychiatr Epidemiol 33 (suppl):S95–S101, 1998

Fazel S, Lubbe S: Prevalence and characteristics of mental disorders in jails and prisons. Curr Opin Psychiatry 18:550–554, 2005

Glen S: Dangerous and severe personality disorder: an ethical concept? Nurs Philos 6:98–105, 2005

Goodwin FK, Jamison KR: Manic-Depressive Illness. New York, Oxford University Press, 1990

Goss JR, Peterson K, Smith LW, et al: Characteristics of suicide attempts in a large urban jail system with an established suicide prevention program. Psychiatr Serv 53:574–579, 2002

Grover S: Reification of psychiatric diagnosis as defamatory: implications for ethical clinical practice. Ethical Hum Psychol Psychiatry 7:77–86, 2005

Gutheil TG: Forensic psychiatry as a specialty. Psychiatr Times 21:2–3, 31–36, 2004

Hare RD, Hart SD: Psychopathy, mental disorder and crime, in Mental Disorder and Crime. Edited by Hodgins S. Newbury Park, CA, Sage Publications, 1993, pp 104–115

Hodgins S: The criminality of mentally disordered persons, in Mental Disorder and Crime. Edited by Hodgins S. Newbury Park, CA, Sage Publications, 1993, pp 1–21

Holley H, Arboleda-Flórez JE: Hypernomia and self-destructiveness in penal settings. Int J Law Psychiatry 11:167–178, 1988

Jones R, Gruer L, Gilchrist G, et al: Recent contact with health and social services by drug misusers in Glasgow who died of a fatal overdose in 1999. Addiction 97:1517–1522, 2002

Konrad N: Prisons as new asylums. Curr Opin Psychiatry 15:583–587, 2002

Konrad N, Arboleda-Florez J, Jager AD, et al: Prison psychiatry. Int J Prison Health 3:111–113, 2007

Levav I: Terrorism and its effects on mental health. World Psychiatry 5:35–36, 2006

Lovgren S: Drug resistant staph infection spreads to gyms, day care. National Geographic News, April 25, 2006. Available at: http://news.nationalgeographic.com/news/2006/04/0425_060425_staph.html. Accessed October 17, 2009.

McKay RD, Wright RE: Schizophrenia and anti-social (criminal) behavior: some responses from sufferers and relatives. Med Sci Law 24:192–198, 1984

Monahan J, Steadman HJ: Crime and mental disorder: an epidemiological approach, in Crime and Justice: An Annual Review of Research. Edited by Tonry M, Morris N. Chicago, IL, University of Chicago Press, 1983, pp 145–189

Penrose LS: Mental disease and crime: outline of a comparative study of European statistics. Br J Med Psychol 18:1–15, 1939

Pffefer E: Código Procesal Penal Anotado y Concordado. Santiago, Editorial Jurídica de Chile, 2001, p 28

Pinals DA: Where two roads meet: restoration of competence to stand trial from a clinical perspective. N Engl J Crim Civ Confin 31:81–108, 2006

Ribé J, Martí Tusquets JL: Psiquiatría Forense, 2nd Edition. Barcelona, Spain, ESPAXS, 2002

Sepúlveda E: Forensic psychiatry in Chile: basic laws, penal process reform and operational aspects. Paper presented at 30th International Congress of Law and Psychiatry, Padua, Italy, 2007

Steadman HJ, McCarty DW, Morrisey JP: Developing Jail Mental Health Services: Practice and Principles (DHS Publication No. ADM 86–1458). Rockville, MD, U.S. Department of Health and Human Services, 1986

Stuart H: Suicide behind bars. Curr Opin Psychiatry 16:559–564, 2003

Stuart H, Arboleda-Flórez JE: A public health perspective on violence offenses among persons with mental illness. Psychiatr Serv 52:654–659. 2001

Stueve A, Link BG: Violence and psychiatric disorders: results from an epidemiological study of young adults in Israel. Psychiatr Q 66:327–342, 1997

Swanson JW, Holzer CE 3rd, Ganju VK, et al: Violence and psychiatric disorder in the community: evidence from the Epidemiologic Catchment Area surveys. Hosp Community Psychiatry 41:761–770, 1990

Swanson JW, Estroff S, Swartz M, et al: Violence and severe mental disorder in clinical and community populations: the effects of psychotic symptoms, comorbidity, and lack of treatment. Psychiatry 60:1–22, 1997

Taylor PJ: Schizophrenia and crime: distinctive patterns in association, in Mental Disorder and Crime. Edited by Hodgins S. Newbury Park, CA, Sage Publications, 1993, pp 63–85

Toch H, Adams K: The Disturbed Violent Offender. New Haven, CT, Yale University Press, 1989

Travin S: History of correctional psychiatry, in Principles and Practice of Forensic Psychiatry. Edited by Rosner R. New York, Chapman & Hall, 1994, pp 369–374

United Nations: Declaration for the Treatment of Prisoners: 663 C (XXIV), 1977

Weisstub D: Inquiry on Mental Competency. Toronto, Ontario, Canada, Queen's Printer, 1994

Wessely S: Violence and psychosis, in Violence: Basic and Clinical Science. Edited by Thompson C, Cowen P, Mental Health Foundation of Ontario. Oxford, UK, Butterworth-Heinemann, 1993, pp 119–134

World Health Organization: Preventing Suicide: A Resource for Prison Officers. Geneva, World Health Organization Department of Mental Health, 2000. Available at: http://www.who.int/mental_health/media/en/60.pdf. Accessed October 18, 2009.

World Health Organization: International Classification of Functioning, Disability and Health. Geneva, World Health Organization, 2001. Available at: http://apps.who.int/classifications/icfbrowser/. Accessed October 18, 2009.

World Health Organization: Mental Health of Populations Exposed to Biological and Chemical Weapons. Geneva, World Health Organization, 2005. Available at: http://www.who.int/mental_health/media/bcw_and_mental_heath_who_2005.pdf. Accessed October 18, 2009.

Yarvis RM: Axis I and Axis II diagnostic parameters of homicide. Bull Am Acad Psychiatry Law 18:249–269, 1990

5

ECONOMIC CONSEQUENCES OF REVISING THE DIAGNOSTIC NOMENCLATURE FOR MENTAL DISORDERS

Howard H. Goldman
Marcela V. Horvitz-Lennon
Teh-wei Hu
Margarita Alegría
Daniel H. Chisholm
Gerhard Heinze
Frank G. Njenga
Darrel A. Regier
Liz Sayce

Setting the Context

WHAT ARE THE KEY ISSUES?

Major policy issues come to the forefront when the diagnostic nomenclature changes. Among the more important questions that arise are: Who defines mental disorders? and How are the definitions used? The broad policy and public health implications of a change in the *International Classification of Diseases* (ICD; World

Health Organization 1992) or the *Diagnostic and Statistical Manual* (DSM; American Psychiatric Association 2000) are the focus of this Conference Expert Group. In this chapter, we focus on only the economic and financing policy implications of a revision of the diagnostic nomenclature.

One of the most important reasons a policy maker might be interested in changes in the diagnostic nomenclature is that assigning a diagnosis is an important step in documenting need for a particular service or resource. Demonstrated need for services or resources is often a basis for making decisions about allocation of and eligibility for benefits, such as transfer payments for income loss due to work disability or housing subsidies. Diagnosis is often used in policy formulation and implementation as a proxy for need.

What is the relation of diagnosis to need? This is the most significant overarching question affecting economic and financing policy. A clear answer to this question requires further specification of the basic question. Assessing need—for what? Assigning a diagnosis might be a valid proxy for establishing a need for any mental health service, but is it as good a proxy for determining the need for a specific level of service, such as hospitalization? Is the presence of a mental disorder alone a sufficient condition for receipt of income supports because of a work disability, for compensation for a loss due to impairment, or for a food subsidy? The next logical step in this decision-making process is usually to consider whether diagnosis is sufficient for determining the severity of impairment. If, and when, the diagnostic nomenclature is revised, the answers to these questions would change. The use of diagnosis as a guide to decision making and policy formulation and implementation is affected by every change in the diagnostic nomenclature. These issues are discussed in several articles published in *Health Affairs* in 2003 (Mechanic 2003; Regier 2003) and elsewhere (Regier et al. 2000).

Diagnosis has been used repeatedly as a proxy for need. Many diagnostic tools focus mainly on symptoms, and Mechanic argued that these symptom measures are not a good marker for the need for treatment. Regier responded by reminding us that the DSM uses clinical distress and poor functioning, along with specific descriptive symptoms and syndromes, to define mental disorders. These basic measures might justify the use of prevalence estimates as indicators of need for care. Changes in the nomenclature might improve or degrade the connection between disease prevalence and need for care. This is a critical issue in economic policy because resources are often allocated according to perceived needs. Advocates repeatedly point to reports from governments, such as the report of the U.S. Surgeon General (U.S. Department of Health and Human Services 1999) and the World Health Organization (2001); both reports indicated that the use of services falls far below projected need, based on mental disorder prevalence estimates. Advocates use these data to apply pressure to governments and the private sector to allocate more resources to bring treated prevalence in line with the true prevalence of mental disorders.

A historical article published in *Health Affairs* (Goldman and Grob 2006) described in detail how diagnosis has figured in policy determinations and debates in the United States since World War II. Some of these instances are presented in the pages that follow. The main point of the 2006 article was to indicate how policies have changed depending on whether society took a broad definition of *mental disorders* (e.g., focusing on anxiety and depression in primary care settings or preventing mental illness by early intervention in mild conditions) or a narrow definition, focusing only on those with disabling mental disorders.

For example, national policy might establish criteria for service in a community mental health center as "all conditions in the mental disorders section of the *International Classification of Diseases*" (World Health Organization 1992), or a policy might restrict access to include only a subset of the disorders, such as the psychoses, or exclude individuals with dementias or developmental disabilities.

WHAT IS ECONOMIC POLICY?

According to a conceptual framework for defining social policy (Gil 1973), all policy focuses on three key issues: division of labor, distribution of rights, and allocation of resources. In this section, we explain each of them and discuss their relation to economic policy, in particular.

Division of labor has economic consequences. For example, if individuals with certain mental disorders are assigned as a priority to the specialty mental health care sector but others are assigned to primary health care, a host of questions related to production and efficiency arise. Which sector can produce better outcomes and at what cost? Which providers are best suited to deliver cost-effective care to which individuals? Changes in the diagnostic nomenclature would alter the decision rules for treatment of specific conditions in such a situation. Furthermore, a change in the nomenclature that expands the number of diagnoses or broadens diagnostic criteria may legitimize treatments for more people with more conditions.

Introduction of new diagnostic categories, such as social phobia, creates more indications for older medications, thereby expanding markets, with economic impact. It also could lead to greater demand for mental health services. To counter the demand for treatment for new conditions, health care delivery systems have introduced additional mechanisms for rationing resources. For example, in the United States, health insurance policies insist that treatment meet criteria of "medical necessity," and managed behavioral health care companies are hired to make such determinations on a case-by-case basis.

How resources are allocated is often related to how rights are distributed in the society, so these two aspects of social policy are linked and have obvious economic consequences. For example, if only individuals with the most severe mental disorders have rights to disability payments, and disability payments are linked to health insurance, then health care resources will be allocated according to rules about rights of access. In this example, individuals with less-disabling conditions would have fewer rights and would be allocated fewer resources from society. This might be justified, according to a redistributive principle of allocating the most resources to those with the greatest need. On the other hand, it might violate a principle of allocating resources to those with the greatest chance of improvement or productivity.

In another example, parity in insurance coverage is both an issue of resource allocation and a question of fairness. This policy is designed to make insurance coverage the same for mental disorders as for other health conditions. The insurance rules often are determined by having been given a specific diagnosis as a basis for the discriminatory policy. Changes in the diagnostic nomenclature could change the definition of who has better insurance coverage and who has worse coverage. In this way, policies related to parity also raise concerns about equity—both in terms of health benefits and in terms of the distribution of benefits.

In the context of low- and middle-income countries where levels of national, social, and private insurance are low, the question would be whether the cost of needed care is somehow subsidized or waived by state providers. Although there is a lack of research on this issue, it is likely that for a significant proportion of households in those countries containing someone with a chronic mental health condition, the costs of seeking and obtaining mental health care services and goods will represent a significant drain on family resources (or assets/savings). This is because persons with mental health problems are expected to pay out of pocket for their care and treatment. In most of these countries, a person with a substance use disorder would be less likely to receive subsidized care than would someone with psychosis. So decisions about what diagnostic categories are to be included in, for example, an essential or extended package of health services could result in catastrophic expenditures (>10% of household income) and associated impoverishment. For example, in the country of Georgia, the State Medical Insurance Company will reimburse inpatient and outpatient costs only for individuals with diagnosed psychosis; no other mental health problems are covered (Georgian Association for Mental Health 2000, quoted in Dixon et al. 2006). In another example, conditions such as anorexia nervosa are virtually unknown in Sub-Saharan Africa (Njenga and Kangethe 2004). For whatever reason, globalization and other economic pressures from the West could "create" a new disease in that region.

Most of the examples offered thus far have come from high-income countries such as the United States. However, these examples apply to low- and middle-income countries as well, wherever diagnoses are assigned in treatment settings. Unfortunately, many individuals in low- and middle-income countries never receive a formal diagnosis or treatment. There are profound economic consequences to such lack of treatment, but changes in the diagnostic nomenclature are unlikely to affect this fundamental problem in health care delivery and economics.

In the following sections, we explore the role that diagnosis plays in allocation of resources and financing mechanisms. The focus is on potential effects from a change in the diagnostic nomenclature. The first discussion concerns the effect of changes in ICD and DSM on cost-of-illness studies and on treated-prevalence data. The second discussion focuses on three specific economic and fiscal policies that will be affected by changes in the diagnostic nomenclature: eligibility criteria for services and resources, insurance coverage policy, and case-mix adjustments. Each of these specific policy areas will be affected by changes in the ICD and DSM diagnostic nomenclature.

Cost-of-Illness Studies and Changes in the Diagnostic Nomenclature

Cost-of-illness studies describe the economic burden of a disease to society. This information is useful to policy makers and health professionals because it provides 1) the quantity of resources (in monetary terms) used to treat a disease and 2) the size of the negative economic impact (in terms of lost productivity) of an illness to society.

The empirical estimate of the magnitude of an illness depends on many key factors, such as the definition of disease category; the definition and measurement of cost, which includes the service mode and unit costs; and the methods of cost estimation.

Revising the diagnostic nomenclature for mental disorders would have economic cost consequences. First, a new classification of disease codes would change the prevalence rate or the treated prevalence rate. A change in the treated prevalence rate could also affect 1) the size of the potential patient population and treated population; 2) the mode of treatment pattern (i.e., outpatient, inpatient, medication, and others); and 3) the amount of services provided. Because the method of cost estimation—either top-down or bottom-up—requires information about the number of patients using the services and the type and amount of services patients receive, the magnitude of cost-of-illness estimates would change accordingly.

Even with no change in the diagnostic nomenclature, cost estimates may vary from one study to another because of differences in methods for identifying diagnostic categories. For instance, in reviewing the costs of depression, one study included major depression and dysthymia in its estimates of the cost of mood disorders, whereas other studies separated anxiety disorders from depression (Hu 2006). The inclusion or exclusion of different depression disease codes results in different magnitudes of the cost of illness. For instance, a study of the cost of nine common mental disorders in the Netherlands (Smit et al. 2006) included cost estimates for each detailed diagnostic category under anxiety disorder (such as panic disorder, agoraphobia, social phobia, simple phobia, and general anxiety disorder). Prevalence rates of the DSM-III-R (American Psychiatric Association 1987) Axis I disorder were obtained from a large epidemiological study of the noninstitutionalized population. Under a general code of anxiety disorder, the prevalence rate was 11.3% of the population; when these five detailed disease codes were combined, without unduplicating for multiple disorders in the same person, the prevalence rate became 16.9%. Similarly, the cost of anxiety would be 405 million Euros under the general code but would reach nearly 575 million Euros if these five individual costs of illness were combined. This example illustrates the effect of disorder classification on cost.

Sources of prevalence rate can be taken from a population survey or from administrative data on use of services. Prevalence rates from these two sources are not always consistent. Thus, it is especially important to specify data sources and detailed disease codes in estimation of cost of illness. A change in DSM or ICD codes will present a potential problem in assessing trends over time. It is possible that if a new condition were identified, such as social anxiety disorder, or if a new medication were introduced to treat the condition, either could cause the treatment rate to increase for anxiety disorder in outpatient clinics or primary care practice. Creating a new disorder condition may cause an increase in prevalence rate and related cost. Therefore, how mental disorders are defined and classified determines data collection and subsequent magnitudes of cost-of-illness estimates.

We could extend these arguments to epidemiological burden-of-disease studies, such as those carried out by the World Health Organization (Murray and Lopez 1996). As with cost-of-illness studies, burden-of-disease studies would be affected by changes in the diagnostic nomenclature. These studies would yield varying numbers of disability-adjusted life-years associated with various mental disorders, depending on criteria for inclusion and exclusion. This would affect advocacy with governments and donors as well as governmental planning for mental health services. This could influence changes in resource allocation and resource distribution (see World Health Organization 2006).

Economic Consequences of the Diagnostic Nomenclature Reflected in Financing Policy

As noted in the introduction to this chapter, changes in the diagnostic nomenclature could have an economic impact in several ways, through the division of labor or the distribution of rights, but the main economic effect of the changes would be on allocation of resources. Financing policy includes consideration of several important questions with economic consequences: Who will use which services? Who will perform which roles?

Changes in diagnostic nomenclature affect planning for use of resources and rules for eligibility for services and transfer payments as well as the right or opportunity to perform certain roles in society (e.g., employment), all of which have economic consequences. The most significant potential economic impact of changes in diagnostic nomenclature is on allocation of resources. In the next section of this chapter, we focus on several areas of financing policy, including eligibility criteria for use of behavioral health services, insurance regulations, and case-mix adjustment. In each section, we discuss ways in which changes in the diagnostic system might affect financing policy.

ELIGIBILITY CRITERIA

Service Eligibility

Diagnosis is a central feature of the criteria used to determine who is eligible for services. Priorities often are established for serving and treating individuals with certain conditions or groups of conditions. In such situations, diagnosis serves as a proxy for need or as a target for specific treatments or services. When diagnostic nomenclature changes, criteria for service eligibility might also change.

The definition of *serious mental illness* has enormous significance for policy making, research, and service planning and evaluation activities (Goldman and Grob 2006; Peck and Scheffler 2002). In the United States, meeting the federal definition of serious mental illness (or serious emotional disturbance among children and adolescents) is a critical component in the process of eligibility determination for public supports, including health insurance programs (Medicaid) and income support programs (Social Security). Serious mental illness involves a "diagnosable mental, behavioral, or emotional disorder of sufficient duration to meet DSM-IV or ICD-9 diagnostic criteria" (exceptions are DSM-IV (American Psychiatric Association 1994) or ICD-9 [World Health Organization 1977] "V" codes, substance use disorders, and developmental disorders), and a resulting "functional impairment which substantially interferes with or limits one or more major life activities."

Although the terms *serious mental illness* and *severe and persistent mental illness* are often used interchangeably, the latter also has been conceptualized as a more severely ill subset of the former (Goldman and Grob 2006). Diagnosis is the centerpiece of the operationalization of *severe and persistent mental illness,* but only half the definitions available by 1990 specified the disorders (Schinnar et al. 1990). Whenever specified, nonorganic psychoses, such as schizophrenia and major affective disorders, are always included; some definitions also include other disorders (Schinnar et al. 1990). It has been established that differences in the operational definitions of eligible diagnoses, functional disability, and illness associated with these definitions result in vastly different prevalence estimates (Ruggeri et al. 2000; Schinnar et al. 1990). The influential 1987 definition of severe (and persistent) mental illness issued by the National Institute of Mental Health (1987) in the United

States required a diagnosis of nonorganic psychosis or personality disorder; a duration determined by "prolonged illness and long term treatment"; and disability as determined by deficits in three of five functional areas.

In many states, eligibility for Medicaid services hinges on meeting the definition of serious mental illness as operationalized by the state. To exemplify, the state of Pennsylvania uses a definition that includes the federal definition *and also* requires 1) a diagnosis of schizophrenia, major affective disorder, psychosis not otherwise specified, *or* borderline personality disorder *and* 2) meeting criteria associated with treatment history (e.g., resided at a state mental hospital up until 2 years ago or less), low functional level (i.e., a Global Assessment of Functioning Scale score of 50 or less), *or* coexisting condition (e.g., homelessness or substance abuse comorbidity).

Differences in definitions used for purposes of benefit eligibility and clinical research can be problematic. A case in point is the difference in diagnoses included in the state or federal definitions of serious mental illness reviewed earlier and the narrower set of diagnoses—largely limited to schizophrenic and major affective disorders—included in studies that provided the supporting evidence for the evidence-based practices for people with severe mental illnesses (Drake et al. 2001; Goldman et al. 2001). In what perhaps constitutes the most salient example of this mismatch, there is plenty of anecdotal evidence that individuals with borderline personality disorder, without schizophrenic or major affective disorders comorbidity, are treated within programs of assertive community treatment, despite a dearth of evidence that it is an effective treatment for persons with these disorders.

An example from a middle-income country is also illustrative of this issue: the Republic of Chile's health care system consists of a public sector that serves 7 out of 10 Chileans and is financed through tax revenues and individual contributions and a network of private providers and for-profit health insurance companies. The country implemented a comprehensive health reform in 2005 aimed at increasing publicly and privately insured individuals' access to health care for the most common conditions (Apablaza et al. 2006). The main component of the reform is the "Plan for Universal Access With Explicit Guarantees"—or AUGE, its Spanish acronym—which, as its name implies, aims to ensure unfettered access to timely, guideline-driven, and equitable services for people diagnosed with health problems from an expanding list (25 in 2005, 40 in 2006, and 56 in 2007). The selection of conditions to be covered by AUGE was based on criteria of prevalence; significance (years of life lost, ability to address equity issues, preferences by various stakeholders); availability of effective care; and societal burden. Currently, AUGE covers three mental disorders: schizophrenia (comprehensive services for all patients diagnosed at first onset), depression in persons older than 14 years (comprehensive services for mild to moderate and severe cases), and a limited package of services for substance use disorders in persons younger than 20 years. Others being considered are attention-deficit/hyperactivity disorder, depression in persons younger than 15 years, chronic suicidal behavior, dementia, domestic violence, and child abuse and neglect (Alberto Minoletti, M.D., Director, Mental Health Department, Ministry of Health, personal communication, June 19, 2007).

The 2007 decree that articulates the reach of the AUGE law refers to health problems and pathological processes diagnosed through "the usual medical terminology" (Republic of Chile 2007). However, the government-sponsored treatment guidelines make reference to ICD-10 signs and symptoms and use the related ICD-10 nomenclature to refer to the selected mental disorders. Although lacking legal standing, private insurance companies have attempted to deny coverage because providers have not used an ICD-10 diagnostic formulation (A. Minoletti, Director, Mental Health Department, Ministry of Health, personal communication, June 26, 2007). Despite these appealable decisions by private industry, it may be said that the Chilean health reform has chosen to steer away from a specific diagnostic system in favor of a more inclusive diagnostic process, with the goal of ensuring greater access to the benefits of this particular reform.

Examples from low-income countries illustrate this issue further. In the Volta region of the Republic of Ghana, psychiatric patients are among those groups that qualify for complete exemption from user fees for locally provided health care (Nyonator and Kutzin 1999). However, such exemption mechanisms may not be implemented. In the United Republic of Tanzania, the traditional healers are the first, and often the last, port of call for persons with mental illness. They treat 45% of persons with mental illness in primary care (Ngoma et al. 2003). Inclusion of their patients in the definitions and benefits of those receiving mental health services would have far-reaching financing costs.

Eligibility for Disability Benefits

Another area of financing policy that potentially would be affected by changes in the diagnostic system is eligibility for disability benefits, or other transfer payments, that might be conferred along with disability status, such as access to housing, clothing allowances, or vouchers for services such as rehabilitation. The definition of *disability* often includes a requirement that an individual must have been diagnosed with an impairment or a health condition. Diagnosis is often used to establish the presence of impairment. Changes in the diagnostic nomenclature can put pressure on a disability determination system to alter its policies about which conditions to include and how to define them. For example, during a period of controversy about disability determinations in the United States in the early 1980s, the Social Security Administration incorporated diagnostic criteria from the then-new DSM-III (American Psychiatric Association 1980) into its regulations for defining mental impairments for purposes of determining disability. At the time, having specific criteria for mental disorders was important in increasing the credibility of the determination regulations and guidelines (Goldman and Grob 2006).

The Social Security Administration regulations for determining mental impairment include diagnostic criteria taken directly from DSM. The operational definition of disability due to specific categories of mental impairment includes Criterion A, which determines whether impairment exists, and Criteria B and C, which determine whether the mental impairment is associated with significant functional limitation. Together, these criteria establish a disability due to mental impairment. When DSM-IV supplanted DSM-III, the Social Security Administration changed its regulations.

Other countries may have related issues. For example, in most low-income countries, only persons who are in formal employment are eligible (often public employees based in urban areas), thus excluding the poor, informal workers and most of the rural population. Thus, access to effective treatment is partly conditional on employment status, and most individuals with a diagnosed mental disorder are not in the labor force.

INSURANCE REGULATIONS

In countries with health insurance coverage of mental health treatments and services, specific financing policies may circumscribe the types of conditions and disorders that are eligible for treatment. These conditions and disorders may be defined by a standardized diagnostic system, such as ICD or DSM, or they might be defined idiosyncratically. Where such health insurance coverage policies use specific diagnostic codes, any change in the nomenclature will affect who is covered and for what conditions. This financing policy concern is similar to the eligibility criteria issue raised in the previous discussion of eligibility for behavioral health services and for disability payments and benefits.

Insurance coverage policies may be designed to pay for services delivered to individuals, with all conditions listed in a specific diagnostic coding system, so the boundaries of that diagnostic system are critical. Will coverage include substance use disorders and developmental disabilities? Will services for individuals with a diagnosis of personality disorders be covered? What about coverage for specific personality disorders, such as antisocial personality? If a policy is to be inclusive, then it will be important for the diagnostic system used in making coverage decisions also to be inclusive.

In countries where health insurance has been restrictive, behavioral health services have not been covered universally. (The history of health insurance parity for behavioral disorders in the United States is reviewed in Grob and Goldman 2006.) In some U.S. states, efforts to expand health insurance coverage for behavioral health conditions focus on specific conditions rather than on all conditions in a diagnostic system. Some insurance policies have included coverage only for "biologically based disorders" from a specified list. Others cover all conditions listed in DSM-IV. Changes in diagnostic nomenclature may result in changes in access to specific treatments and services for certain individuals. The economic consequences, in terms of limited access to services and higher out-of-pocket payments by service users, can cause catastrophic financial losses for individuals and families.

Examples from several other countries illustrate this point. In Malaysia, health is predominantly financed through private health insurance schemes. However, all private insurers exclude mental health services from their plans, leaving those services to be financed through general taxation and out-of-pocket payments (Parameshvara Deva 2004). The Mental Health Act of 1989 in the Republic of Kenya makes it a criminal offense to exclude from coverage persons defined as having mental illness. The definition of what is, and what is not, a mental illness is as defined in classification systems such as ICD-9 and DSM-IV. Changes in diagnostic nomenclature will, in turn, change insurance coverage policy.

CASE-MIX ADJUSTMENT

In setting payment levels for services, it is important to be able to adjust for differences in patient needs. This allows payers to make valid comparisons between populations with diverse clinical complexity levels and diverse resource utilization needs or between providers serving these populations. Such adjustments are a critical component of contracting decisions, formulating payment schemes, administrating performance-based financial rewards and penalties, choosing targets for quality improvement, and making public reports (Berlowitz et al. 1998; Frank et al. 1997; Hendryx and Teague 2001). Hence, there is a need for *risk adjustment methodologies* that account for differing patient and environmental characteristics, which may affect treatment needs, health care resource utilization and costs, and patient outcomes (Dunn 1998; Ettner et al. 1998, 2001; Iezzoni 1994). Commonly used risk adjustors include health status, age, sex, and geographic location. Although used interchangeably with risk adjustment by some, the term *case-mix adjustment* is considered a specific case of risk adjustment in which adjustors are exclusively health-related patient characteristics (Hendryx and Teague 2001).

Here is a hypothetical example: The Ministry of Health in a country wished to establish a rate of payment for every visit to a primary care provider by individuals who have mental disorders. If the Ministry established only one rate for every patient visit, that might underpay for visits for complex problems and overpay for very routine care. The Ministry decided to adjust the payments according to a simple diagnostic scheme, paying more for visits by patients in some diagnostic categories and less for others.

Diagnosis and Case-Mix Adjustment

Case-mix adjustment methods are frequently used in environments where available data are largely limited to claims collected for administrative purposes, with scarce patient-related information beyond diagnosis and demographic variables.

As a result, *health status* is usually described through *diagnosis,* the underlying assumption being that diagnosis is predictive of treatment needs, resource utilization, and outcomes.

A specific case of the use of diagnosis for case-mix adjustment is the Diagnosis-Related Group (DRG) system instituted in the United States by Medicare in 1983 with passage of the inpatient Prospective Payment System (Fetter et al. 1980; Iglehart 1982). (Medicare is a health insurance program in the United States for individuals who have achieved retirement age, typically 65 years, or who have retired from work because of a disability.) The Prospective Payment System involved a major transformation in the financing of Medicare. Cost-based payments to acute-care hospitals were replaced by prospective payments at a rate calculated on the basis of typical charges associated with the care of *case types* defined by ICD-9 diagnosis (Ashcraft et al. 1989). The driving assumptions in the application of the DRG system were that inpatient resource use, length of stay, and hospitalization-associated costs may be sufficiently explained by diagnosis—a readily available and hard-to-game data element—and that each case type was a clinically meaningful grouping of disease conditions characterized by within-group homogeneity and between-group heterogeneity (Ashcraft et al. 1989; Taube et al. 1984).

Although 15 of the 486 DRGs are psychiatric, most inpatient psychiatric providers were exempted from the Prospective Payment System. (Some groups are very diverse, including all of the psychotic disorders, whereas others are narrower, including substance use disorders.) This decision was based on several factors. One was the acknowledgment that psychiatric diagnosis was only imperfectly associated with course of treatment and resource utilization (American Psychiatric Association 1983; Lave 2003). Psychiatric patients' treatment needs are influenced by other aspects of the presentation, including clinical characteristics (e.g., severity, degree of impairment, responsiveness to treatment); social characteristics (e.g., availability of social supports); and legal characteristics (e.g., potential for harm to self and others) (Lave 2003). Furthermore, actual treatment is influenced by factors, such as treatment goals and availability of treatment alternatives, that are not captured by diagnosis (Goldman et al. 1984; Mitchell et al. 1987).

A related factor entering into the exemption decision was the fact that psychiatric DRGs were found to have lower explanatory power *vis-à-vis* length of stay and costs compared with medical and surgical groups. Whereas psychiatric DRGs have been found to explain 2%–7% of variance in length of stay or costs (Cromwell 2001; English et al. 1986; Frank and Lave 1985; Hirdes et al. 2002; Schumacher et al. 1986; Taube et al. 1984), medical-surgical DRGs explain more than 30% of variation (Pettengill and Vertrees 1982). Adding other claims-based data elements does not significantly improve their explanatory power (Frank and Lave 1985; Taube et al. 1984).

Attempts to design a better claims-based classification system that would allow Medicare to extend the Prospective Payment System to exempted psychiatric inpatient providers were not met with success, because none of the alternative classification systems proved to be a significant improvement over DRGs (McGuire et al. 1987; Mitchell et al. 1987). Psychiatric DRGs were recently revised as part of a new effort to extend the Prospective Payment System to all psychiatric inpatient facilities (U.S. Department of Health and Human Services 2003, 2004). Unfortunately, the new DRGs are not that different from the groupings generated in 1983; new additions are age, medical comorbidity, and an adjustment for electroconvulsive therapy use (U.S. Department of Health and Human Services 2004).

It has been posited that the inadequacy of psychiatric DRGs as predictors of resource utilization is due partly to the diagnostic system on which they are based (Mitchell et al. 1987). The ICD-9 nomenclature for mental disorders is scarcely prescriptive, and it also includes symptoms and pathological processes, thus burdening the coding process (Mitchell et al. 1987). Studies have shown that DRGs would be substantially improved if risk adjustors not typically found in claims data were a part of the model (illness severity, social supports, dangerousness, assistance with activities of daily living) (Ashcraft et al. 1989; Fries et al. 1990; Horn et al. 1989; Mezzich and Coffman 1985). It follows that if the psychiatric diagnostic system captured these dimensions, the DRG classification system would be substantially improved.

Use of Diagnosis-Related Groups Around the World

The impetus for a DRG-based Medicare Prospective Payment System in the United States was to decrease costs associated with acute-care inpatient services and increase the efficiency of the most expensive sector of health care (Lave 2003). Over the past 20 years, Canada, New Zealand, Australia, and most European Union countries have also adopted DRG-based financing of inpatient services, although not all at a national level (Forgione and Vermeer 2002; Roger France 2003; Schreyögg et al. 2006). In socialized-medicine systems, like those of the Scandinavian countries, DRGs were implemented as a means to achieve greater cost-effectiveness and equity in the allocation of public resources (Mikkola et al. 2002). A recent study of 25 countries using, or planning to use, DRG-based payment systems found that ICD-10 is used more widely than ICD-9 (Roger France 2003). The Australian DRG system (AR-DRG), adopted by the Federal Republic of Germany and the Republic of Singapore, is a refined DRG based on ICD-10 diagnoses because it incorporates other health-related patient variables, such as clinical complexity (Antioch and Walsh 2004). Phelan and McCrone (1995) also reported on the effectiveness of DRGs in the United Kingdom of Great Britain and Northern Ireland.

It seems clear that any attempt to alter diagnostic nomenclature would alter existing diagnosis-based case-adjustment systems. Although this might be disruptive to existing payment systems that use diagnosis-based measures, there are severe limitations in the ability of current diagnoses to predict resource utilization and to estimate need for services, as has been shown. Perhaps newer diagnostic systems for mental disorders will be better at predicting the need for, and utilization of, mental health services.

Conclusions

Changes in the diagnostic nomenclature may have a wide range of economic consequences, from the impact on studies of cost of illness and burden of disease to eligibility policies for mental health services and insurance and disability compensation. Most of our examples come from high-income, and high-resource, countries, but the general principles apply across the board. Rather, they apply with one very salient proviso. They can only have meaning in countries where individuals in distress or experiencing dysfunction from a mental disorder have sufficient access to diagnostic assessment to be diagnosed. Unfortunately, this is not true for many individuals in low- and middle-income countries.

References

American Psychiatric Association: Statement to the House Ways and Means Subcommittee on Health, 15 February 1983. Washington, DC, American Psychiatric Association, 1983

American Psychiatric Association: Diagnostic and Statistical Manual of Mental Disorders, 3rd Edition. Washington, DC, American Psychiatric Association, 1980

American Psychiatric Association: Diagnostic and Statistical Manual of Mental Disorders, 3rd Edition, Revised. Washington, DC, American Psychiatric Association, 1987

American Psychiatric Association: Diagnostic and Statistical Manual of Mental Disorders, 4th Edition. Washington, DC, American Psychiatric Association, 1994

American Psychiatric Association: Diagnostic and Statistical Manual of Mental Disorders, 4th Edition, Text Revision. Washington, DC, American Psychiatric Association, 2000

Antioch KM, Walsh MK: The risk-adjusted vision beyond casemix (DRG) funding in Australia: international lessons in high complexity and capitation. Eur J Health Econ 5:95–109, 2004

Apablaza RC, Pedraza CC, Roman A, et al: Changing health care provider incentives to promote prevention: the Chilean case. Harv Health Policy Rev 7:102–112, 2006

Ashcraft M, Fries BE, Nerenz DR, et al: A psychiatric patient classification system: an alternative to diagnosis-related groups. Med Care 27:543–557, 1989

Berlowitz DR, Ash AS, Hickey EC, et al: Profiling outcomes of ambulatory care: casemix affects perceived performance. Med Care 36:928–933, 1998

Cromwell J: Report on the Feasibility of a Per Diem Prospective Payment System for Psychiatric Facilities Excluded From PPS. Draft Report. Waltham, MA, Health Economics Research, 2001

Dixon A, McDaid D, Knapp M, et al: Financing mental health services in low- and middle-income countries. Health Policy Plan 21:171–182, 2006

Drake RE, Goldman HH, Leff HS, et al: Implementing evidence-based practices in routine mental health service settings. Psychiatr Serv 52:179–182, 2001

Dunn DL: Applications of health risk adjustment: what can be learned from experience to date? Inquiry 35:132–147, 1998

English JT, Sharfstein SS, Scherl DJ, et al: Diagnosis-related groups and general hospital psychiatry: the APA Study. Am J Psychiatry 143:131–139, 1986

Ettner SL, Frank RG, McGuire TG, et al: Risk adjustment of mental health and substance abuse payments. Inquiry 35:223–239, 1998

Ettner SL, Frank RG, McGuire TG, et al: Risk adjustment alternatives in paying for behavioral health care under Medicaid. Health Serv Res 36:793–811, 2001

Fetter RB, Shin Y, Freeman JL, et al: Case mix definition by diagnosis-related groups. Med Care 18(suppl):iii, 1–53, 1980

Forgione DA, Vermeer TE: Toward an international case mix index for comparisons in OCED countries: Organization for Economic Cooperation and Development. J Health Care Finance 29:38–52, 2002

Frank RG, Lave JR: The psychiatric DRGs: are they different? Med Care 23:1148–1155, 1985

Frank R, McGuire TG, Bae JP, et al: Solutions for adverse selection in behavioral health care. Health Care Financ Rev 18:109–122, 1997

Fries BE, Nerenz DR, Falcon SP, et al: A classification system for long-staying psychiatric patients. Med Care 28:311–323, 1990

Gil D: Unraveling Social Policy: Theory, Analysis, and Political Action Towards Social Equality. Cambridge, UK, Schenkman, 1973

Goldman HH, Grob GN: Defining "mental illness" in mental health policy. Health Aff (Millwood) 25:737–749, 2006

Goldman HH, Pincus HA, Taube CA, et al: Prospective payment for psychiatric hospitalization: questions and issues. Hosp Community Psychiatry 35:460–464, 1984

Goldman HH, Ganju V, Drake RE, et al: Policy implications for implementing evidence-based practices. Psychiatr Serv 52:1591–1597, 2001

Grob GN, Goldman HH: The Dilemma of Federal Mental Health Policy: Radical Reform or Incremental Change. Piscataway, NJ, Rutgers University Press, 2006

Hendryx MS, Teague GB: Comparing alternative risk-adjustment models. J Behav Health Serv Res 28:247–257, 2001

Hirdes JP, Fries B, Botz C, et al: A system for classification of in-patient psychiatry (SCIPP): a new case-mix methodology for mental health. Paper prepared for the Psychiatric Working Group, Joint Policy and Planning Committee. Waterloo, Ontario, Canada, University of Waterloo, 2002

Horn SD, Chambers AF, Sharkey PD, et al: Psychiatric severity of illness: a case mix study. Med Care 27:69–84, 1989

Hu TW: Perspectives: an international review of the national cost estimates of mental illness, 1990–2003. J Ment Health Policy Econ 9:3–13, 2006

Iezzoni LI: Using risk-adjusted outcomes to assess clinical practice: an overview of issues pertaining to risk adjustment. Ann Thorac Surg 58:1822–1826, 1994

Iglehart JK: Health policy report: the new era of prospective payment for hospitals. N Engl J Med 307:1288–1292, 1982

Lave JR: Developing a Medicare prospective payment system for inpatient psychiatric care. Health Aff (Millwood) 22:97–109, 2003

McGuire TG, Dickey B, Shively GE, et al: Differences in resource use and cost among facilities treating alcohol, drug abuse, and mental disorders: implications for design of a prospective payment system. Am J Psychiatry 144:616–620, 1987

Mechanic D: Is the prevalence of mental disorders a good measure of the need for services? Health Aff (Millwood) 22:8–20, 2003

Mezzich JE, Coffman GA: Factors influencing length of hospital stay. Hosp Community Psychiatry 36:1262–1264, 1270, 1985

Mikkola H, Keskimaki I, Hakkinen U: DRG-related prices applied in a public health care system: can Finland learn from Norway and Sweden? Health Policy 59:37–51, 2002

Mitchell JB, Dickey B, Liptzin B, et al: Bringing psychiatric patients into the Medicare prospective payment system: alternatives to DRGs. Am J Psychiatry 144:610–615, 1987

Murray CJL, Lopez AD (eds): The Global Burden of Disease: A Comprehensive Assessment of Mortality and Disability From Diseases, Injuries, and Risk Factors in 1990 and Projected to 2020. Cambridge, MA, Harvard School of Public Health, World Health Organization, World Bank, Harvard University Press, 1996

National Institute of Mental Health: Towards a Model for a Comprehensive Community-Based Mental Health System. Washington, DC, U.S. Department of Health and Human Services, National Institutes of Health, National Institute of Mental Health, 1987

Ngoma C, Prince M, Mann A: Common mental disorders among those attending primary health clinics and traditional healers in urban Tanzania. Br J Psychiatry 183:349–355, 2003

Njenga F, Kangethe RN: Anorexia nervosa in Kenya. East Afr Med J 81:188–193, 2004

Nyonator F, Kutzin J: Health for some? The effects of user fees in the Volta region of Ghana. Health Policy Plan 14:329–341, 1999

Parameshvara Deva M: Malaysia mental health country profile. Int Rev Psychiatry 16:167–176, 2004

Peck MC, Scheffler RM: An analysis of the definitions of mental illness used in state parity laws. Psychiatr Serv 53:1089–1095, 2002

Pettengill J, Vertrees J: Reliability and validity in hospital case-mix measurement. Health Care Financ Rev 4:101–128, 1982

Phelan M, McCrone P: Effectiveness of diagnosis-related groups in predicting psychiatric resource utilization in the U.K. Psychiatr Serv 46:547–549, 1995

Regier DA: Mental disorder diagnostic theory and practical reality: an evolutionary perspective. Health Aff (Millwood) 22:21–27, 2003

Regier DA, Narrow WE, Rupp A, et al: The epidemiology of mental disorder treatment need: community estimates of "medical necessity," in Unmet Need in Psychiatry. Edited by Andrews G, Henderson S. Cambridge, UK, Cambridge University Press, 2000, pp 41–58

Republic of Chile, Ministry of Health, Department of Judicial Affairs: Explicit Health Guarantees of the General Program of Health Guarantees. Decreto No. 44 of 2007, 2007. Available at: http://www.supersalud.cl/normativa/571/articles-3174_recurso_1.pdf. Accessed October 21, 2009.

Roger France FH: Case mix use in 25 countries: a migration success but international comparisons failure. Int J Med Inform 70:215–219, 2003

Ruggeri M, Leese M, Thornicroft G, et al: Definition and prevalence of severe and persistent mental illness. Br J Psychiatry 177:149–155, 2000

Schinnar AP, Rothbard AB, Kanter R, et al: An empirical literature review of definitions of severe and persistent mental illness. Am J Psychiatry 147:1602–1608, 1990

Schreyögg J, Stargardt T, Tiemann O, et al: Methods to determine reimbursement rates for diagnosis related groups (DRG): a comparison of nine European countries. Health Care Manag Sci 9:215–223, 2006

Schumacher DN, Namerow MJ, Parker B, et al: Prospective payment for psychiatry: feasibility and impact. N Engl J Med 315:1331–1336, 1986

Smit F, Cuijpers P, Oostenbrink J, et al: Costs of nine common mental disorders: implications for curative and preventive psychiatry. J Ment Health Policy Econ 9:193–200, 2006

Taube C, Lee ES, Forthofer RN: Diagnosis-related groups for mental disorders, alcoholism, and drug abuse: evaluation and alternatives. Hosp Community Psychiatry 35:452–455, 1984

U.S. Department of Health and Human Services: Mental Health: A Report of the Surgeon General. Rockville, MD, Substance Abuse and Mental Health Services Administration, Center for Mental Health Services, National Institute of Mental Health, 1999

U.S. Department of Health and Human Services, Centers for Medicare and Medicaid Services: Medicare program; prospective payment system for inpatient psychiatric facilities; proposed rule. Fed Regist 68:66919–66978, 2003

U.S. Department of Health and Human Services, Centers for Medicare and Medicaid Services: Medicare program; prospective payment system for inpatient psychiatric facilities; final rule. Fed Regist 69:66921–67015, 2004

World Health Organization: International Classification of Diseases, 9th Revision. Geneva, World Health Organization, 1977

World Health Organization: International Statistical Classification of Diseases and Related Health Problems, 10th Revision. Geneva, World Health Organization, 1992

World Health Organization: The World Health Report 2001—Mental Health: New Understanding, New Hope. Geneva, World Health Organization, 2001. Available at: http://www.who.int/whr/2001/en/whr01_en.pdf. Accessed October 22, 2009.

World Health Organization: Dollars, DALYS, and Decisions: Economic Aspects of the Mental Health System, Geneva, World Health Organization, 2006. Available at: http://www.who.int/mental_health/evidence/dollars_dalys_and_decisions.pdf. Accessed October 25, 2009.

6

EDUCATION AND TRAINING

Horst Dilling
Aksel Bertelsen
John Cooper
Patricia Esparza
Michael B. First
Rafia Gubash
Fritz Hohagen
Alexander Kornetov
Srinivasa Murthy
Olabisi Odejide

General Considerations

CONFERENCE EXPERT GROUP FOR EDUCATION AND TRAINING

The Conference Expert Group (CEG) for Education and Training is in a different situation compared with most of the other CEGs. Whereas other groups discuss clinical studies and systematic descriptive evidence, this CEG discusses education and training activities that can facilitate introduction of the new and revised diagnostic and classification systems into the field, activities that tend to be subject to local policy and clinical customs and practices. At the moment, little scientific evidence exists on the effectiveness of educational and training activities pertaining to diagnostic and classification systems. Hence, this chapter details a descriptive and historical account of education and training activities pertaining to earlier diagnostic and classification systems.

For this CEG, the primary consideration in the revisions to ICD-10 (World Health Organization [WHO] 1992a) Chapter V, on "Mental and Behavioural Disorders," and DSM-IV (American Psychiatric Association 1994) is the processes by which these new systems will be introduced to the medical, professional, and research fields across countries. In particular, the planning of education and training in the content and use of the new classification systems needs to be part of the processes of introducing these systems into the field to facilitate the efficiency and proper utilization of the systems across professional, community, and clinical settings. For this reason, we propose that systematic planning and programs on education and training of these new systems be created before actual completion of the revisions takes place and be included as integral components of the revision processes.

When ICD-10 was first introduced in 1993 and 1994, no recommendations were provided on education and training or on how to present the new classification system to the medical community. A few years later, in 1996, the "Educational Kit," set up in collaboration with the WHO and the World Psychiatric Association, was handed out to participants of the World Congress of Psychiatry in Madrid, Spain, at a time when many institutions and several countries were already working with the new classification. Unfortunately, the only comprehensive review of the educational activities related to Chapter V (F), by Jenny J. van Drimmelen-Krabbe, medical officer at WHO Geneva, was never published (van Drimmelen-Krabbe, unpublished data, 1997). Apart from questionnaires handed out after the training course, no research (e.g., follow-up) took place (Janca 2001), and no scientific account was written as to the efficiency of any ICD-10 training.

We propose that a program of education and training concerning the new classification be prepared before the arrival of ICD-11 and that the necessary scientific studies recording the efficiency of this education and training program also be planned in advance.

POLICIES AND PUBLICATIONS

A difficult question concerning planning of education and training for the new classification will be its relevance for different fields, such as clinical use, research, primary care, international statistics, and public health. The interest and vigor with which the existing medical and psychiatric organizations support the introduction of a new psychiatric classification will depend on existing policies. The experience of the past 15 years has shown that results of the international introduction of the diagnosis and classification system can differ surprisingly in many countries. For instance, in the United States, virtually all clinical and research psychiatrists have to use DSM-IV, and most are barely aware of the existence of ICD-10. In Australia and New Zealand, psychiatrists are not equally under pressure to use DSM, but many prefer to use this classification under the mistaken impression that ICD-10 is the inferior classification. In the United Kingdom of Great Britain and Northern Ireland, ICD is recommended for clinical work, yet for research papers, either DSM or both classifications are used in parallel. In Western Europe and many Asian countries, usage is very mixed. In a few Eastern European countries, DSM is not used for political reasons, except for publications aimed at the top few international journals. These differences are the result of a variety of policies, beliefs, and influences (including economic) that have nothing to do with psychiatry or scientific and clinical knowledge. Our recommendations concerning the goals of education and training will be successful only if these issues connected to policies are decided on beforehand and if the goal is that both classifications—without any diagnostic differences between them—will find their own fields of action, without competition.

Another "political" question that is important for education and training concerns the distribution of WHO publications. In the past, governments of member nations have been informed about new revisions of the classification, but not the professional corporations, to stimulate sales and to suggest use of the publications in professional education. For ICD-10, in several European countries, such as the Kingdom of Denmark, the French Republic, the Federal Republic of Germany, the Republic of Italy, the Kingdom of Spain, and the United Kingdom, the various collaborating centers accepted this task, together with publishing houses and sometimes pharmaceutical companies, and played an important role in promulgating the sales of publications and use of the classification.

Two options should be discussed: 1) WHO could openly adopt a much more-active role in the advertising and general promulgation of ICD-11, or 2) WHO Geneva could reactivate its worldwide set of collaborating centers and request them to publicize ICD-11 in general as well as communicate with professional organizations in national and local mental health services to encourage use of ICD-11 in professional education at various levels.

Implementation of the ICD-10 Classification of Mental and Behavioral Disorders

With regard to preparing the necessary steps for implementation of the new diagnostic and classification systems, we describe earlier experiences with the implementation of ICD-10, with the intent to avoid former errors and detours in implementing the upcoming systems. Thus, we begin with a description of how ICD-10 was introduced, using experiences of the German-speaking countries as examples, followed by a description of the implementation process in several other countries. In addition, the introduction of DSM is discussed, and in the last section, we make suggestions and recommendations regarding implementation of the new diagnostic and classification systems.

After several years of preliminary work by the WHO, and a WHO conference held in Copenhagen, Denmark, in 1982 with representatives from the United States, an international expert group constituted itself in Geneva in 1984 under the chairmanship of the late Erik Strömgren. Within the framework of this CEG, a number of national centers were represented that discussed an initial draft of the new classification written by experienced psychiatric specialists. The planning and scientific responsibility on the part of the WHO were in the hands of Norman Sartorius, who initiated several worldwide field studies to gain experience on the design of the new classification, and as a result, drafts were changed considerably. In May 1990, ICD-10 was officially adopted by the World Health Assembly, and since January 1993, it has been used in various countries.

In preparation for the joint WHO and American Psychiatric Institute for Research and Education (APIRE) meeting, scheduled for September 2007, we gathered reports on the topic "education and training" from various countries and discussed them during a preparatory meeting held in Lübeck, Germany, on November 2–3, 2006. Although the general picture about the introduction of Chapter V (F) resembles, to a large degree, that of the German-speaking countries, experiences from a variety of countries were also mentioned. The reports and discussions at this meeting were the basis for joint recommendations.

INTRODUCTION INTO GERMAN-SPEAKING COUNTRIES

In the next paragraphs, we first describe the introduction of ICD-10 in German-speaking countries, followed by a description of the implementation process in other countries. This, of course, is the program which I, the present lead of the CEG, am most familiar with, and thus, with the help of Harald Freyberger, the German experience is given here as an example for ICD-11. The lead of this CEG "Education and Training" at that time had assumed chairmanship of the German Commission on Psychiatric Diagnoses of the DGPPN (German Society of Psychiatry and Psychotherapy) and since then had been involved in implementing and introducing ICD-10 into German-speaking countries. (The position of the chairman presently is held by Prof. H. Freyberger, Greifswald, who at the time of the introduction of ICD-10 also was working at Lübeck University.) Thus, in the 1980s and 1990s, the University Department of Lübeck, in cooperation with WHO, was the center (Field Trial Coordinating Centre) responsible for the introductory studies, implementation, and introduction of the German-language version.

Scientific Studies and Translations

Following several international studies on the development of structured, standardized diagnostic instruments—the Composite International Diagnostic Interview (CIDI) and Schedules for Clinical Assessment in Neuropsychiatry (SCAN) (World Health Organization 1990, 1992c), among others—our center, in connection with other psychiatric hospitals, carried out a study of the penultimate edition of the guidelines, the 1987 version (Dilling et al. 1990; Freyberger et al. 1990, 1992), and then also a study of the ICD-10 research criteria (Freyberger et al. 1992; Stieglitz et al. 1996). These studies tested the feasibility, applicability, goodness-of-fit, and reliability of the diagnostic categories and texts in ICD-10. Participating in the German-language part of the study on research criteria were 14 hospitals or departments for adult psychiatry (Basel, Berlin, Essen, Freiburg, Göttingen, Hamburg, Hannover, Homburg, Kaufbeuren, Lübeck, Mainz, Mannheim, Munich, Vienna); 11 hospitals of psychosomatic medicine (Berus, Bochum, Essen, Geldern, Giessen, Göttingen, Hannover, Heidelberg, Lübeck, Mannheim, Stuttgart); and 5 hospitals for child and juvenile psychiatry (Frankfurt/Main, Cologne, Lübeck, Mannheim, Marburg). Worldwide, a total of 112 centers in 39 countries took part in this study. The German contribution to the studies had to wait until the preliminary texts had been translated. The joint international findings (Sartorius et al. 1993) were then incorporated into the final versions of the English-language texts.

Published first in 1991–1992, the English (World Health Organization 1992a) and German (Dilling et al. 2008) editions of the Chapter V (F) "Clinical Descriptions and Diagnostic Guidelines" were followed in 1992 by the systematic complete edition of the ICD-10, with short psychiatric descriptions (Deutsches Institut für Medizinische Dokumentation und Information 1994; World Health Organization 1992b), and finally in 1993 by the English-language (World Health Organization 1993) and in 1994 by the German-language editions of the Diagnostic Criteria for Research (Dilling et al. 2006). The translations were carried out by the working group in Lübeck, in cooperation with the centers in Munich, Mannheim, and Marburg. Through the translation work and empirical studies, there grew a network of centers in the German-speaking countries. Long before the official German introduction of ICD-10 on January 1, 2000, area-wide ICD-10 seminars at numerous hospitals—also for physicians in private practice—had been carried out within this continuously growing network. The introduction of the new ICD-10 coding in our psychiatric hospital took place January 1, 1994. Various central psychiatric meetings were held, including an international diagnostic congress in Lübeck in 1992 (Dilling et al. 2006). In the annual German Society {Deutsche Gesellschaft} for Psychiatry, Psychotherapy and Neuropsychiatry congress, corresponding events took place.

In Germany, this initial involvement of field testing the ICD-10 diagnostic categories and texts by a network of hospitals, as well as the translation of these texts by centers and working groups, created an established network that served to facilitate the introduction of ICD-10 via individual/independent seminars even before the official German introduction took place.

Introductory Courses and Seminars

Before the official German introduction, the individual implementation of education and training in the institutions was carried out at the discretion of a hospital's medical director. Thus, the transfer of information and experience connected with individual diagnostic exercises for the learners could be carried out over an extended period without time pressure.

At the beginning, training courses were generally offered at the centers previously listed and gradually moved to other institutions over time. In preparation, overhead transparencies were produced that listed both the general questions with regard to the ICD-10 (history, preliminary studies, definitions, structure) and the diagnostic criteria, especially in abbreviated form, yet, in substance, complete texts. We produced videos of 20-minute diagnostic interviews for the most common disorders as well as selected videos of case histories from field studies. The courses lasted from 1.5 to 2.5 days and corresponded to the familiarization workshops (J. van Drimmelen-Krabbe, unpublished data, 1997). Following a 3-hour introduction, the individual subchapters (F1–F7) were systematically addressed in an additional 10–12 hours. The videos were shown, and participants were required not only to form a diagnostic evaluation but also to document the case in terms of psychopathology and the contents in terms of operational diagnostics, after which a general discussion was held.

After some years, the basic training needs of the clinical institutions had more or less been fulfilled, and there were requests for advanced seminars that would provide more detail. Further introductory courses for new beginners were still offered once or twice a year. This demand was met by the Lübeck Days of Diagnostics (Lübecker Diagnostiktage), which were held regularly once or twice a year. The courses were taught by external lecturers as well as numerous employees of our psychiatric department, who took part in the various familiarization training sessions. Seminars on diagnostic interviews were held in parallel (e.g., SCAN or CIDI).

An expansion of teaching activity in this area developed according to the expressed wish of WHO to further disseminate knowledge of ICD-10 Chapter V (F) in Eastern Europe. Together with his colleagues, Jenny van Drimmelen from WHO Headquarters in Geneva and Aksel Bertelsen from Denmark, Horst Dilling took part in a group that carried out joint seminars in St. Petersburg, Kiev, Minsk, Tartu, Riga, and Vilnius from 1994 to 1996.

Teaching Materials and Study Instruments

In addition to the videos and overhead transparencies mentioned earlier, further teaching materials were needed. An expanded edition of the easy-to-read pocket guidelines, originally edited by John Cooper (1994), was translated and published (Dilling and Freyberger 2008). Several casebooks were compiled, among them an international casebook edited by WHO (Üstün et al. 1996), which was translated into German (Dilling 2000), and a German publication with cases of adult patients (Freyberger and Dilling 1993). An additional casebook was published by the child and juvenile psychiatrists Poustka and van Goor-Lambo (2000), and finally, together with the German DSM Working Group, a casebook with comparative case evaluation according to DSM and ICD was also published (Zaudig et al. 1998).

To compare the diagnostic coding of ICD-9 with that of ICD-10, bidirectional reference tables were constructed to maintain continuity in case histories and for administrative tasks (Cooper 1994; Dilling and Freyberger 2008). In addition, reference tables between DSM-IV-TR and ICD-10 were published (American Psychiatric Association 2000; Dilling and Freyberger 2008; Schulte-Markwort et al. 2002; van Drimmelen-Krabbe et al. 2001). Moreover, books and essays in manuals and journals were compiled to facilitate the implementation (Dilling 2001; Sartorius 1995). On the basis of several texts by the WHO, a lexicon on ICD-10 was produced (Dilling 2000), as well as a computerized tutorial (Malchow et al. 1995). The transfer of diagnostic contents into the instruction of medical students was also surveyed (Lencer et al. 1997; Müssigbrodt and Dilling 1994).

For scientific purposes, WHO recommended instruments compiled by international research teams, among them the CIDI and SCAN, and an inventory of personality traits (International Personality Disorder Examination; Loranger 1996). The German-speaking regions contributed the Structured Interview for Diagnosis of Dementia of Alzheimer Type, Multi-Infarct Dementia, and Dementia of other Aetiology According to ICD-10 and DSM-III-R (Zaudig and Hiller 1996), the Munich Diagnostic Check List for DSM-III-R (Hiller et al. 1995), and the ICD-10-Features List (ICD-10-Merkmalsliste) (Dittmann et al. 1992).

Primary Health Care—Operationalized Psychodynamic Diagnostic

A particularly important area of research is the recognition and treatment of mental disorders in primary health care. A handbook providing descriptions and treatment alternatives for the main mental disorders was published by WHO in 1996 (World Health Organization 1996a) as well as a German translation by our group (Dilling 2001) and a slightly expanded version for the "coat pocket" (Müssigbrodt et al. 2006), which was met with a great deal of interest.

The ICD-10 field studies in the area of psychoanalytical psychotherapy and psychosomatics were a primary impetus for the subsequent development of the multiaxial system of "operational psychodynamic diagnostics" (OPD) (Arbeitskreis OPD 2001; Dahlbender et al. 2004; Schauenburg et al. 1998). The OPD system supplements traditional multiaxial approaches with features relevant to therapy and results and has led to remarkable research innovations (Operationalized Psychodynamic Diagnostics Task Force 2007). The original multiaxial system introduced by Rutter and colleagues (World Health Organization 1996b) in the field of child and juvenile psychiatry (Remschmidt et al. 2005) has thus been supplemented by an operationalized psychodynamic approach.

A different group cooperated with the Danish center in Århus to study transculturally, in 10 countries, the successful (or unsuccessful) introduction of the

ICD-10—primarily the use of diagnostic options and diagnoses that were never needed (Müssigbrodt et al. 2000) and might be omitted.

INTRODUCTION OF ICD-10 CHAPTER V IN ENGLISH-SPEAKING COUNTRIES

In many English-speaking countries, the "Educational Kit PC Version" of ICD-10 Chapter V (F), produced by WHO and the World Psychiatric Organization in 1996, was a helpful resource during the introduction process even if it appeared too late for many countries to put to use. The (undated) diskette contains materials useful for training, transparencies, and case histories as well as assistance for designing a training program for different professionals in the mental health field.

United Kingdom

The Royal College of Psychiatrists organized a set of seminars for local clinical tutors, guided by Professors Michael Gelder and John Cooper. A package of about 25 transparencies was prepared for these seminars, and the transparencies were then used locally by clinical tutors for training of other tutors and then psychiatric trainees. The efficiency of this snowball system was not formally tested, but it was popular with both tutors and trainees. An advantage was that, as in other English-speaking countries, the necessary texts were already available and did not require translation. In addition to the WHO publications, John Cooper (1994) published and edited a practical ICD-10 pocket guide containing introductory definitions, research criteria, the most important somatic categories of ICD-10, and reference tables. This guide was produced for use by any English-speaking country or by any English-speaking psychiatrist and has been translated into French, Italian, Spanish, and German.

Australia

In Australia, for a long time, mainly the DSM classification was used. Aleksandar Janca, Director of the WHO collaborating center in Perth, Australia, stated in 2001:

> Although numerous Australian psychiatric research institutions have actively participated in the development and field trials of the ICD-10 section on mental and behavioural disorders, its use for coding of psychiatric diagnoses by clinicians in Australia has just begun. One reason for the slow implementation was the lack of organized ICD-10 educational and training programmes at state and national levels. (Janca et al. 2001)

After introducing ICD-10 to the professionals through 12 workshops and seminars in the densely populated area around Perth in Western Australia, Janca organized telepsychiatry training in the countryside, with evaluations of the immediate success through before-and-after comparisons in knowledge (Janca and Gillam 2002). A further training, based on the Primary Health Care (PHC) version (World Health Organization 1996a), was started as a next step. Workshops also took place outside of Western Australia in Hanoi; Hong Kong; Sydney; Cambridge, Massachusetts; and Russia.

The aforementioned examples of education and training activities in English-speaking countries illustrate the importance of targeting clinical tutors and psychiatric trainees in the introduction process as well as the need for implementing training and educational programs at state and national levels that include before and after evaluations to assess their effectiveness (as was done in Western Australia).

INTRODUCTION OF ICD-10 CHAPTER V IN OTHER COUNTRIES

The introduction of ICD into other countries took many forms, but one notable strategy was the use of existing structures to educate psychiatrists-in-training about the new system. Established educational structures were used to target groups of psychiatrists-in-training and incorporate education about the new system as a requirement in their training (e.g., Denmark), and international conferences were used to target professional psychiatrists. In line with this strategy, a national network of "quality circles" was accessed to target family physicians in Spain, for example, and trans-Atlantic links and networks were used to reach psychiatrists in Latin American countries.

The Kingdom of Denmark and Other Scandinavian Countries

ICD-10 Chapter V (F) was introduced in Scandinavia by the WHO Collaborating Centre for Research and Training in Mental Health at the Århus University Hospital, Risskov, a WHO Field Trial Coordinating Centre headed by Aksel Bertelsen. The classification was introduced in a fashion similar to that described earlier for the German-speaking countries. A difference, however, was that the Danish Psychiatric Society more strictly demanded participation in the training courses and obligatory training in psychiatry, including a course of psychopathology. In addition, regular refresher courses were given at 1- or 2-year intervals. With regard to the acceptance of the new classification, it is reported that older specialists reacted tentatively, whereas younger psychiatrists were highly enthusiastic.

The interest of the pharmaceutical industry and its support of the introduction of ICD-10, such as through distribution of the Danish translation of the classification of mental disorders, ought to be mentioned. The attempt to introduce the PHC version among general practitioners was less successful, because that group preferred the International Classification of Primary Care. Based on the WHO classification, a lexicon of psychiatric terms was written in Danish (Bertelsen and Jörgensen 2000). The WHO center in Århus organized many postgraduate training courses and diploma courses, during different international congresses, and participated actively in workshops in Scandinavia and in eight introductory courses and workshops in Eastern Europe between 1994 and 1997.

The Kingdom of Spain

The WHO collaborating center in Madrid, Spain (Juan J. Lopez-Ibor, Director), with support from the pharmaceutical industry (GKB, Pfizer), translated the different versions of Chapter V (F) and coordinated the field trials in Spain and Latin America. The center distributed the pocketbook edition of the guidelines to 4,000 psychiatrists in Spain and 2,000 in Latin America and offered familiarization seminars—with high participation rates—in Spain (1,900 psychiatrists, or two-thirds of the total), the Republic of Ecuador, the Bolivarian Republic of Venezuela, the United Mexican States, and the Argentine Republic. In Spain, the PHC version was distributed to two-thirds of the family physicians (20,000 copies), and 7,000 family physicians attended 1-day seminars. In addition, 54 quality circles were organized in which one psychiatrist worked with 20–30 family physicians.

The Russian Federation

In different places in Russia—for example, Moscow, St. Petersburg, Irkutsk, Novosibirsk, Omsk, and Tomsk—seminars and workshops were organized by Professors Krasnow (Moscow) and Kornetov (Tomsk), with visiting psychiatrists from the Geneva ICD-10 advisory group (Professors Cooper, Janca, and Sartorius) representing different countries. In particular, the younger generation of Russian psychiatrists welcomed the opportunity to discuss ICD-10. Implementation in Russia was difficult, because an influential group of psychiatrists opposed the new system of classification on the grounds that it was less nosological than the traditional system; thus, the introduction there has been only partially successful.

ICD-10 seminars also were held in other Eastern countries, including parts of the former Soviet Union (e.g., White Russia [Minsk], Ukraine [Kiev], the Republic of Estonia [Tartu], the Republic of Latvia [Riga], and the Republic of Lithuania [Vilnius]).

The People's Republic of China

In China, translation of the ICD-10 is apparently complicated and very difficult to apply in practice. As a result, the Chinese classification, although in a revised version that approximates the ICD-10, continues to be used.

The Republic of India, Arabic Countries, and Central African Countries

In India, Arabia, and Central African countries, a major point of criticism is the failure of the "European" system of classification to consider particular features of the disorders, especially among rural populations. To address this concern, acute and transient psychotic disorders (F 23) were included in the ICD-10. Many professionals in the health care system do not require the complete version of the classification, but the more practical texts of the useful PHC version were, unfortunately, not easily available in many African countries. Arab countries criticized the fact that the coexistence of DSM and ICD had a negative effect on motivation to use the ICD-10 in practical psychiatry, such as in Bahrain, where most psychiatrists of the teaching faculty at the university are Americans.

This survey about the introduction of Chapter V (F) indicates that a wide variety of tasks and activities ensued with the implementation of the new classification. Thus, one cannot speak of a planned procedure with regard to this process. The success (or lack thereof) of efforts within the various countries was subject to extremely heterogeneous international, national, regional, or local conditions.

DSM and Training

When DSM-III was published in the United States in 1980 (American Psychiatric Association 1980), it was regarded as a significant paradigm shift in psychiatric nosology and classification (Spitzer et al. 1980). Several new features were introduced that distinguished it from its predecessors, DSM-II (American Psychiatric Association 1968) and ICD-8 (World Health Organization 1967). New features included the 1) adoption of an atheoretical approach regarding etiology; 2) provision of operationalized diagnostic criteria for every disorder; 3) introduction of new terminology and disorders (e.g., posttraumatic stress disorder, somatization disorder, attention-deficit disorder) and elimination of familiar terminology (e.g., neurosis); 4) large expansion in the number of disorders, including new sections on psychosexual dysfunctions, gender identity disorders, eating disorders, and so on; and 5) provision of a multiaxial system for psychiatric evaluation (i.e., Axis I for clinical syndromes, Axis II for personality disorders and specific developmental disorders, Axis III for physical disorders and conditions, Axis IV for rating the severity of psychosocial stressors, and Axis V for indicating the highest level of adaptive functioning in the past year).

The depth and breadth of these changes necessitated the provision of an intensive training effort in order to bring clinicians up to speed. In response to various demands for training programs, both the American Psychiatric Association and the Columbia University Department of Psychiatry organized national symposia and continuing-education workshops in the United States to teach DSM-III (Skodol 1989). Skodol et al. (1981) recommended a curriculum for a six-session didactic training course on DSM-III that focused on the elements of descriptive psychopathology, principles of classification, and differential diagnosis. Various training materials were also developed in the wake of DSM-III. These included

1. *DSM-III Institutional Instruction Kit,* developed by the American Psychiatric Association's Task Force on DSM-III Educational Activities, which included audiocassette recordings, written transcripts, and slides of lectures delivered at a national DSM-III symposium that emphasized the transition from DSM-II to DSM-III and the multiaxial diagnostic system.

2. *DSM-III for Clinicians,* a self-study audiocassette program aimed at an individual clinician's need for training on the DSM-III. This program was a recording of a lecture series that the developers of DSM-III presented at the 1980 annual meeting of the American Psychiatric Association.

3. *DSM-III Case Book* (Spitzer et al. 1981), assembled by the developers of DSM-III, a collection of more than 200 written case vignettes covering the entire range of DSM-III categories and including a series of famous cases from the psychiatric literature.

4. *DSM-III Training Guide* (Webb et al. 1981b), developed by the Office of Continuing Education, Texas Department of Mental Health and Mental Retardation, and Texas Research Institute of Mental Sciences (TRIMS). Designed to assist trainers in training for DSM-III, it included both slides and written and videotaped case vignettes for practice and was based on a 2.5-day training program. The effectiveness of the training program was evaluated by examining the accuracy of DSM-III diagnoses made by 251 clinicians who participated in the training program but who had no prior exposure to DSM-III (Webb et al. 1981a). They were each asked to diagnose three cases from a series of five videotaped case vignettes, and their ratings were compared with ratings made by the course faculty. Although the degree of agreement varied across the five cases, the overall level of agreement was reported to be high (74.2%), suggesting that the Texas training program was effective in training participants in the basic concepts and use of DSM-III.

In contrast to the seismic shift in classification practices entailed by the adoption of DSM-III, subsequent revisions of the DSM—that is, DSM-III-R (American Psychiatric Association 1987), DSM-IV (American Psychiatric Association 1994), and the latest text revision, DSM-IV-TR (American Psychiatric Association 2000)—have been relatively minor, mostly encompassing modifications in diagnostic criteria and additions of new disorders. Given that the fundamental features of the DSM (i.e., the descriptive approach, provision of diagnostic criteria, and use of a multiaxial system for recording the assessment) remained relatively unchanged, the changes in DSM-III-R and DSM-IV were able to be presented in the context of relatively short grand rounds presentations and workshops generally lasting 1–2 hours. Instead of providing training to the participants on an entirely new diagnostic approach, these presentations started from the perspective that the attendees were already familiar with the DSM-III system and would therefore focus only on the changes in diagnostic criteria and terminology and on the new disorders that had been introduced.

Each subsequent edition of the DSM has seen simultaneous revision and updating of the DSM-III materials—for example, *DSM-III-R Casebook* (Spitzer et al. 1989), *DSM-III-R Training Guide* (Reid and Wise 1989), *DSM-IV Casebook* (Spitzer et al. 1994), and *DSM-IV Training Guide* (Reid and Wise 1995)—as well as the development of new training materials such as the *DSM-III-R Training Guide for Diagnosis of Childhood Disorders* (Rapoport and Ismond 1990); *DSM-IV Handbook of Differential Diagnosis* (First et al. 1995); and *DSM-IV Guidebook* (Frances et al. 1995). It is likely that these books are primarily used for purposes of training students, interns, residents, and other new clinicians about psychiatric diagnosis rather than for purposes of transitioning clinicians from one edition of DSM to the next.

Suggestions and Recommendations

The implementation of ICD-11 and DSM-5 will be accompanied by recommendations for education, teaching, and training. For ICD, these recommendations will refer, in large part, to experiences with the implementation of ICD-10. Although education and training activities were discussed among commissions and working groups, neither the German-speaking nor any other countries produced a comprehensive and scientific report on the efficacy and effectiveness of such activities. Nonetheless, the introduction of the diagnostic and classification systems was managed in a variety of different ways, some of which were highly satisfactory.

GENERAL PRELIMINARY IDEAS

Teaching and training in basic psychiatric education and advanced and continuing education are bound together through numerous learning processes between teachers and students. The premise of advanced professional training is the prior basic education on the part of learners that links knowledge to thought and personal opinions and emotions and causes a certain formation of personality. The willingness and capacity to achieve special training goals must be accompanied by an increasing proportion of training that in turn is accompanied by an increasing inception of knowledge on the part of the student. *Training* can be defined as the acquisition of knowledge or skills, often taught by a teacher, so that the trainee learns to fulfill certain tasks.

The application of psychiatric classificatory systems, meaning well-founded diagnostics, is not possible without a fundamental professional education followed by corresponding specialization and a solid knowledge of the possibilities and limits connected with the respective classification. Because diagnosis is prerequisite to all successful therapeutic work, it is a medical focus. In preparation, this area must continually be addressed during our studies, by presenting either biological models of classification or the taxonomy of somatic pathology, before moving on to teach the more complicated psychiatric classification. With respect to the self-evident topic of continuous education, diagnostics ought to be continuously anchored to advanced education. Learners who are trained in this manner will more easily recognize and accept the advantage and necessity of a new system of classification and will support the transition.

Education and training in the upcoming systems of classification should not apply only to those individuals currently receiving advanced professional education or to specialists in psychiatry and psychotherapy and clinical psychologists. In the same manner, other members of the health care services, who are involved in the treatment and rehabilitation of mental disorders, as well as individuals in the corresponding administrations, should be included in education and training programs. With regard to rehabilitation, there will be much overlap with the International Classification of Functioning, Disability and Health created by the WHO (World Health Organization 2001). A fundamental condition, in addition to the availability of experienced teachers, is the supply of texts and learning materials. Material should be attractive, practical, and learner friendly and, above all, not too expensive. In great measure, the acceptance of the new system of classification will depend on the initial interest and motivation of users. In this context too, the current diagnostic and classification systems of the WHO and the American Psychiatric Association should, it is hoped, become harmonized (Regier et al. 2002).

SCIENTIFIC STUDIES

In the run-up to ICD-11, which is evolving in parallel to DSM-5 (Kupfer et al. 2002), a number of preliminary ideas and suggestions have been published (Cooper 2003; Schmidt 2007) that are to flow into the preliminary drafts of the new classifications. The compilation, implementation, and introduction of ICD-11 should be accompanied by national and international studies. Initially, one could start with a study that would correlate the items or criteria, in practical work currently used, with the diagnoses of the mental disorders according to Chapter V (F) (Dittmann et al. 1992). Field studies will be carried out to test the validity, reliability, and goodness-of-fit of individual categories as well as the acceptance of the classification draft by members from other language and cultural regions. Computer technology, along with the World Wide Web and an e-mailing system, can be used to communicate drafts to the professional public for discussion. This will stimulate scientific interest in the topic of diagnostics, simplify the implementation, and promote the worldwide use of ICD-11. Evaluation of the training success during the introductory process could be linked to other studies of outcome and could contain a renewed evaluation and refreshment training for a later time.

According to past experiences, clinical guidelines and diagnostic criteria should not diverge, because this increases unwanted separation of these areas for researchers and clinicians. Nonetheless, for certain scientific studies, it might be recommendable to define individual categories according to special criteria, which—in the case of pharmacological studies, for example—would include only a definitively diagnosed core group. However, generally speaking, research and clinical work should be linked as closely as possible. At the specialist level of psychiatric or psychosomatic professionals, everything points in favor of a uniform system of scientific classification, but for other professionals (e.g., primary caregivers, administrators, and statisticians) there have to be several versions at different levels.

INDIVIDUAL RECOMMENDATIONS

Discrete recommendations from the CEG on Education and Training include the following:

- Preparation and publication of educational and training materials for use in practice (inpatient, semiambulatory, and ambulatory institutions) and research will be very important. The lion's share of this work will have to be performed by centrally guided, but differently focused, expert groups of the World Health Organization and the American Psychiatric Association. Texts will be written, such as a complete version of the ICD-11; special texts for psychiatric diagnoses in practice and research; brief versions; texts for the primary health care sector and for the language of public health; Internet and personal-computer versions; lexica; conversion tables; casebooks or case collections; diagnostic videos with presentation of differences between the versions (e.g., ICD-10 and -11); structured clinical interviews; and other instruments.
- Initial seminars for trainers at the international, national, regional, and institutional levels (teaching the teachers) should be organized.
- At the national, regional, and (where appropriate) language levels, *responsible specialists* must be found and appointed who will continuously advise, plan, structure, and guide the introductory processes. Perhaps some of the earlier training centers can be reactivated, but in most cases new centers will have to be established. These, in turn, will activate networks of further centers in order to carry out multicenter studies and parallel programs of education and training that are the prerequisite for scientific diagnostic work.
- Types of education and training required include lectures, seminars, and controlled reading, as well as perhaps Internet conferences and interactive learning programs.
- Groups that should be targeted in the introduction process include

   Group A: psychiatrists, psychologists, psychotherapists, and other physicians (specialists) in close contact with the care of mentally ill patients; also members of the groups named who are receiving their basic education or continuing education.

Group B: occupational therapists, social workers, nursing personnel, general practitioners, and other medical specialists.

Group C: administrative personnel (e.g., in institutions of health care provision and in government ministries) and health-insurance personnel.

Group D: those affected and their social environment (relatives, partners, friends).

Group E: the general public.

- Training modules for the various targeted groups should include

Group A: fundamental knowledge of the classification and diagnostic systems in hospital and practice.

Group B: knowledge of how to apply the diagnostic systems in practice.

Group C: general basic knowledge.

Group D: general information and a deeper knowledge with regard to interesting topics.

Group E: information by general scientific journals and by mass media; campaigns explaining facts about psychiatric disorders.

- Quality assurance of the introduction processes at different levels will be necessary, including evaluation at the scientific and individual levels; evaluation of training events, with renewed evaluation following a defined period; and evaluation of prejudice in public opinion.
- Flexibility of introduction will be important; the structures should be flexible and capable of being modified according to national or regional, or even language and geographical, particularities.
- A decisive precondition for a successful implementation of the new systems of classification is, in many parts of the world, the degree of political support. The responsible governments should know the necessity of implementation and be motivated to support it. If, in addition, those who are professionally responsible for the provision of health care also support the plan, one can reckon with its success.

RECOMMENDATIONS TO OTHER CONFERENCE EXPERT GROUPS AND AMERICAN PSYCHIATRIC ASSOCIATION OR WORLD HEALTH ORGANIZATION WORKING GROUPS

For education and teaching purposes, as a basic rule, a classification has to be constructed logically. Every disorder should appear only once, and overlapping of criteria of several disorders should be avoided. Such overlapping is sometimes difficult to avoid because of the current limited knowledge about certain disorders, but in at least two sections, eating disorders and personality disorders, there is, without discussion of the problem, considerable overlap in the list of symptoms given as identifiers of the constituent disorders. A simple rearrangement could have made these sections easier to use and to understand. If, in the new revisions, taxonomic principles are not sufficiently observed, this should be stated, and any necessary compromises should be reported. In an overall descriptive classification, each disorder should have its place, but only one place. Otherwise it might be difficult to teach and learn. Finally, statements about what a disorder *is not* can be very important; "exclusion clauses" should be provided, in addition to a more considered discussion of this principle, in order to educate and help the user.

Very often cultural differences of disorders are mentioned, and separate diagnoses are claimed. Only cases for which there are clear phenomenological criteria should be taken into consideration. In most cases, they can be assigned to already existing diagnoses. The main goal should be "one common language in psychiatry" (Lopez-Ibor 2003).

Conclusions

In contrast to the introduction of DSM-III, which also is described in this chapter, the subject of education and training was not systematically considered in the implementation of earlier versions of ICD or in the implementation of Chapter V (F) of ICD-10. Nonetheless, the introductory process of ICD-10 was carried through in different ways, and often very successfully. As an example, the introduction of the psychiatric chapter of the ICD-10 in the German-speaking countries is described in detail here, followed by a description of this process in other countries. Finally, our CEG on Education and Training presents recommendations for the future introduction of the new classification and diagnostic systems of mental and behavioral disorders.

References

American Psychiatric Association: Diagnostic and Statistical Manual of Mental Disorders, 2nd Edition. Washington, DC, American Psychiatric Association, 1968

American Psychiatric Association: Diagnostic and Statistical Manual of Mental Disorders, 3rd Edition. Washington, DC, American Psychiatric Association, 1980

American Psychiatric Association: Diagnostic and Statistical Manual of Mental Disorders, 3rd Edition, Revised. Washington, DC, American Psychiatric Association, 1987

American Psychiatric Association: Diagnostic and Statistical Manual of Mental Disorders, 4th Edition. Washington, DC, American Psychiatric Association, 1994

American Psychiatric Association: Diagnostic and Statistical Manual of Mental Disorders, 4th Edition, Text Revision. Washington, DC, American Psychiatric Association, 2000

Arbeitskreis OPD (ed): Operationalisierte Psychodynamische Diagnostik [Operationalized Psychodynamic Diagnostics], 3. Bern, Switzerland, Hans Huber, 2001

Bertelsen A, Jörgensen OS: Psykiatrisk Ordbog [Psychiatric Dictionary]. Copenhagen, Denmark, Hans Reitzels Förlag, 2000

Cooper JE (ed): Pocket Guide to the ICD-10 Classification of Mental and Behavioural Disorders. Edinburgh, UK, Churchill Livingstone, 1994

Cooper JE: Prospects for chapter V of ICD-11 and DSM-V. Br J Psychiatry 183:379–381, 2003

Dahlbender RW, Buchheim P, Schüssler G (eds): Lernen an der Praxis: OPD und Qualitätssicherung in der Psychodynamischen Psychotherapie [Learning by Experience. OPD and Quality Assurance in Psychodynamic Psychotherapy]. Bern, Switzerland, Hans Huber, 2004

Deutsches Institut für Medizinische Dokumentation und Information (DIMDI) (ed): Internationale Statistische Klassifikation der Krankheiten und Verwandter Gesundheitsprobleme, 10 Revision, Band I: Systematisches Verzeichnis [International Statistical Classification of Diseases and Related Health Problems, 10th Revision, Vol: Tabular List]. Heidelberg, Germany, Springer, 1994

Dilling H (ed): Weltgesundheitsorganisation. Die vielen Gesichter Psychischen Leids: Das Offizielle Fallbuch der WHO zur ICD-10 Kapitel V(F). Falldarstellungen von Erwachsenen. [The Many Faces of Mental Distress: The Official Casebook of WHO ICD-10 Chapter V (F). Adult Disorders]. Bern, Switzerland, Hans Huber, 2000

Dilling H (ed): Weltgesundheitsorganisation Psychische Störungen in der Primären Gesundheitsversorgung. Diagnostik und Behandlungsrichtlinien. 25-Karteikartensystem. [Diagnostic and Management Guidelines for Mental Disorders in Primary Care: 25 Index Card System]. Bern, Switzerland, Hans Huber, 2001

Dilling H, Freyberger HJ (eds): Taschenführer zur ICD-10-Klassifikation Psychischer Störungen [Pocket Guide to the ICD-10 Classification of Mental and Behavioural Disorders], 4th Edition. Bern, Switzerland, Hans Huber, 2008

Dilling H, Freyberger HJ, Malchow CP: Design of the ICD-10 field trial in German-speaking countries. Pharmacopsychiatry 23:142–145, 1990

Dilling H, Mombour W, Schmidt MH, et al (eds): Internationale Klassifikation Psychischer Störungen. ICD-10 Kapitel V (F). Diagnostische Kriterien für Forschung und Praxis [The ICD-10 Classification of Mental and Behavioural Disorders: Diagnostic Criteria for Research and Practice], 4th Edition. Bern, Switzerland, Hans Huber, 2006

Dilling H, Mombour W, Schmidt MH, (eds): Internationale Klassifikation Psychischer Störungen. ICD-10 Kapitel V(F). Klinisch-Diagnostische Leitlinien [The ICD-10 Classification of Mental and Behavioural Disorders: Clinical Descriptions and Diagnostic Guideline], 6th Edition. Bern, Switzerland, Hans Huber, 2008

Dittmann V, Dilling H, Freyberger HJ: Psychiatrische Diagnostik Nach ICD-10: Klinische Erfahrungen bei der Anwendung. Ergebnisse der ICD-10 Merkmalslistenstudie [Psychiatric Diagnostics According to ICD-10: Clinical Experiences in Its Use. Results of the ICD-10 Study Concerning the Lists of Clinical Criteria]. Bern, Switzerland, Hans Huber, 1992

First M, Frances A, Pincus H: DSM-IV Handbook of Differential Diagnosis. Washington, DC, American Psychiatric Association, 1995

Frances A, First M, Pincus H: DSM-IV Guidebook. Washington, DC, American Psychiatric Association, 1995

Freyberger HJ, Dilling H (eds): Fallbuch Psychiatrie. Kasuistiken zum Kapitel V(F) der ICD-10 [Case Book Psychiatry: Case Studies Concerning the Chapter V(F) of ICD-10]. Bern, Switzerland, Hans Huber, 1993

Freyberger HJ, Dittmann V, Stieglitz RD, et al: ICD-10 in der Erprobung: Ergebnisse Einer Multizentrischen Feldstudie in den Deutschsprachigen Ländern [Trials With ICD-10: Results of a Multicenter Field Study in German Speaking Countries]. Nervenarzt 61:271–275, 1990

Freyberger HJ, Stieglitz RD, Dilling H: Ergebnisse Multizentrischer Diagnosenstudien zur Einführung des Kapitels V(F) der ICD-10 [Results of Diagnostic Multicenter Studies for the Introduction of Chapter V(F) of ICD-10]. Fundamenta Psychiatrica 6:121–127, 1992

Hiller W, Zaudig M, Mombour W (eds): WHO ICD-10 Checklisten [ICD-10 Checklists]. Bern, Switzerland, Hans Huber, 1995

Janca A: ICD-10 as a coding tool in psychiatry. Australas Psychiatry 9:358–363, 2001

Janca A, Gillam D: Development and evaluation of an ICD-10 telepsychiatry training programme in Western Australia. J Telemed Telecare 8:120–122, 2002

Janca A, Ahern K, Rock D: Introducing ICD-10 into psychiatric coding practice: a WA experience. Aust N Z J Public Health 25:376–377, 2001

Kupfer DJ, First MB, Regier DA: A Research Agenda for DSM-V. Washington, DC, American Psychiatric Association, 2002

Lencer R, Malchow CP, Dilling H: Qualitätssicherung in der Lehre am Beispiel der Vorlesung und Kasuistik im Fach Psychiatrie [Quality assurance in teaching: example of lecture and case presentation in the subject of psychiatry]. Medizinische Ausbildung 14:26–32, 1997

Lopez-Ibor JJ: Cultural adaptations of current psychiatric classifications: are they the solution? Psychopathology 36:114–119, 2003

Loranger AW, World Health Organization: International Personality Disorder Examination. IPDE. ICD-10 Modul. Bern, Switzerland, Hans Huber, 1996

Malchow CP, Kanitz R-D, Dilling H: ICD-10 Computer Tutorial: Psychische Störungen. Bern, Switzerland, Hans Huber, 1995

Müssigbrodt H, Dilling H: Studentenunterricht im fach psychiatrie. Erwartungen und einschätzungen [Teaching medical students in the subject of psychiatry: expectations and evaluations]. Medizinische Ausbildung 11:61–69, 1994

Müssigbrodt H, Michels R, Malchow CP, et al: Use of the ICD-10 classification in psychiatry: an international survey. Psychopathology 33:94–99, 2000

Müssigbrodt H, Kleinschmidt S, Schürmann A, et al: Psychische Störungen in der Praxis. Leitfaden zur Diagnostik und Therapie in der Primärversorgung nach dem Kapitel V(F) der ICD-10 [Psychiatric Disorders in Practice: Manual for Diagnosis and Therapy in Primary Care According to Chapter V (F) of ICD-10], 3rd Edition. Bern, Switzerland, Hans Huber, 2006

Operationalized Psychodynamic Diagnostics Task Force (ed): Operationalized Psychodynamic Diagnostics OPD-2: Manual for Diagnosis and Treatment Planning. Göttingen, Germany, Hogrefe, 2007

Poustka F, van Goor-Lambo G: Fallbuch Kinder- und Jugendpsychiatrie. Erfassung und Bewertung belastender Lebensumstände von Kindern nach Kapitel V(F) der ICD-10 [Casebook for Child and Youth Psychiatry: Recording and Evaluation of Children in Burdened Life Situations According to Chapter V(F)]. Bern, Switzerland, Hans Huber, 2000

Rapoport JL, Ismond DR: DSM-III-R Training Guide for Diagnosis of Childhood Disorders. New York, Brunner/Mazel, 1990

Regier DA, Narrow WE, First MB, et al: The APA classification of mental disorders: future perspectives. Psychopathology 35:166–170, 2002

Reid W, Wise M: DSM-III-R Training Guide. New York, Brunner/Mazel, 1989

Reid W, Wise M: DSM-IV Training Guide. New York, Brunner/Mazel, 1995

Remschmidt H, Schmidt M, Poustka F (eds): Multiaxiales Klassifikations-Schema für Psychische Störungen des Kindes- und Jugendalters Nach ICD-10 der WHO [Multiaxial Classification According to ICD-10 Concerning Child and Youth Age], 5th Edition. Bern, Switzerland, Hans Huber, 2005

Sartorius N: Understanding the ICD-10 Classification of Mental Disorders. London, Science Press, 1995

Sartorius N, Kaelber CT, Cooper JE, et al: Progress toward achieving a common language in psychiatry: results from the field trials of the clinical guidelines accompanying the WHO classification of mental and behavioural disorders in ICD-10. Arch Gen Psychiatry 50:115–124, 1993

Schauenburg H, Freyberger HJ, Cierpka M (eds): OPD in der Praxis. Konzepte, Anwendungen, Ergebnisse der Operationalisierten Psychodynamischen Diagnostik [OPD in Practice: Concepts, Applications, Results of Operationalized Psychodynamic Diagnostics]. Bern, Switzerland, Hans Huber, 1998

Schmidt LG: Substanzbezogene Störungen: auf dem weg zu ICD-11 und DSM-V [Mental disorders due to psychoactive substance use: on the road to ICD-11 and DSM-V]. Fortschritte der Neurologie und Psychiatrie 11:634–642, 2007

Schulte-Markwort M, Marutt K, Riedesser P (eds): Cross-Walk ICD-10: DSM-IV. Bern, Switzerland, Hans Huber, 2002

Skodol A: Problems in Differential Diagnosis: From DSM-III to DSM-III-R in Clinical Practice. Washington, DC, American Psychiatric Association, 1989

Skodol AE, Spitzer RL, Williams JB: Teaching and learning DSM-III. Am J Psychiatry 138:1581–1586, 1981

Spitzer RL, Williams JB, Skodol AE: DSM-III: the major achievements and an overview. Am J Psychiatry 137:151–164, 1980

Spitzer RL, Skodol AE, Gibbon M, et al: DSM-III Case Book: A Learning Companion to the Diagnostic and Statistical Manual of Mental Disorders, 3rd Edition. Washington, DC, American Psychiatric Association, 1981

Stieglitz RD, Freyberger HJ, Malchow CP, et al: Design of the ICD-10 field trial of the Diagnostic Criteria for Research in German-Speaking Countries. Psychopathology 29:260–266, 1996

Üstün TB, Bertelsen A, Dilling H, et al (eds): The Many Faces of Mental Disorders: Adult Case Histories According to ICD-10. Washington, DC, American Psychiatric Association, 1996

van Drimmelen-Krabbe J, Bertelsen A, Pull C: International psychiatric classification: ICD-10 and DSM-IV, in Contemporary Psychiatry, Vol 1. Edited by Henn FA, Sartorius N, Helmchen H, et al. Heidelberg, Germany, Springer, 2001

Webb LJ, Gold RS, Johnstone E, et al: Accuracy of DSM-III diagnoses following a training program. Am J Psychiatry 138:376–378, 1981a

Webb LJ, DiClemente CC, Johnstone EE, et al: DSM-III Training Guide. New York, Brunner/Mazel, 1981b

World Health Organization: International Classification of Diseases, 8th Revision. Geneva, World Health Organization, 1967

World Health Organization: Composite International Diagnostic Interview (CIDI). Geneva, World Health Organization, 1990

World Health Organization: The ICD-10 Classification of Mental and Behavioural Disorders: Clinical Descriptions and Diagnostic Guidelines. Geneva, World Health Organization, 1992a

World Health Organization: International Statistical Classification of Diseases and Related Health Problems, 10th Revision. Geneva, World Health Organization, 1992b

World Health Organization: Schedules for Clinical Assessment in Neuropsychiatry (SCAN). Interview and Manual. Geneva, World Health Organization, 1992c

World Health Organization: The ICD-10 Classification of Mental and Behavioural Disorders: Diagnostic Criteria for Research. Geneva, World Health Organization, 1993

World Health Organization: Diagnostic and Management Guidelines for Mental Disorders in Primary Care: ICD-10 Chapter V Primary Care Version. Göttingen, Germany, Hogrefe and Huber, 1996a

World Health Organization: Multiaxial Classification of Child and Adolescent Psychiatric Disorders. Cambridge, UK, Cambridge University Press, 1996b

World Health Organization: International Classification of Functioning, Disability and Health. Geneva, World Health Organization, 2001

Zaudig M, Hiller W: SIDAM. Strukturiertes Interview für die Diagnose einer Demenz Nach DSM III R, DSM IV und ICD 10 [SIDAM. Structured Interview for the Diagnosis of Dementia According to DSM III, DSM IV and ICD-10]. Bern, Switzerland, Hans Huber, 1996

Zaudig M, Wittchen H-U, Sass H: DSM IV und ICD-10 Fallbuch, Fallübungen zur Differentialdiagnose [DSM IV and ICD-10 Casebook: Case Exercises for Differential Diagnosis]. Göttingen, Germany, Hogrefe, 1998

7

STATISTICS AND INFORMATION SYSTEMS

Walter Gulbinat
Francesco Amaddeo
María Elena Icaza Medina-Mora
Malik Mubbashar
David M. Ndetei
Robert M. Plovnick

The World Health Organization (WHO) defines a *Mental Health Information System* (MHIS) as a "system for collecting, processing, analyzing, disseminating and using information about a mental health service and the mental health needs of the population it serves" (World Health Organization 2005). A *system* is seen as "a collection of components that work together to achieve a common objective" (World Health Organization Regional Office for the Western Pacific 2004). The objective of an MHIS is to serve as a tool for improving the mental health of a population and its individual members. The question we discuss here is how issues of classification and diagnosis may contribute to this objective. Before we undertake this, we identify the main uses of an MHIS, review the information and data typically processed in such a system, and analyze the role of a common language aimed at facilitating communication and understanding among users of such systems.

Main Uses of Mental Health Information Systems

An MHIS is used primarily for patient management, program and policy management, administrative purposes, and in support of research programs:

- A system for patient management is expected to provide information about a patient for use by the clinician or treatment team.
- Systems for policy and program management should be capable of handling information for planning, resource allocation, and reporting to governing, regulatory, and funding bodies. Information is required not only for assessing mental health needs but also for suitable program monitoring and evaluation.
- An administrative information system should provide data for purposes of accounting or reimbursement of provided services. Such information typically is needed by payers, such as government and insurance companies.

Psychiatric case registers deserve special mention. In addition to the uses just listed, such registers have been used for a variety of research purposes since the 1960s (ten Horn et al. 1986). Today, psychiatric case registers are used mainly in three fields of epidemiological research: studies on mental health services utilization patterns (including health economics studies); studies on the effect that clinical and social variables have on services' utilization and planning; and studies that integrate geographical information with register data, using a health-geography approach.

The ultimate use of an MHIS determines the information and data requirements. It goes without saying that a country (or region or community) will not run four separate information systems. However, an MHIS, which in most situations is embedded in a general health information system, may provide data elements that can be used for some or all of the purposes outlined here.

Information and Data to Be Processed

Before we approach the problem of classification of information, we review the information and data items that are typically considered in an MHIS.

Categories of information relevant for patient management include identification (e.g., name), patient demographic characteristics, patient history, family history, psychopathology, functioning (such as disabilities, impairments, handicaps), laboratory tests, diagnosis, treatment, procedures, prognosis, and outcome.

For policy and program management, there are two types of data: individual and population-based data (Table 7–1). Individual data are derived from individual patients and include diagnosis, treatment, outcome, and length of stay. These data can be aggregated and provide information for regional or national program manage-

TABLE 7–1. Data needed for policy and program management

Type	Characteristics	Examples
Individual	Aggregated data are derived from data of individual patients	Diagnosis Treatment Number of admissions Number of involuntary admissions Number of physical restraints or seclusions Length of stay
Population based	Data are essentially rate based and derived independently for numerator and denominator	Admission rate Attendance rate Bed occupancy rate Percentage with symptom relief Percentage with improved level of functioning Percentage of health budget allocated to mental health Number of mental health staff per population

ment. Population-based data have two characteristics. First, these data are essentially rate based and are calculated using denominator and numerator, including admission rates, attendance rates, and bed-occupancy rate. Second, aggregated individual data can be used as population-based data. For example, aggregated diagnosis data of a health care facility can be incorporated into a larger database of multiple facilities.

The Need for a Common Language

Interventions for prevention and treatment of mental disorders, as well as for promotion of mental health, typically require intersectoral and interdisciplinary collaboration, regardless of whether such interventions are patient- or program-management oriented or are research oriented. This means that information generated at various entrance points to the health and social system will have to be shared by many users, including people representing different professional groups. Such information is increasingly used for comparison of data within populations over time, and between populations at the same point in time, as well as for compilation of nationally consistent data. The unprecedented studies on the burden of disease conducted by the World Bank (1993) and WHO (Murray and Lopez 1996) are based on such data.

A prerequisite for a smooth exchange of information among all those who need the data is that such information is valid and accessible. Both *validity* and *accessibility* of information have several dimensions.

The *validity* of information may be compromised at times of data generation, storage, transfer, and use. At the time of generation, the data may be wrong, ill defined, or incomprehensible. At times of storage or transfer, data may be lost or corrupted. At the time of use, information may be misunderstood.

Data accessibility has functional as well as physical components. *Functional accessibility* pertains to access rights and ease of access (e.g., defined by the format in which data are stored) as well as the professional capacity to understand the content and significance of the data (i.e., appropriate training programs). Physical access, both at data entry and during data use, may be manual or computer assisted (Drake et al. 2005) or a combination of both methods. Again, training of personnel is an important component for facilitating physical access to the MHIS.

A prerequisite for meaningful use of information generated from different sources by different people representing different professions is an agreement on the use of a *common language*. Important elements of such a common language are definition of terms, nomenclatures, dictionaries, classification, and taxonomies. To date, there is no common language to cover all the different types of information entered into and processed by MHISs. Examples of such types of information are clinical data (personal and medical history, symptomatology, diagnosis, treatment, course, and outcome); laboratory data (including imaging); social data (including family history, occupational information); administrative information (including finances, insurance); and data on the health and social system (including data on system performance). Nevertheless, great efforts have been devoted to developing classifications for international use in a great number of domains relevant to health and mental health.

The Family of International Classifications

WHO, over the past four decades, has been very active in developing a common language pertaining to psychiatric diagnosis, embedded in the *International Classification of Diseases* (ICD; Papart 2004; Sartorius 1989; Sartorius and Shapiro 1973; Weitzel et al. 1974). However, there are numerous international classifications in fields other than diagnosis that are of high relevance to mental health.

WORLD HEALTH ORGANIZATION CLASSIFICATIONS

The WHO constitution mandates production of international classifications on health (see www.who.int/classifications/en/; www.who.int/classifications/en/

WHOFICFamily.pdf) so that there is a consensual, meaningful, and useful framework that governments, providers, and consumers can use as a common language. In particular, WHO maintains three *core* or *reference* classifications that have been approved by its governing bodies for international use:

- *International Classification of Diseases* (World Health Organization 2007b). The ICD has become the international standard diagnostic classification for all general epidemiological and many health-management purposes. These include the analysis of the general-health situation of population groups and monitoring of the incidence and prevalence of diseases and other health problems in relation to other variables, such as the characteristics and circumstances of the individuals affected. The ICD is used to classify diseases and other health problems recorded on many types of health and vital records, including death certificates and hospital records. In addition to enabling the storage and retrieval of diagnostic information for clinical and epidemiological purposes, these records also provide the basis for the compilation of national mortality and morbidity statistics by WHO Member States (see www.who.int/classifications/icd/en/).
- *International Classification of Functioning, Disability and Health (ICF;* World Health Organization 2001a). The ICF is WHO's framework for measuring health and disability at both individual and population levels.
- *International Classification of Health Interventions (ICHI;* World Health Organization 2007a). The purpose of this classification is to provide a common tool for reporting and analyzing the distribution and evolution of health interventions for statistical purposes. It is structured with various degrees of specificity for use at the different levels of the health system and uses a common accepted terminology in order to permit comparison of data between countries and services.

In addition to reference classifications, the WHO family includes *derived* classifications. Derived classifications are based on the reference classifications (i.e., ICD and ICF). Derived classifications may be prepared by adopting the reference classification structure and categories, by providing additional detail beyond that provided by the reference classification, or by rearranging or aggregating items from one or more reference classifications. Examples of derived classifications are

- *The ICD-10 Classification of Mental and Behavioural Disorders: Clinical Descriptions and Diagnostic Guidelines* (World Health Organization 1992)
- *The ICD-10 Classification of Mental and Behavioural Disorders: Diagnostic Criteria for Research* (World Health Organization 1993)
- *Application of the International Classification of Diseases to Neurology (ICD-NA;* World Health Organization 1997a)

A third category of classifications in the WHO family of classifications comprises the *related* classifications. Related classifications are those that partially refer to reference classifications or are associated with the reference classification at specific levels of structure only. Examples of related classifications of particular importance to the mental health field are

- *International Classification of Primary Care (ICPC-2;* World Organization of Family Doctors [WONCA] International Classification Committee 1998). ICPC-2 classifies patient data and clinical activity in the domains of general/family practice and primary care. It allows classification of the patient's reason for an encounter, the problems/diagnosis managed, interventions, and the ordering of these data in an episode-of-care structure.
- *International Classification of External Causes of Injury (ICECI;* World Health Organization Working Group on Injury Surveillance Methods 2000). The purpose of ICECI is to enable classifying external causes of injuries. It is designed to help researchers and prevention practitioners to describe, measure, and monitor the occurrence of injuries and to investigate their circumstances of occurrence using an internally agreed-upon classification.
- *Assistive Products for Persons With Disability: Classification and Terminology* (International Organization for Standardization 2007). The international standard establishes a classification of assistive products for persons with disabilities. It is restricted to assistive products intended mainly for the use of an individual.

UNITED NATIONS CLASSIFICATIONS

The United Nations (UN) Statistical Commission maintains a registry of classifications of direct relevance to health and mental health or, more specifically, to MHISs, *The International Family of Economic and Social Classifications.* This family comprises *reference* classifications that have been registered into the UN Inventory of Classifications and reviewed and approved as guidelines by the UN Statistical Commission—or other competent intergovernmental board—on matters such as economics, demographics, labor, health, education, social welfare, geography, environment, and tourism. It also includes those classifications on similar subjects that are registered into the inventory and are *derived from,* or *related to,* the reference classifications. The family of UN classifications is primarily, but not solely, used for regional or national purposes (United Nations Statistical Commission 1999).

The following examples are taken from the classifications registry and have been selected to illustrate their relevance for MHISs:

- *International Standard Industrial Classification of All Economic Activities, Revision 4* (United Nations Statistics Division 2006). Wide use has been made of this classification in organizing data according to kind of economic activity. It may be used to code a patient's occupation and provides guidance for classifying human health and social work activities, such as hospital activities, medical practice activities, and other human-health activities. The latter includes activities of nurses, midwives, physiotherapists, or other paramedical practitioners in the field of optometry, hydrotherapy, medical massage, occupational therapy, speech therapy, chiropody, homeopathy, chiropractic, acupuncture, and others.

- *Central Product Classification, Version 1.1* (United Nations Statistics Division 2002). This constitutes a comprehensive classification of all goods and services—including health and social services, such as hospital services—as well as services provided by medical laboratories (e.g., diagnostic imaging services).
- *International Classification of Status in Employment* (United Nations Statistics Division 1993). An important objective of this classification is to serve as model for the development of national standard classifications of status in employment.
- *International Standard Classification of Occupations* (United Nations Statistics Division 1988). This classification facilitates international communication about the types of work carried out by persons in different jobs, including both individual jobs and statistics on jobs, their pay, and so forth, and serves as a model for the development of national standard classifications of occupations.
- *International Standard Classification of Education 1997* (United Nations Statistics Division 1997). This classification is designed to serve as an instrument suitable for assembling, compiling, and presenting comparable indicators and statistics of education, both within individual countries and internationally.
- *International Classification of Activities for Time-Use Statistics* (United Nations Statistics Division 2009). This classification deals with assessment of the time people spend on various activities. This is quite important not only in regard to patients with psychiatric problems but also for members of a patient's family or other caregivers. It provides a tool for classifying such time-use activities. Examples for categories of direct relevance to the mental health fields include work in "formal sector" employment; work for household in primary production activities (such as farming of animals, collecting water); and core activities, such as time spent in socializing and community participation, providing unpaid caregiving services to household members, providing community services and help to other households, and in personal care and maintenance.
- *Classification of the Functions of Government* (United Nations Statistics Division 1999). Coding information on government activities is particularly important for mental health policy and program management. Data items for this classification include provision of pharmaceutical products, other medical products, and therapeutic appliances and equipment; administration and operation of government agencies engaged in applied research and experimental development related to health; and provision of grants, loans, and subsidies by nongovernment bodies to support applied research and experimental development related to health, such as research institutes and universities.

It is likely that data of the kind described in the first five of these classifications are to be recorded in most MHISs, regardless of their ultimate use. For example, knowledge about a patient's education, occupation, status of employment, or economic activities may be as important as knowledge about the activities and services of the health and social services and their personnel. Although not all such information may be needed in each particular MHIS, subsets are typically recorded in MHISs used for patient or service management, administration, or research. The usefulness of international classifications increases with the need of sharing information with others, whether at local, regional, or global level. There may be little need, if any, to use international classifications for recording patient data in an isolated (geographically and functionally) specialized mental hospital with only one or two psychiatrists. On the other hand, even highly specialized mental health research may benefit from the use of international classifications, if the research is to be published and thus compared internationally. Furthermore, data validity and reliability are likely to increase if internationally accepted classifications are applied, because such classifications are developed with the involvement of many experts and according to established methodological procedures (such as extended feasibility testing).

OTHER CLASSIFICATIONS OF INTERNATIONAL USE

Other classifications and nomenclatures of wide international distribution and acceptance bear directly on mental health and MHISs. Just three of those should be mentioned here.

The most important one in the mental health field is DSM-IV (American Psychiatric Association 1994). It lists different categories of mental disorder and the criteria for diagnosing them according to the publishing organization, the American Psychiatric Association. Like ICD, DSM-IV is used worldwide by clinicians and researchers as well as insurance companies, pharmaceutical companies, and policymakers.

The *International Classification of Nursing Practices* is maintained by the International Council of Nurses (www.icn.ch/publications/international-classification-for-nursing-practice/classification-of-nursing-practice.html). The classification allows description of patient phenomena of concern to nurses and the nurse-specific interventions, with their attendant patient outcomes. More specifically, a shared terminology is used to express the elements of nursing practice (what nurses do, relative to certain human needs or patient conditions, to produce certain outcomes) and allows description of nursing practice in such a way as to be able to compare practice across clinical settings, patient populations, geographic areas, or time. The shared terminology also identifies the particular contribution of the nurse to the multidisciplinary health care team and differentiates the practices of expert professional nurses and other health care providers.

The *Systematized Nomenclature of Medicine* is maintained by the International Health Terminology Standards Development Organization (www.ihtsdo.org). It is a dynamic, clinical health care terminology and infrastructure developed to make health care knowledge more usable and accessible. It provides a common language that enables a consistent way of capturing, sharing, and aggregating health data across specialties—including psychiatry—and sites of care. Particular benefits of recording information in a standard terminology are linked to the use of the electronic care record (see section "Electronic Health Records for Mental Health" later in this chapter).

There are many classifications of regional importance or of use in particular countries or language groups. For illustrative purposes, the *Chinese Classification of Mental Disorders* (CCMD), published by the Chinese Society of Psychiatry, should be mentioned. It is a clinical guide used in the People's Republic of China for diagnosis of mental disorders. It is currently on a third version, the CCMD-3, written in Chinese and English. It is intentionally similar in structure and categorization to ICD and DSM, although it includes some variations on their main diagnoses and around 40 culturally related diagnoses (Lee 2001).

In Latin America, two adaptations of the international psychiatric classification have emerged: the *Cuban Glossary of Psychiatry* and the project of the *Latin American Guide for Psychiatric Diagnosis.* Keeping ICD-10 as the basis for nosological organization, the latter is being developed with contributions by mental health professionals from Latin American countries (Berganza et al. 2002).

The *French Classification of Child and Adolescent Mental Disorders* has been used since 1983. It is the classification of reference for French child psychiatrists (Mises et al. 2002).

Table 7–2 provides a summary of the classifications of mental health importance referred to in the previous paragraphs.

Compatibility of Classifications

With the advancement of knowledge, with changing needs, and for many other reasons, any classification will need to be updated from time to time or may need substantial revision. For example, the ICD has undergone nine revisions since publication of ICD-1 in 1900, at intervals shown in Figure 7–1 (Üstün 2005).

Any change in reporting into an MHIS raises a question of compatibility between the old and the new classifications. As discussed earlier, MHISs may provide information for important and far-reaching decisions on heath policy and programs. Incompatibility of different versions of a diagnostic classification—that is, *vertical incompatibility*—may jeopardize the very basis for evidence-based decision making.

Incompatibility of different classifications of the same phenomena, such as diagnosis—*horizontal incompatibility*—may also cause problems in comparing and interpreting information. For example, ICD and DSM are different diagnostic classifications that are both suitable for classifying mental disorders. Some countries use

TABLE 7–2.   Selected international classifications of importance in the mental health field

Steward	Classification	Abbreviation
Family of WHO classifications	International Classification of Diseases	ICD
	The ICD-10 Classification of Mental and Behavioural Disorders: Clinical Descriptions and Diagnostic Guidelines	—
	The ICD-10 Classification of Mental and Behavioural Disorders: Diagnostic Criteria for Research	—
	Application of the International Classification of Diseases to Neurology	ICD-NA
	International Classification of Functioning, Disability and Health	ICF
	International Classification of Health Interventions	ICHI
	International Classification of Primary Care	ICPC
	International Classification of External Causes of Injury	ICECI
	Assistive Products for Persons With Disabilities: Classification and Terminology	ISO/DIS 9999
Family of UN classifications	International Standard Industrial Classification of All Economic Activities	ISIC
	Central Product Classification	CPC
	International Classification of Status in Employment	ICSE
	International Standard Classification of Occupations	ISCO
	International Standard Classification of Education	ISCED
	International Classification of Activities for Time-Use Statistics	ICATUS
	Classification of the Functions of Government	COFOG

TABLE 7–2. Selected international classifications of importance in the mental health field *(continued)*

Steward	Classification	Abbreviation
Other classifications of international use	*Diagnostic and Statistical Manual of Mental Disorders*	DSM
	International Classification of Nursing Practices	ICNP
	The Systematized Nomenclature of Medicine	SNOMED
	Chinese Classification of Mental Disorders	CCMD
	Cuban Glossary of Psychiatry	GC
	Latin American Guide for Psychiatric Diagnosis	GLADP
	French Classification of Child and Adolescent Mental Disorders	CFTMEA

Note. UN = United Nations; WHO = World Health Organization.

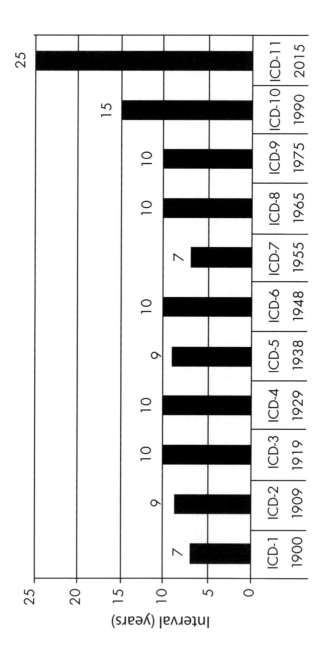

FIGURE 7–1. Revisions of the *International Classification of Diseases.*

ICD, others DSM. However, ICD and DSM may even be used at the same time in the same country but for different purposes. A survey on ICD-10 and related systems in 205 psychiatrists from 66 different countries found that ICD-10 was more frequently used, and preferred, for clinical diagnosis and training, whereas DSM-IV was considered more appropriate for research (Mezzich 2002; Nakane and Nakane 2002). This difference will be reflected in the information systems. Therefore, great care is indicated when data originating from such information systems are being compared or even merged.

Compatibility is also an issue for classifications with partially overlapping themes, such as ICD, ICF, ICHI, and ICPC-2.

COMPATIBILITY BETWEEN DIFFERENT VERSIONS OF THE SAME CLASSIFICATION

Different versions of the ICD may illustrate the problems of vertical compatibility. The time between official releases of two successive versions of ICD has been approximately 10 years in the past and will be more than 20 years in the future. Furthermore, countries may decide to skip a particular version of ICD; for example, they might switch from ICD-8 to ICD-10 without ever using ICD-9. Many of the differences between the old and new versions of ICD have been substantial and conceptual in nature. For example, the number of three-digit categories given to mental disorders doubled from 30 in ICD-6 (1948 revision) to 60 in ICD-10 (1989 revision).

In order to achieve compatibility of longitudinal data based on two different revisions of ICD, it is essential to agree on clearly defined rules of transformation from old to new categories, and vice versa. Methodologically, this does not cause problems for conditions that appear in both classifications and are identically defined, regardless of whether they have the same or a different code. Neither does the addition of new categories present any particular difficulty. Of course, such changes will require some training of staff involved. When data are processed automatically, appropriate computer programs can be written to deal with the transition to the new revision.

The situation is more difficult in cases of reassignments of rubrics and inclusion terms. There may be conditions that have been collapsed into a single category in the old version but recorded under separate codes in the new version. Other conditions have a single code in the new version but were classified under different codes in the previous version. This means that no general transformation rule can be given on how to convert numbers of cases or rates for conditions classified under one rubric in one revision into numbers or rates for conditions classified under several rubrics in another revision of ICD. The only method for maintaining the comparability of data recorded by different revisions of the ICD may be to code the conditions according to both revisions for a certain period of time (e.g., 6–12 months).

In this way, baseline figures can be established that indicate the proportions of cases of the single category of one ICD revision to be placed in several categories of the other ICD revision. When necessary, such baseline figures will have to be computed for individual facilities, because they depend on diagnostic patterns that may vary not only between countries but also among areas and individual facilities within countries (Kramer et al. 1979).

An example may illustrate the issue: Kessing (1998) presented the diagnostic concordance between ICD-8 diagnoses given in 1993 and ICD-10 diagnoses given in 1994 to the same patients admitted in both years, according to the Danish register of psychiatric admissions. In total, 1,487 patients received an ICD-8 diagnosis of manic-depressive psychoses in 1993 and were readmitted in 1994. The majority of patients (84.0%) with a manic-depressive diagnosis according to ICD-8 received a diagnosis of affective disorder according to ICD-10. Patients with a diagnosis of affective disorder according to ICD-10 had previously been diagnosed as having manic-depressive (69.6%), psychogenic psychoses (8.7%), personality disorders (5.5%), or neurosis (3.2%) according to ICD-8. The ICD-10 concept of affective disorder thus appeared broader and more comprehensive compared with ICD-8.

Other methodologically more sophisticated methods, such as interactive conversion from ICD-9 to ICD-10, have also been suggested (Schulz et al. 1998).

COMPATIBILITY BETWEEN DIFFERENT CLASSIFICATIONS WITH OVERLAPPING COVERAGE

The concept of the "Family of International Classifications" has been created to have a common framework and language to report, compile, use, and compare health information at the national and international level (Madden et al. 2007). The family brings together different health classifications dealing with various dimensions of health and health care, so as to present a more comprehensive picture of health care. It covers the areas of death and disease, disability, and health interventions. Other members cover fields such as drugs, causes of injury, and reasons for encounter. These classifications represent the building blocks of health information required in order to be able to provide the best possible health to all people.

WHO's core classifications are the ICD (World Health Organization 2007b); ICF (World Health Organization 2001a); and ICHI (World Health Organization 2007a). Historically, these classifications were developed at different points in time, by different expert groups ("stewards"), and with limited cross-fertilization.

For example, the introductions to the 2004 edition of ICD-10 and the ICF both explicitly recognize ICD and ICF as members of the WHO Family of International Classifications (WHO-FIC). However, ICD-10 was finalized before the ICF development process got under way, so there has been no opportunity as yet to consider the implications of the ICF for the ICD.

The concepts of disease, health, disability, functioning, and interventions are intrinsically linked to one another as well as to outcome. Clinical treatment, health systems, and research all increasingly require that pertinent classifications be far more integrated than they are presently.

It is to be expected that all those dimensions of health will be routinely recorded in MHISs. Consequently, they should be covered by the same common language and by classifications that are compatible.

Madden et al. (2007) compared ICD-10 and ICF and pointed to a few inconsistencies. Dementia may serve as an example. In ICD, *dementia* is described as a "disturbance of functions," such as memory, thinking, orientation, comprehension, calculation, learning capacity, judgment, consciousness, emotion (emotional control), social behavior, and motivation. Various qualifiers, such as disturbance, deterioration, and clouded, are used. Most, but not all, of these terms also appear in Chapter 1 of the ICF. Furthermore, ICF includes additional domains, such as temperament and personality, energy and drive functions, attention, psychomotor, perceptual, and higher-level cognitive functions. It seems that such discrepancies are not determined by the nature of the syndrome or the disability but are rather arbitrary. Madden et al. concluded that there should be an explicit decision about the ICF domains to be included in the definition of the syndrome. In addition, the ICD user should be referred to the ICF for more information on the various functioning domains.

Other examples of compatibility problems have been observed in relation to body functions and pain. Compatibility problems pertaining to international classifications developed and maintained by different UN organizations are not discussed here. However, the situation is considerably more complex.

Time Lag Between Revision and Use of Revised Classifications

The release of a new or revised classification does not coincide with the time of its implementation at country level; the time lag between release and use may be considerable. As mentioned earlier, countries may even decide to skip a particular revision. ICD-10 was officially released by WHO for use in member countries in 1989. Although the number of countries reporting data by ICD-10 codes has been increasing steadily (Figure 7–2), some countries still use ICD-9 codes, and some use both ICD-9 and ICD-10. According to WHO, among countries reporting ICD in information gathering systems, 86% used ICD-10, but 14% still used ICD-9 (World Health Organization 2005).

There are various obstacles in the transition from ICD-9 to ICD-10. For example, an alphanumeric coding scheme is used in ICD-10, based on codes with a single letter followed by two numbers (A00–Z99), whereas numeric codes are used

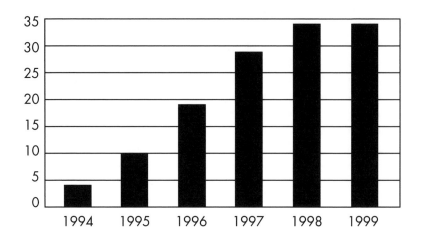

FIGURE 7–2.   Number of countries reporting data by ICD-10 codes.

Note.   There are 47 countries listed on the World Health Organization Web site (http://www.who.int/classifications/icd/).

in ICD-9 (001–999). The number of codes available for classification is significantly increased in ICD-10. There are conceptual changes as well. All this implies that personnel need to be trained in use of the new version of ICD. As a consequence, costs entailed in the transition may be considerable.

Implementation of ICD-10 for coding morbidity is slower than that for mortality. The coding system for morbidity is often related to reimbursement, and it makes the conversion more complicated due to a magnitude of the effect in different stakeholders.

In Australia, the Epidemiology and Surveillance Branch of the New South Wales Department of Health maintained a collection of databases called *Health Outcomes and Information Statistical Toolkit* (HOIST). Many of the datasets in the HOIST used ICD-9 in 2001, because "there is a time lag between the introduction of a new revision and the release of data collections that use the new standard" (Muscatello and Travis 2001, p. 289). The Australian Bureau of Statistics has used ICD-10 to code causes of death in the bureau's mortality data collection since 1997. Interestingly, causes of death were coded using both ICD-9 and ICD-10 for deaths registered in 1997 and 1998 (Muscatello and Travis 2001).

In the United Kingdom of Great Britain and Northern Ireland, ICD-10 codes are mandatory for use across its national health system. In contrast, since 1999 the United States has used ICD-10 for mortality reporting but not for morbidity. ICD-9 Clinical Modification (ICD-9-CM) codes are being applied for purposes of reimbursement on individual inpatient cases. The transition process is still being debated, but modification of ICD-10 will eventually be applied according to the recommendations of the American Health Information Management Association.

Although developing countries recognize the importance of international data comparability, a lack of manpower and resources causes delays of updating health information systems (Fekadu 1999). Such countries need simpler diagnostic systems that are easy to use and have clear relevance to practice (Murthy 2004). This issue is discussed in more detail later in the next section.

Many internal and external problems emerge from the time lag in implementing a new version. For example, using outdated terminology and classification may entail difficulties in meeting data standards for quality assurance, reimbursement, and administration, in view of the fact that coding systems are fundamental for medical recording. Using ICD-10 for mortality and ICD-9 for morbidity is likely to cause confusion when comparing data within the country over time. At the international level, countries using data that are incompatible with the rest of the world will fall behind and may not be eligible for international collaboration. International data incompatibility may result in information systems of limited utility in clinical care, research, and training.

Classifications for Use at Different Levels of the Health Services

Most patients with mental disorders are treated by health professionals at primary- or general-care level. This is true not only in developing countries but also in the industrialized world (Goldberg and Huxley 1992; Regier et al. 1993). The Republic of Kenya may serve as an example for the situation in many developing countries: Prevalence of mental health problems has been shown to be in the region of 25%–30% at the primary health care level and in most general outpatient clinics in all hospitals (Ndetei and Muhangi 1979). For inpatients in general hospitals, the prevalence of mental health disorders is even higher, up to 50% in a recent survey in Kenya (Ndetei et al. 2006). This high prevalence is found in adults, children, and adolescents attending these facilities. In all these situations, the conditions go unnoticed. For example, in a recent survey at Kenyatta National Hospital, fewer than 5% of patients had been suspected by nonpsychiatrist clinicians to have a mental disorder, whereas diagnostic tests were able to detect a prevalence of nearly 50%.

There is a dearth of mental health personnel across Africa, a situation likely to persist for many years to come. The ratio of psychiatrists to population in 10 countries in Sub-Saharan Africa varies from 1:500,000 in Kenya and 1:1,600,000 in the Federal Republic of Nigeria to 1:9,600,000 in the Rwandese Republic (Ndetei et al. 2007). Even in countries with more favorable psychiatrist-to-population ratios, ratios vary greatly from urban to rural areas. The ratio has hardly changed in the past 10 years and in some cases is getting worse with time because of migration. Therefore, for a long time to come, the care of mentally ill patients in Africa will have to be delegated to general doctors and nurses, social workers, and counseling and clinical psychologists.

In such situations, the problem is not so much how to best choose a diagnostic code; the problem is to recognize a mental condition and how to deal with it. Lack of manpower in low-resource settings, resulting in work overload, is a main reason for a rather restricted use of classification systems, often limited only to tertiary-care settings. Although there is general agreement that adequate planning is impossible without appropriate information systems in primary care, the reason usually given for the lack of such data and information systems is that there is no time to treat thousands of patients and keep accurate data at the same time (Jenkins et al. 2002).

In response to such restrictions, special classifications were developed for use at the primary health care level. The ICD-10 Primary Health Care version (ICD-10-PHC; World Health Organization 1996) is a very simplified system that is considered suitable for primary care personnel. Its 20 categories look simple compared with the full classification. However, experience in developing countries has shown that even this system of classification is difficult to use. Therefore, for multipurpose workers, an even simpler version is available that consists of only six categories: cognitive disorders, alcohol and drug use disorder, psychotic disorders, depression, anxiety disorders, and unexplained somatic complaints.

The classification corresponds to ICD-10 categories. It is linked to the different types of management, including drug treatment, that the various conditions require. It also provides information about each disorder that should be given to a patient and family, and it points to situations that require specialist referral. However, only diagnostic categories are entered into health information systems used at primary health care level. Conceptual linkage of the diagnostic categories to patient management—including treatment, family involvement, or referral—is not translated into coding instructions. Other key tasks inherently need to be linked to a classification of mental disorders and need to be recorded: disability is an important predictor of health and social service use, and mental health outcomes should be linked to broad categories of disorder.

Jenkins et al. (2002) insisted that for a classification and information system to become meaningful for the daily work of a primary health care worker, it has to be simple and address issues beyond diagnosis, such as severity and chronicity, disability assessment, training, and the supply of essential medication.

However, there is still a long way to go. One reason for this is that mental health categories need to be integrated into health information systems for primary health care. Because of competing demands on the general information system, only a small number (usually four to six) of psychiatric items can be accommodated (Murthy and Wig 2002). Nevertheless, one would not have to start from scratch, given the work that has been accomplished by the international family of classifications referred to earlier. It may thus be indicated that mental health research on classifications at the primary health care level should broaden its scope beyond diagnosis and include, more vigorously than in the past, disability, procedures, interventions, outcome, and so on.

The need for classifications for use in the mental health field at the primary health care level is not limited to low-resource settings. In industrialized countries, the move to primary care is a way of extending the reach of mental health services, whereas in developing countries it is the primary and often the only method of providing mental health care. Primary care workers in industrialized countries, very often general practitioners and family doctors, are quite sophisticated in regard to both training and the use of technical equipment. Although the ICD-10-PHC is the most widely used system in primary care settings around the world, it is not the only one. Three classification systems are available for primary care workers to diagnose, label, and classify mental disorders: the ICD-10-PHC, the primary care version of DSM-IV (American Psychiatric Association 1995), and ICPC-2. Although it is unlikely that a particular family physician will use the three systems simultaneously, it may still be important to pool diagnostic data from various sources and thus assess the comparability of the diagnostic categories emanating from the different systems. It has been shown that, for common mental disorders, it is possible to choose codes from one system while maintaining compatibility with the other two. Comparability as to the diagnostic content of the different classes, however, is more difficult to establish. The different classification systems give both primary care physicians and psychiatrists options to diagnose, label, and classify mental disorders from their own perspectives, but once a system has been chosen, the clinical comparability of a patient with the same diagnosis in other systems is limited. Compatibility among systems can be optimized by strictly following a number of rules (Lamberts et al. 1998). This is of particular interest for computer-based patient records in primary care. The clinical comparability of the same diagnosis in different systems, however, is limited.

Methods of Classification

Multiaxial classification is used in mental health to capture the complexity of a clinical situation and to succinctly represent several domains of information. WHO suggested using three axes in connection with ICD-10: mental and general medical disorders; disabilities; and contextual factors (World Health Organization 1997b). DSM-IV describes a five-domain multiaxial classification: Axis I (clinical disorders, other conditions that may be a focus of clinical attention); Axis II (personality disorders, mental retardation); Axis III (general medical conditions); Axis IV (psychosocial and environmental problems); and Axis V (global assessment of functioning) (American Psychiatric Association 2000).

More recently, the World Psychiatric Association section on classification developed a multiaxial schema based on the WHO-FIC. Four axes are proposed: Axis I on clinical disorders; Axis II on disabilities; Axis III on contextual factors; and Axis IV on quality of life (Kastrup 2002). Other proposals for multiaxial classification in mental health were made by WHO (for use in general health; Clare et al. 1992) and Rutter et al. (1969) (for use in child mental health). Even though the multiaxial approach has been widely taught, and surveys report on its international acceptability, daily use by clinicians of the "nondiagnostic" axes has, until now, been limited. In fact, MHISs usually use uniaxial versions of classification systems.

There are several reasons for this. The heterogeneity of information structure of the various classification systems could lend itself to variable implementation in different settings, minimizing the ability of an MHIS to aggregate or share this rich information consistently. If individual clinicians are not consistent in their use of multiaxial classification versus uniaxial classification to record diagnoses, an MHIS may not be able to capture information that is comparable. A survey study showed that psychiatrists in New Zealand, for example, made limited use of multiaxial systems (Mellsop et al. 2007). Additional complications will occur if attempts are made to translate multiaxial diagnoses to uniaxial diagnoses, or vice versa, because information may be lost or degraded in the MHIS. Incompatible or inconsistent uses of these methods of information classification may present challenges to MHISs.

Availability, Reliability, and Validity of Information

A prerequisite for an MHIS to be useful is that the data recorded must be available and valid and can be assessed reliably. It is thus important to analyze to what extent these criteria may be affected by the choice and characteristics of classification.

AVAILABILITY

One of the major advantages of information systems is making health information more readily available to those who can use it for clinical service delivery, service needs assessment, and other purposes. Service users with mental health conditions are often treated in multiple environments for the same condition, and clinical information systems can make data simultaneously available, in multiple settings, to members of the multidisciplinary treatment team, potentially reducing fragmentation.

Availability of information may be hindered when different settings that use the same MHIS use different classification systems. Mapping information from one classification to another, a complicated undertaking that may lead to inaccuracy or loss, may be required in order to aggregate or transmit effectively. A survey study of maternity data collection in England showed that several factors—such as variations in data definitions, data recording methods (e.g., paper vs. electronic), and data analysis—negatively affected the availability of this information at a national level (Kenney and Macfarlane 1999). These principles would extend to mental health information as well. Also, technical limitations in some settings may hinder availability of information to some stakeholders, particularly in "paper and pencil" information system models (World Health Organization 2005).

The increased availability of potentially sensitive and stigmatizing mental health information raises concerns about privacy and inappropriate access. These issues are discussed in a later section of this chapter, "Confidentiality of Information."

RELIABILITY

To provide information meaningful for aggregated analysis and clinical purposes, data elements, such as diagnosis and psychiatric ratings scales, need to be recorded with high reliability across settings. Several potential barriers to reliability within an MHIS exist.

Because of its narrative nature, mental health documentation is often communicated in an unstructured, "free text" form (Lewis 2002). Because of great variation in the way "free text" information is represented, it is unlikely that it will be transmitted, or aggregated, reliably beyond its origin. Classification and coding systems introduce limits to information, encouraging reliability by imposing structure and limiting a user's options. However, a classification system that allows complex combinations of terms, such as the Systemized Nomenclature of Human and Veterinary Medicine, may still introduce inconsistency, because a single concept can be validly expressed in many different ways (Lewis 2002). Reliability of diagnosis reporting may also depend on the nature of the condition. A study comparing the reliability of recording schizophrenia and major depressive disorder in clinical records (hospital and outpatient) with administrative databases used for epidemiological study showed high concordance for specific and severe diagnoses such as schizophrenia but less agreement for depressive disorder (Rawson et al. 1997).

There may be many users who report information to an MHIS (e.g., local providers, specialized clinicians, and service users), encompassing a wide range of experience and training and thus introducing the possibility of inconsistency. Variation at the local health worker's level of training may affect information reliability. A study of the record-keeping practices of health workers in Nigeria noted that factors associated with variation included availability of official data collection instruments, training history, and feedback received (Umar et al. 2003).

MHIS users may use different methods of data recording and reporting (e.g., paper-based and computerized records) that may adversely affect reliability. To illustrate, a neurology department in a Norwegian hospital that used parallel paper and electronic patient records reported that these two systems were inconsistent, with data often missing from one system or the other. Incorporating multiple methods of record keeping may decrease the reliability of the system (Mikkelsen and Aasly 2001). Agreement on comorbid diagnoses between local clinical records and a computerized MHIS also has been shown to be reduced, compared with agreement on the primary diagnosis (Robinson and Tataryn 1997; Stausberg et al. 2003). In general, the longer and more complex the problem list, the more likely that reliability will be lowered across settings.

Intra- and interrater reliabilities are factors considered in mental health assessment and rating scales. Most survey instruments, research questionnaires, and psychiatric assessment instruments have a test-retest agreement in the 80% range (Robinson and Tataryn 1997). It is to be expected that there always will be a degree of disagreement when this information is captured in an MHIS, a fact that should be considered in the analysis and use of data for clinical purposes.

VALIDITY

An MHIS will be optimally useful only if the information is valid—that is, it closely reflects the true clinical situation. The level of training of the clinician reporting information and the complexity of the clinical picture represented are among the factors that will affect information validity. Again, however, data structured according to rules of a common language may be recorded with higher validity than unstructured, free-text information.

Research on the validity of administrative registers for use in psychiatric research is sparse (Byrne et al. 2005). Validity measures vary widely and lack methodological rigor. Nevertheless, several themes regarding the validity of an MHIS can be identified. The training level of users reporting to the MHIS may vary widely, from local workers with little training to highly specialized clinicians. Training discrepancies may affect the degree of validity of information contained in an MHIS. In the United States, there is much activity around the concept of Personal Health Records, in which individuals maintain control of a personal health care record that may be accessed by clinicians or linked to an official record. Patients may be able to accurately report information, such as symptoms and simple objective parameters, but may not accurately report more complex information, including laboratory values (Tang et al. 2006). Patient-entered information may, therefore, affect negatively the validity of information contained in an MHIS.

Accuracy of information is likely to be enhanced if the purpose for which information is gathered and analyzed is clear and analyses are made readily available to the staff reporting the information (World Health Organization 2005). Conversely, an information system that is difficult to use may decrease the accuracy of information collected. A report on an early automated health information system in Papua New Guinea concluded that software design, focus on user friendliness, and hands-on training were critical aspects to successful maintenance of the information system and the accuracy of the data collected (Vickers and Vickers 1993). In another example, the quality of data collected in an electronic medical record in the Kingdom of the Netherlands was shown to improve after the software was upgraded. The completeness and accuracy of recording indications for certain medications increased markedly when the system was redesigned to make entering this information more intuitive (Hiddema-van de Wal et al. 2001). Features of computerized clinical information systems may also reduce information validity. A study of the accuracy of a computerized clinical information system in an intensive care unit in the United States noted that both human-entered and automatically generated data were prone to error, particularly when entered by overburdened clinicians. Discrepancies were observed for data elements related to time (such as length of stay), inaccuracy of medications administered, and diagnoses (Ward 2004).

Another factor that may affect information validity is the specificity allowed at the point of data collection. If limited specificity is permitted, the information collected will not accurately reflect the true situation. For example, the form used for the health management information system in the Republic of Zambia only allows for the general categorization of "mental disorder"—rather than allowing for specifying the nature of the disorder—which negatively affects the validity and utility of information collected in this system (World Health Organization 2005). If a classification system is too narrow or restrictive, it might not be able to accurately capture the full clinical picture as well as narrative text would. The clinical terms classification system, for example, restricts how terms may be combined and may force the user to choose a term that may not entirely reflect the clinical picture (Lewis 2002).

Among the mental health data elements that may be difficult to represent accurately in MHISs are "first contact" and "dropout." A study of continuity of care of psychiatric services in the Republic of Italy, which used a computerized health information system, noted that a study limitation was system inaccuracy of these elements. Service users were incorrectly recorded as dropped-out if a follow-up appointment was not properly recorded in the information system, and service users who dropped out of treatment were missed when the system did not capture an appointment that was scheduled but for which the patient did not show up. Determination of first contact was difficult because settings did not have access to each other's service utilization data (Percudani et al. 2002). These and other mental health data elements may, therefore, not be reflected accurately in MHISs.

Linking Mental Health to Other Information Systems

Integrating mental health services into general health care is an important goal in many countries. Moreover, it is widely accepted that mental health promotion—as well as prevention, treatment, and management of mental disorders—requires multisectoral and multidisciplinary involvement. It would be counterproductive to build and run MHISs in isolation. There are several ways of linking them with other information sources.

An MHIS may be integrated into the general health information system. If mental health services are fully integrated, mental health information is gathered as part of general health information. This is possible when mental health services are provided at different care levels, for example, when primary health care programs are provided at a general health center or hospital beds are available in general hospitals. Information from specialized mental health facilities can be collected separately, and subsequently integrated, or both information sources may be linked to each other. In situations in which mental health care is not integrated into general health services, special efforts have to be made and resources allocated to collect data, which, ideally, would then be integrated into, or linked to, a general health information system.

The integration of an MHIS into a health information system can support integration policies, help meet the needs of patients with comorbidity, and reduce costs, because it takes advantage of existing infrastructure in terms of manpower and equipment. It can also increase the awareness of mental health needs, such as for substance use disorders, among planners, service providers, and health system users.

On the other hand, integration can limit the amount of mental health information that can be incorporated; particularly, when a limited number of indicators have been defined for all disorders.

Parallel systems may be needed to enable more in-depth information to be gathered. In order to avoid segregation from general health, it is crucial that compatible designs are used for all systems involved.

Drug and HIV surveillance systems are good examples of parallel systems because they typically cover all levels of health care, from the community or individual facility to the national or, indeed, global levels. Specified sources of data include health facility records, laboratory reports, case reports, and surveys, all of which are used to identify disease outbreaks, monitor trends, determine the characteristics of those affected (such as age, sex, and location), and produce mapping of disease incidence. Such surveillance systems collect more in-depth information, ideally covering all levels of the health care system, although their scope is considerably narrower than that of health information systems as a whole.

The use of computer technology facilitates widespread sharing and linkage of electronic health care data. MHISs can be linked with health and nonhealth electronic databases. Linkage studies allow investigation of risk factors for mental illnesses or investigation of the pathways of care among several sources of care. For example, important studies have been published on the increased risk of depression and anxiety in patients with stroke (Dam et al. 2007; Driessen et al. 2001) or the increased risk of cancer in patients with schizophrenia (Gulbinat et al. 1992). Other examples are mortality studies, in which MHISs are linked with "causes of death" databases (Amaddeo et al. 1995, 2007; Laursen et al. 2007), or ecological studies on the effects of deprivation or environmental factors on incidence, prevalence, and services utilization (Tello et al. 2005).

A key problem in linking data sets from different registers or, more generally, information systems is correct identification of each patient in each of the sets to be linked. This more technical problem should not be further discussed here. Crucially important for the correct interpretation of the results of these studies is that the data items, including diagnoses, but also other patient characteristics, are correctly assigned and have the same meaning. This will be facilitated if the information systems to be linked use the same classification systems for all information dimensions (e.g., clinical data, data on procedures, sociodemographic data, administrative data), which may be best achieved if internationally accepted classifications are used throughout, as much as possible. The themes of most of such international classifications are much broader than mental health. In view of their potential relevance for mental health, it is thus important that mental health expertise enters into the development of such classifications. Appropriate mechanisms to ensure that this takes place should be developed.

Electronic Health Records for Mental Health

Electronic health records (EHRs) deserve particular attention in view of the fact that the baseline information that is aggregated for a variety of public health purposes is increasingly derived from such records. Furthermore, several large-scale, nation-level initiatives are under way to expand or nationalize the use of information systems for health care, including ones in the United Kingdom (National Programme for IT, www.connectingforhealth.nhs.uk/); the Netherlands (National IT Institute for Healthcare [NICTIZ], http://www.nictiz.nl); Australia (HealthConnect, www.health.gov.au/internet/hconnect/publishing.nsf/Content/home); and the United States (National Health Information Infrastructure, Office of the National Coordinator for Health Information Technology, www.hhs.gov/healthit/). A large component of these programs is expanded use of EHRs as a tool for patient management. The usefulness of EHRs, to a very large extent, depends on availability of a common language by which the data can be represented.

The Healthcare Information and Management Systems Society (2009) defined an EHR as

> a longitudinal electronic record of patient health information generated by one or more encounters in any care delivery setting.... The EHR automates and streamlines the clinician's workflow. The EHR has the ability to generate a complete record of a clinical patient encounter—as well as supporting other care-related activities directly or indirectly via interface—including evidence-based decision support, quality management, and outcomes reporting.

Mental health documentation is often narrative in nature. Narrative text is less computer readable than structured data such as laboratory test results. Therefore, there has been less focus on the use of information technology in mental health than in other disciplines of health care. Nevertheless, there are several documented examples of successful use of information technology for patient management in mental health. Young et al. (2004) described use of the Medical Informatics Network Tool, a software system used in the U.S. Department of Veterans Affairs, with patients with schizophrenia. Clinicians were provided with clinical reminders and links to guidelines at the point of care and used the system for electronic messaging between members of the clinical team. Use of this system led to identification of previously unrecognized trends, such as a high prevalence of obesity within the patient population, and to actions taken to improve quality, such as modifications in prescribing practices and an increase in the offering of family intervention. Modai et al. (2002) described the implementation of an electronic patient record in an inpatient hospital in the State of Israel and reported improvements in the quality of care, such as rapid adjustments in medications made in response to automated alerts triggered by blood lithium–concentration results.

Specific benefits have been attributed to the use of information systems for patient management. Benefits include documentation, communication, representation of clinical information, and point-of-care clinical decision support.

DOCUMENTATION AND REPRESENTATION OF CLINICAL INFORMATION

Templates and structured data can be used to encourage ordered and consistent documentation. Electronic representation of clinical information also eliminates issues of illegible handwriting.

Information systems also aid the automated generation of graphical views of clinical information (e.g., charting of medication blood concentrations or outcome measures over time).

COMMUNICATION

Mental illness is often chronic in nature, and treatment may involve many care providers in a variety of settings over time. Access to paper-based records is often limited to the individual who has physical possession of the chart, but electronic health information can often be accessed by authorized health care providers with network-enabled computers, from any location, at any time. This feature facilitates continuity (e.g., exchange of information during transitions of care) and coordination of care (e.g., general practitioners, psychiatrists, psychologists, nurses, and others caring for a patient all have concurrent access to the same information). Privacy concerns tied to greater access to clinical information are addressed in the next section.

POINT-OF-CARE CLINICAL DECISION SUPPORT

EHRs can be used to introduce point-of-care interactive alerts, reminders, and prompts to providers (e.g., medication interaction or allergy warnings, preventive care reminders, guideline-based prompts). EHRs can also provide case-specific links to relevant literature, including journal articles and practice guidelines.

Although much of the movement toward EHRs has been reported from resource-rich nations, Fraser et al. (2005) noted that, with decreasing hardware costs and increased Internet availability, developing countries are also able to implement and realize the benefits of these systems. For example, in Kenya, the Academic Model for the Prevention and Treatment of HIV Medical Record System is an electronic record used in a rural primary care health care center. This system has yielded decreased patient waiting times and has facilitated the generation of reports used for public health.

For the advantages of electronic patient management to be fully realized, clinical information must be structured so that it can be read, analyzed, and manipulated by computers. This is a challenge facing all aspects of health care, but it is particularly relevant in mental health, where there is a large role for narrative information. Even for systems that have applied a degree of structure to clinical documentation, inconsistent terminologies require mapping of concepts to allow communication with other systems, again limiting the clinical advantages introduced by information technology. Widespread use of generally accepted definitions, nomenclature, and classification of data elements commonly used in mental health could accelerate realization of the potential benefits of information systems in mental health.

Confidentiality of Information

MHISs may facilitate service needs analysis, service delivery, and quality improvement by making information available to a wider pool of stakeholders. However, the increased access to potentially stigmatizing information that is afforded by MHISs may increase the risk of loss of privacy of health care participants. This is particularly true for populations that are vulnerable as a result of particular circumstances or cognitive disability. Prisoners are considered vulnerable as a result of their circumstances, whereas children and mentally disadvantaged persons are considered vulnerable because of their youth and because of cognitive disabilities, respectively.

Trust is an essential element in the treatment of mental health conditions. Service users may withhold information if they feel it will not be kept confidential by an MHIS, which could negatively influence treatment effectiveness. Several polls in the United States have illustrated this concern: one poll found that 17% of patients withheld information from their health care providers because of worries the information might be disclosed (Harris Interactive 2007); another survey found that

13% of patients engaged in behavior to protect personal health information (e.g., asking a physician to forgo reporting a health condition or avoiding diagnostic tests because of concern about privacy of results) (California HealthCare Foundation 2005); and a third survey found that 33% of patients cited medical information being made accessible on the Internet as a primary reason for feeling less comfortable about sharing information with primary care physicians (Press release 2007). Steps must be taken to ensure that service users' information is protected and that they are made aware of all privacy protection mechanisms.

When MHISs are computerized, it is important to take steps to ensure the information is secured from risks such as theft, loss, unauthorized access, or modification (World Health Organization 2005). Protection may also be needed against inappropriate access by authorized users of the system. Identifying information should be removed when information is accessed by non–service providers (e.g., for service-needs assessment). Classification systems and standard definitions introduce structure to mental health information. This feature could be capitalized on to implement sophisticated privacy protection. Structured data can be parsed, and unique access and sharing rules can be applied to specific data elements, whereas unstructured information can be shared or withheld in its entirety. For example, clinical information systems may restrict access using a matrix of user roles and data types (Barrows and Clayton 1996). Also, patient-controlled records allow individuals to set granular access rights to specific users at the data-element level (Simons et al. 2005). Features such as these may increase trust and improve privacy protection in MHISs.

Recommendations

The Statistics and Information Systems Conference Expert Group summarized nine principal recommendations for those responsible for revising classifications of mental disorders, such as DSM-5 and ICD-11. These recommendations are listed here (numerical order does not necessarily indicate ranking in order of importance):

1. Awareness among mental health professionals of the existence of a wide range of international classifications of direct relevance for use in MHISs should be heightened, and the use of such classifications should be promoted. This applies in particular to WHO's family of classifications and WHO-FIC, for which the UN Statistical Division serves as steward.
2. Professional organizations in the mental health field should actively increase their involvement in the processes of development and revision of classifications of mental health importance, such as the families of international classifications.

3. Efforts should be intensified for improving the following:

- Compatibility of successive revisions of mental health classifications ("vertical compatibility"). For example, whenever a classification is revised, methods and instruments should be provided for translating the categories of the old version into categories of the new version, and vice versa.
- Mutual compatibility of classifications pertaining to mental health issues, such as those belonging to the WHO and UN families of international classifications ("horizontal compatibility").

4. Developers of the ICD and DSM should consider electronic applications of diagnosis and classifications and the use of computerized ontologies in health records and information systems as a part of the revision process.

5. Particular attention should be paid to the adaptability of classifications of mental health importance for use at different levels of health care and in low-resource countries or situations. Also, provisions should be taken for allowing uniaxial recording of multiaxial classifications. Corresponding research programs should be strengthened.

6. Awareness of governments, or other pertinent bodies, should be sharpened for the importance of minimizing the time lag between release and the actual use of a new version of a classification; for example, by making the new classifications available in the languages required.

7. A number of measures should be considered and aimed at further increasing the quality of data of a (mental) health information system, including

- Use of the same classification system (e.g., ICD, DSM, Chinese Classification of Mental Disorders, Latin American Guide for Psychiatric Diagnosis) should be encouraged as well as use of uniform definitions for representing and recording clinical data.
- Adoption, validation, and standardization of tests—screening, diagnostic, and psychometric—should be conducted in various social-cultural contexts in developing countries to create databases comparable across facilities, across countries, and within developed countries.
- Care should be taken to ensure that systems that incorporate multiple methods of record keeping or reporting (e.g., both paper-based and electronic) are compatible.
- Information systems must be designed to ensure they are "user friendly" and intuitive.
- The source of information must be taken into account when assessing validity and reliability (e.g., service user, local provider, specialized clinician).
- Training and feedback should be provided on proper use of classifications and definitions and record keeping for MHIS users. In this context, technical support should be provided to low-resource countries.

8. MHISs should not be seen in isolation but rather as elements of a country's network of information sources. Consequently, they should be developed with due regard to the characteristics of existing systems within the health sector and sectors other than health, such as the definitions and classification systems used. Corresponding research programs should be strengthened.

9. Information must be protected to avoid inappropriate access to information that may be afforded by MHISs. It is recommended that classification systems and definitions be used to introduce data-element-level privacy protection to limit access to information to those that require it. Corresponding research programs should be strengthened.

Conclusions

The objective of a mental health information system is to serve as a tool for improving the mental health of a population and its individual members. We have shown how issues of classification and diagnosis may contribute to this objective. In this context, we have reviewed the main uses of MHISs: patient management, policy and program management, administration, and research. We have discussed the information and data typically processed in such a system and analyzed the role of a common language in facilitating communication and understanding among users.

In view of the crucial role classifications play, both in development of a common language and in recording data in (mental) health information systems, we provided an overview of the international family of classifications developed and maintained under the aegis of WHO, the UN, and professional groups. For example, WHO maintains the ICD, ICF, and ICHI as well as a number of classifications directly related to or derived from them. Examples of the UN family of international classifications include those dealing with economic activities, employment, education, and activities for time-use. Other classifications of international use include DSM, the International Classification of Nursing Practices, and the Systematized Nomenclature of Medicine.

Subsequently, we showed that the usefulness of classifications for recording data in (mental) health information systems may be hampered unless a number of precautions are taken. Those are discussed in some detail.

We emphasized that a revision of a classification should be compatible with its predecessor. It is of equal importance that different classifications that are part of the same family—for example, those that deal with health topics in a wider sense, such as diseases, disability, or medical procedures—be compatible with one another. The time lag between release of a new version of a classification and its actual use in health information systems may cause problems regarding comparability of data across countries or even across regions within countries. The utility of a classification depends to a large extent on its adaptability for use at different levels of health care and the compatibility of pertinent versions of the classification. Closely related to this issue are problems of multiaxial recording. We discussed factors that may affect the quality of data that are processed in a (mental) health information system. In particular, we analyzed how availability, validity, and reliability of data can be improved. We emphasize that although linking mental health and other information systems may be highly desirable, this may put additional constraints on the classification systems involved.

EHRs are being introduced in an increasing number of countries. Therefore, we have analyzed the roles of diagnostic and other classifications. The increased access to potentially stigmatizing information afforded by MHISs may increase a risk of loss of privacy for health care participants. This is particularly true for populations that are vulnerable because of particular circumstances (such as prisoners) or because of cognitive disability. Linked to this problem are issues of data confidentiality. We end the chapter with a list of recommendations.

References

Amaddeo F, Bisoffi G, Bonizzato P, et al: Mortality among patients with psychiatric illness: a ten-year case register study in an area with a community-based system of care. Br J Psychiatry 166:783–788, 1995

Amaddeo F, Barbui C, Perini G, et al: Avoidable mortality of psychiatric patients in an area with a community-based system of mental health care. Acta Psychiatr Scand 115:320–325, 2007

American Psychiatric Association: Diagnostic and Statistical Manual of Mental Disorders, 4th Edition. Washington, DC, American Psychiatric Association, 1994

American Psychiatric Association: Diagnostic and Statistical Manual of Mental Disorders, 4th Edition, Primary Care. Washington, DC, American Psychiatric Association, 1995

American Psychiatric Association: Diagnostic and Statistical Manual of Mental Disorders, 4th Edition, Text Revision. Washington, DC, American Psychiatric Association, 2000

Barrows RC Jr, Clayton PD: Privacy, confidentiality, and electronic medical records. J Am Med Inform Assoc 3:139–148, 1996

Berganza CE, Mezzich JE, Jorge MR: 2002 Latin American Guide for Psychiatric Diagnosis (GLDP). Psychopathology 35:185–190, 2002

Byrne N, Regan C, Howard L: Administrative registers in psychiatric research: a systematic review of validity studies. Acta Psychiatr Scand 112:409–414, 2005

California HealthCare Foundation: 2005 National Consumer Health Privacy Survey. Oakland, California HealthCare Foundation, 2005. Available at: http://www.chcf.org/topics/view.cfm?itemID=115694. Accessed November 2, 2009.

Clare A, Gulbinat WH, Sartorius N: A triaxial classification of health problems presenting in primary health care: a World Health Organization multi-centre study. Soc Psychiatry Psychiatr Epidemiol 27:108–116, 1992

Dam H, Harhoff M, Andersen PK, et al: Increased risk of treatment with antidepressants in stroke compared with other chronic illness. Int Clin Psychopharmacol 22:13–19, 2007

Drake RE, Teague GB, Gersing K: State mental health authorities and informatics. Community Ment Health J 41:365–370, 2005

Driessen G, Evers S, Verhey F, et al: Stroke and mental health care: a record linkage study. Soc Psychiatry Psychiatr Epidemiol 36:608–612, 2001

Fekadu D: Conforming to the international classification of disease: a critique on health information reporting system in Ethiopia. Ethiopian Journal of Health Development 13:28–30, 1999

Fraser HS, Biondich P, Moodley D, et al: Implementing electronic medical record systems in developing countries. Inform Prim Care 13:83–95, 2005

Goldberg D, Huxley P: Common Mental Disorders: A Bio-Social Model. London, Routledge, 1992

Gulbinat WH, Dupont A, Jablensky A, et al: Cancer incidence of schizophrenic patients: results of record linkage studies in three countries. Br J Psychiatry Suppl 18:75–85, 1992

Harris Interactive: Many U.S. Adults are satisfied with use of their personal health information. Harris Interactive, 2007. Available at: http://www.harrisinteractive.com/vault/Harris-Interactive-Poll-Research-Health-Privacy-2007-03.pdf. Accessed February 6, 2012.

Healthcare Information and Management Systems Society: Electronic Health Record (EHR). Chicago, IL, Healthcare Information and Management Systems Society, 2009. Available at: http://www.himss.org/ASP/topics_ehr.asp. Accessed November 10, 2009.

Hiddema-van de Wal A, Smith RJ, van der Werf GT, et al: Towards improvement of the accuracy and completeness of medication registration with the use of an electronic medical record (EMR). Fam Pract 18:288–291, 2001

International Organization for Standardization: Assistive Products for Persons With Disability: Classification and Terminology (ISO/DIS 9999). Geneva, International Organization for Standardization, 2007. Available at: http://www.iso.org/iso/iso_catalogue/catalogue_tc/catalogue_detail.htm?csnumber=38894. Accessed November 3, 2009.

Jenkins R, Goldberg D, Kiima D, et al: Classification in primary care: experience with current diagnostic systems. Psychopathology 35:127–131, 2002

Kastrup M: Experience with current multiaxial diagnostic systems: a critical review. Psychopathology 35:122–126, 2002

Kenney N, Macfarlane A: Identifying problems with data collection at a local level: survey of NHS maternity units in England. BMJ 319:619–622, 1999

Kessing L: A comparison of ICD-8 and ICD-10 diagnoses of affective disorder: a case register study from Denmark. Eur Psychiatry 13:342–345, 1998

Kramer M, Sartorius N, Jablensky A, et al: The ICD-9 classification of mental disorders: a review of its development and contents. Acta Psychiatr Scand 59:241–262, 1979

Lamberts H, Magruder K, Kathol RG, et al: The classification of mental disorders in primary care: a guide through a difficult terrain. Int J Psychiatry Med 28:159–176, 1998

Laursen TM, Munk-Olsen T, Nordentoft M, et al: Increased mortality among patients admitted with major psychiatric disorders: a register-based study comparing mortality in unipolar depressive disorder, bipolar affective disorder, schizoaffective disorder, and schizophrenia. J Clin Psychiatry 68:899–907, 2007

Lee S: From diversity to unity: the classification of mental disorders in 21st-century China. Psychiatr Clin North Am 24:421–431, 2001

Lewis A: Health informatics: information and communication. Advances in Psychiatric Treatment 8:165–171, 2002

Madden R, Sykes C, Üstün TB: World Health Organization Family of International Classifications: Definition, Scope and Purpose. Geneva, World Health Organization, 2007, pp 1–26. Available at: http://www.who.int/classifications/en/FamilyDocument 2007.pdf. Accessed November 5, 2009.

Mellsop G, Dutu G, Robinson G: New Zealand psychiatrists views on global features of ICD-10 and DSM-IV. Aust N Z J Psychiatry 41:157–165, 2007

Mezzich JE: International surveys on the use of ICD-10 and related diagnostic systems. Psychopathology 35:72–75, 2002

Mikkelsen G, Aasly J: Concordance of information in parallel electronic and paper based patient records. Int J Med Inform 63:123–131, 2001

Mises R, Quemada N, Botbol M, et al: French classification for child and adolescent mental disorders. Psychopathology 35:176–180, 2002

Modai I, Ritsner M, Silver H, et al: A computerized patient information system in a psychiatric hospital. Psychiatr Serv 53:476–478, 2002

Murray CJL, Lopez AD (eds): The Global Burden of Disease: A Comprehensive Assessment of Mortality and Disability From Diseases, Injuries, and Risk Factors in 1990 and Projected to 2020. Harvard School of Public Health on behalf of World Health Organization and the World Bank, Cambridge, MA, Harvard University Press, 1996

Murthy RS: Psychiatric comorbidity presents special challenges in developing countries. World Psychiatry 3:28–30, 2004

Murthy RS, Wig NN: Psychiatric diagnosis and classification in developing countries, in Psychiatric Diagnosis and Classification. Edited by Maj M, Gaebel W, Lopez-Ibor JJ. Chichester, UK, Wiley, 2002, pp 249–279

Muscatello D, Travis S: Using the International Classification of Diseases with HOIST. N S W Public Health Bull 12:289–293, 2001

Nakane Y, Nakane H: Classification systems for psychiatric diseases currently used in Japan. Psychopathology 35:191–194, 2002

Ndetei DM, Muhangi J: The prevalence and clinical presentation of psychiatric illness in a rural setting in Kenya. Br J Psychiatry 135:269–272, 1979

Ndetei DM, Ongecha FA, Mutiso V, et al: The challenges of human resources in mental health in Kenya. South African Psychiatry Review 10:33–36, 2007

Papart JP: [Milestones toward a common language in psychiatry and mental health: what a shared reflection on schizophrenia can offer]. Rev Méd Suisse Romande 124:3–9, 2004

Percudani M, Belloni G, Contini A, et al: Monitoring community psychiatric services in Italy: differences between patients who leave care and those who stay in treatment. Br J Psychiatry 180:254–259, 2002

Rawson NS, Malcolm E, D'Arcy C: Reliability of the recording of schizophrenia and depressive disorder in the Saskatchewan health care datafiles. Soc Psychiatry Psychiatr Epidemiol 32:191–199, 1997

Regier DA, Farmer ME, Rae DS, et al: One-month prevalence of mental disorders in the United States and sociodemographic characteristics: the Epidemiologic Catchment Area study. Acta Psychiatr Scand 88:35–47, 1993

Robinson JR, Tataryn DJ: Reliability of the Manitoba Mental Health Management Information System for Research. Can J Psychiatry 42:744–749, 1997

Rutter M, Lebovici S, Eisenberg L, et al: A tri-axial classification of mental disorders in childhood. J Child Psychol Psychiatry 10:41, 1969

Sartorius N: Making of a common language for psychiatry: development of the classification of mental, behavioural and developmental disorders in the 10th revision of the ICD. World Psychiatric Association Bulletin 1:3–6, 1989

Sartorius N, Shapiro R: A common language: the relevance of epidemiology for psychiatry. World Health, May 1973

Schulz S, Zaiss A, Brunner R, et al: Conversion problems concerning automated mapping from ICD-10 to ICD-9. Methods Inf Med 37:254–259, 1998

Simons WW, Mandl KD, Kohane IS: The PING personally controlled electronic medical record system: technical architecture. J Am Med Informatics Assoc 12:47–54, 2005

Stausberg J, Koch D, Ingenerf J, et al: Comparing paper-based with electronic patient records: lessons learned during a study on diagnosis and procedure codes. J Am Med Inform Assoc 10:470–477, 2003

Tang PC, Ash JS, Bates DW, et al: Personal health records: definitions, benefits, and strategies for overcoming barriers to adoption. J Am Med Inform Assoc 13:121–126, 2006

Tello JE, Jones J, Bonizzato P, et al: A census-based socio-economic status (SES) index as a tool to examine the relationship between mental health services use and deprivation. Soc Sci Med 61:2096–2105, 2005

ten Horn GHMM, Giel R, Gulbinat H, et al: Psychiatric Case Registers in Public Health: A Worldwide Inventory 1960–1985. Amsterdam, The Netherlands, Elsevier, 1986

Umar US, Olumide EA, Bawa SB: Village health workers' and traditional birth attendants' record keeping practices in two rural LGAs in Oyo State, Nigeria. Afr J Med Med Sci 32:183–192, 2003

United Nations Statistical Commission: Preamble: International Family of Economic and Social Classifications. New York, United Nations Statistics Division, 1999, pp 1–5. Available at: http://unstats.un.org/unsd/statcom/doc99/preamble.pdf. Accessed November 5, 2009.

United Nations Statistics Division: International Standard Classification of Occupations (ISCO-88), 1988. Available at: http://unstats.un.org/unsd/class/family/family2.asp?Cl=224. Accessed November 6, 2009.

United Nations Statistics Division: International Classification of Status in Employment (ICSE-93), 1993. Available at: http://unstats.un.org/unsd/class/family/family2.asp?Cl=222. Accessed November 6, 2009.

United Nations Statistics Division: International Standard Classification of Education, 1997. Available at: http://unstats.un.org/unsd/class/family/family2.asp?Cl=223. Accessed November 6, 2009.

United Nations Statistics Division: Classification of the Functions of Government (COFOG). 1999. Available at: http://unstats.un.org/unsd/class/family/family2.asp?Cl=4. Accessed November 6, 2009.

United Nations Statistics Division: Central Product Classification Version 1.1, (CPC Ver. 1.1). 2002. Available at: http://unstats.un.org/unsd/class/family/family2.asp?Cl=16. Accessed November 5, 2009.

United Nations Statistics Division: International Standard Industrial Classification of All Economic Activities, Revision 4 (ISIC Rev. 4), 2006. Available at: http://unstats.un.org/unsd/class/family/family2.asp?Cl=27. Accessed November 5, 2009.

United Nations Statistics Division: International Classification of Activities for Time-Use Statistics (ICATUS), 2009. Available at: http://unstats.un.org/unsd/cr/registry/regcst. asp?Cl=231&Lg=1. Accessed November 6, 2009

Üstün TB: WHO Family of International Classifications. Geneva, World Health Organization, 2005

Vickers P, Vickers S: Developing software in the Third World: Papua New Guinea provincial health information system. J Trop Pediatr 39:322–324, 1993

Ward NS: The accuracy of clinical information systems. J Crit Care 19:221–225, 2004

Weitzel WD, Morgan DW, Robinson JA, et al: Do psychiatrists have a common language? Int J Psychiatry Med 5:223–230, 1974

World Bank: World Development Report 1993: Investing in Health. New York, Oxford University Press, 1993

World Health Organization: The ICD-10 Classification of Mental and Behavioural Disorders: Clinical Descriptions and Diagnostic Guidelines. Geneva, World Health Organization, 1992

World Health Organization: The ICD-10 Classification of Mental and Behavioural Disorders: Diagnostic Criteria for Research. Geneva, World Health Organization, 1993

World Health Organization: Diagnostic and Management Guidelines for Mental Disorders in Primary Care: ICD-10 Chapter V Primary Care Version. Göttingen, Germany, Hogrefe, 1996

World Health Organization: Application of the International Classification of Diseases to Neurology (ICD-NA), 2nd Edition. Geneva, World Health Organization, 1997a

World Health Organization: Multiaxial Presentation of the ICD-10 for Use in Adult Psychiatry. Cambridge, UK, Cambridge University Press, 1997b

World Health Organization: International Classification of Functioning, Disability and Health (ICF). Geneva, World Health Organization, 2001a

World Health Organization: 2005 Mental Health Atlas. Geneva, World Health Organization, 2001b

World Health Organization: Mental Health Information Systems. Geneva, World Health Organization, 2005. Available at: http://www.who.int/mental_health/policy/mnh_info_sys.pdf. Accessed November 5, 2009.

World Health Organization: International Classification of Health Interventions (ICHI), Beta Version Edition. Geneva, World Health Organization, 2007a

World Health Organization: International Statistical Classification of Diseases and Related Health Problems, 10th Revision, Version for 2007. Geneva, World Health Organization, 2007b. Available at: http://apps.who.int/classifications/apps/icd/icd10online/. Accessed November 5, 2009.

World Health Organization Regional Office for the Western Pacific: Developing Health Management Information Systems: A Practical Guide for Developing Countries. Manila, The Philippines, World Health Organization, Regional Office for the Western Pacific, 2004

World Health Organization Working Group on Injury Surveillance Methods: International Classifications of External Causes of Injury (ICECI). Amsterdam, The Netherlands, Consumer Safety Institute, 2000. Available at: http://www.who.int/classifications/icd/adaptations/iceci/en/. Accessed November 5, 2009.

World Organization of Family Doctors (WONCA) International Classification Committee: International Classification of Primary Care ICPC-2, 2nd Edition. Oxford, UK, Oxford Medical Publications, 1998

Young AS, Mintz J, Cohen AN, et al: A network-based system to improve care for schizophrenia: the Medical Informatics Network Tool (MINT). J Am Med Inform Assoc 11:358–367, 2004

8

TRANSLATING PSYCHIATRIC DIAGNOSIS AND CLASSIFICATION INTO PUBLIC HEALTH USAGE

Alberto Minoletti
Margarita Alegría
Hugo Barrionuevo
Dante Grana
John P. Hirdes
Edgardo Perez
Francisco Torres-Gonzalez
Pichet Udomratn

In this chapter, we first describe the public health approach to mental disorders worldwide and summarize four World Health Organization (WHO) public health functions that can be used to reduce the burden of these disorders. We then describe successful experiences and constraints of the current psychiatric diagnosis and classification system with regard to public policy, with an emphasis on low- and middle-income (LAMI) countries. Next, we propose some qualities for the diagnostic and classification system that can help its translation into public health usage. Finally, we suggest some strategies to improve use of the current diagnostic system, from the public health point of view.

A Public Health Approach as the Most Appropriate Response for Reducing Mental Disorders Worldwide

The WHO, in its *World Health Report 2001* (World Health Organization 2001c), made a strong call for an integrated public health approach to reduce the burden of an estimated 450 million people with mental and behavioral disorders worldwide. According to this report, "given the sheer magnitude of the problem, its multifaceted aetiology, widespread stigma and discrimination, and the significant treatment gap that exists around the world, a public health approach is the most appropriate method of response" (p. 16). Some of WHO's public health recommendations were as follows:

- Formulate national policies and plans, as well as legislation, to improve the mental health of populations.
- Ensure universal access to appropriate and cost-effective services, including mental health promotion, prevention services, and primary care.
- Assess and monitor the mental health of communities, including vulnerable populations such as children, women, and the elderly.
- Promote healthy lifestyles and reduction of risk factors for mental and behavioral disorders.
- Enhance research into the causes of mental disorders, development of effective treatments, and evaluation of mental health systems.

Public health, generally speaking, refers to all organized measures—both public and private—to improve and promote health, prevent disease, prolong life, and improve welfare and quality of life among a population as a whole (Khaleghian and Das Gupta 2004; Pan American Health Organization 2002; World Health Organization Regional Office for the Western Pacific 2002; Yach 1996). Although some degree of control has been achieved over communicable diseases, much work remains to be done in mental health, from a public health perspective. Unfortunately, there is evidence that, in most countries, current public health systems and services are not able to cope with public health problems or to have strategic plans to address them in a systematized fashion.

Four WHO Public Health Functions That Can Be Used to Reduce the Burden of Mental Disorders

The WHO is encouraging states to provide more systematic and comprehensive public health actions and has developed an initiative to identify the "essential public health functions" that need to be in place in any health system (World Health

Organization Regional Office for the Western Pacific 2003). These public health functions can also be applied to the field of mental health and mental disorders. Actually, most of them can be encompassed within the recommendations given by the WHO in the *World Health Report 2001* to reduce the burden of mental disorders (World Health Organization 2001c).

According to the literature, four of these essential functions are more closely interrelated with psychiatric diagnosis and classification. First, regarding the function of "health situation monitoring and analysis," many studies have been published about the prevalence of mental disorders, and the demographic correlates and service use of persons with these disorders, in community samples (Kessler et al. 2005a; World Health Organization 2000), and some of these studies have been in LAMI countries (Canino et al. 2004; Kohn et al. 2005a; Medina-Mora et al. 2005; Negash et al. 2005; Vicente et al. 2006). Other surveys carried out in these countries have focused on the prevalence of mental disorders in primary care settings (Üstün and Sartorius 1995), the relation between poverty and prevalence of common mental disorders (Patel and Kleinman 2003; Patel et al. 1998b, 1999), and the outcome of these disorders in primary care attenders (Patel et al. 1998a).

The second function, that of "epidemiological surveillance/disease prevention and control," has been mainly applied in mental health to assess and reduce the psychological impact of natural disasters (Caldera et al. 2001; Kohn et al. 2005b; Kutcher et al. 2005) and armed conflicts, with displacement of people to other regions or countries (refugees) (de Jong et al. 2003; Loza and Hasan 2007; Mufti et al. 2007; Njenga 2007; Thapa and Hauff 2005) and torture (Thapa et al. 2003).

Less has been done regarding the third function, "development of policies and planning in public health" for improvement of mental health status and quality of life, reduction of inequalities, and reduction of the burden of mental diseases. Only a few mental health policies and plans have been developed in LAMI countries (World Health Organization 2001a, 2005a). Several of them have been based on a population's needs, determined by epidemiological studies of mental disorders (Alarcón and Aguilar-Gaxiola 2000; Gureje and Alem 2000; Minoletti and Zaccaria 2005; Udomratn 2007; World Health Organization 2005b).

Finally, the fourth function, that of "strategic management of health systems and services for population health gain," has been applied as a way to access mental health services and decrease the treatment gap for mental disorders, which have been critical issues worldwide. Many studies have been carried out on this function over the past few years (Forsell 2006; Hough et al. 2002; Issakidis and Andrews 2006; Naganuma et al. 2006; Salsberry et al. 2005; Sareen et al. 2005a), and also in LAMI countries (Chien et al. 2004; Demyttenaere et al. 2004; James et al. 2002; Saldivia et al. 2004; Vicente et al. 2005). Less research has been done about the effectiveness and cost-effectiveness of mental health interventions from a public health perspective in these countries, although some promising initiatives have been carried out (Araya et al. 2003, 2006a; Mirza et al. 2006; Shibre et al. 2002).

Adequate implementation of these public health functions in mental health requires reliable diagnostic categories that respond to specific psychosocial and pharmacological interventions (Berganza et al. 2002; Moller 2005; Regier et al. 2002). Health monitoring and epidemiological surveillance produce different estimates of prevalence and incidence of mental disorders, depending on what classification or diagnostic criteria are used (Bye and Partridge 2004; Lewczyk et al. 2003; Rocha et al. 2005). Similarly, variations in diagnostic criteria can affect the outcomes of other public health activities, such as determining what communities identify as mental health problems, understanding help-seeking behaviors, setting priorities for public mental health interventions, and formulating and evaluating mental health policies and plans.

Successful Public Health Experiences With the Current Psychiatric Diagnosis and Classification in Low- and Middle-Income Countries

Psychiatric diagnoses based on standardized criteria, such as the diagnoses defined by ICD or DSM, are useful to support public health decision making. First, the use of a universal language to classify diagnoses in a consistent, meaningful way across countries supports national and cross-national comparative research that can inform policy about prevalence and cost-effectiveness of interventions (Mojtabai and Olfson 2006; Sigman and Hassan 2006), two of the most fundamental cornerstones for setting priorities in public health. Second, ICD-10 (World Health Organization 1992) and DSM-IV (American Psychiatric Association 1994) adaptations for primary care settings, which use simplified large diagnostic categories, have been helpful in developing large-scale public health treatment programs for the most frequent mental disorders in LAMI countries.

IDENTIFICATION OF THE BURDEN OF MENTAL DISORDERS, LEADING TO AN IMPACT ON POLICY

With the advances of the ICD and DSM classifications of mental and behavioral disorders, mental disorders can be identified and diagnosed with clinical methods similar to those used for physical diseases. "Structured interview schedules, uniform definitions of symptoms and signs, and standard diagnostic criteria have now made it possible to achieve a high degree of reliability and validity in the diagnosis of mental disorders" (World Health Organization 2001c, p. 22).

The definitions of Research Diagnostic Criteria for mental disorders and the development of a common format for the diagnostic interview—both translated into several languages—have made it possible to assess the burden of mental disorders with a high degree of reliability and validity. Several community epidemiological surveys that used the Composite International Diagnostic Interview (CIDI) have been carried out in many parts of the world in the past 15 years. Although this type of study still has many limitations, these studies have consistently shown that mental disorders are highly prevalent and often associated with serious role impairment in most countries worldwide (Demyttenaere et al. 2004; World Health Organization 2000).

Both epidemiological surveys and global burden-of-disease studies based on current classifications of mental and behavioral disorders have drawn public health attention to the previously unrecognized burden of these disorders in LAMI countries. The idea that psychiatric diseases are mainly problems of industrialized and relatively richer regions of the world has been proved wrong.

In terms of years lived with disability and premature death in disability-adjusted life-years (DALYs), psychiatric and neurological conditions accounted for 10.5% of the global disease burden in the year 1990, and this figure is projected to rise to 14.7% by the year 2020 (Murray and Lopez 1997). The burden of neuropsychiatric disorders is comparatively lower in developing countries than in developed countries but still high enough to be considered a public health problem. (It is expected to increase to 13.7% of the global disease burden by the year 2020.) Among developing regions, the top leading cause of DALYs, for both sexes, in 2020, is predicted to be unipolar major depression, followed by road-traffic accidents and ischemic heart disease (Murray and Lopez 1997). The results of the 2001 Global Burden of Disease study reinforced the conclusions of the 1990 study about the growing public health importance of neuropsychiatric disorders in LAMI countries (Lopez et al. 2006).

These types of studies provided invaluable evidence to any country for advocating for mental health (Funk et al. 2005; World Health Organization 2003a), as well as for making policy decisions (World Health Organization 2005b) and planning resource allocations (World Health Organization 2003c). For example, in Australia, a high-income country, a national survey was carried out in the mid-1990s that estimated the prevalence of mental disorders and the DALYs linked to them. The findings of this survey are believed to have influenced advocacy from nongovernmental organizations, consumers, and caregivers; the implementation of the National Mental Health Strategy; allocation of funds for mental health services; and the development of mental health literacy programs from federal and state governments (Henderson 2002).

An example from a middle-income country is the process that has been taking place in Chile since 1999. That year, a book summarizing the principal studies about the prevalence and burden of mental disorders in the country was published (Minoletti and López 1999) and widely distributed, and its main data were communicated through the media. The information from this book was influential in development of a new national mental health plan; an increase in health care expenditures directed toward mental health (from 1.20% in 1999 to 3.1% in 2008); and the addition of three mental disorders (schizophrenia, depression, and alcohol and drug abuse and dependence) to the 56 health problems with legal guarantees for access, quality, care opportunity, and financial protection (Minoletti and Saxena 2006; Minoletti and Zaccaria 2005; Minoletti et al. 2009).

IDENTIFICATION OF COST-EFFECTIVE INTERVENTIONS AND PLANNING FOR MENTAL HEALTH SERVICES

The disease burden is not, in itself, sufficient as a public health mechanism for planning services and allocating resources. A more appropriate approach is to set priorities according to the amount of burden from a particular disease that can be avoided through use of evidence-based interventions and the relative cost of implementing those interventions in the target population (World Health Organization 2006b). The definitions of major diagnostic syndromes, according to ICD and DSM, that respond to specific treatment approaches in a manner similar to physical illnesses have been fundamental for carrying out this type of economic analysis in the field of mental health.

The WHO has recently developed a framework for cost-effectiveness analysis, called WHO-CHOICE (Choosing Interventions that are Cost-Effective), that provides public health specialists with a tool for comparative assessment of a wide range of potential strategies for improving mental health (World Health Organization 2006b). WHO-CHOICE has been applied to four mental disorders thus far: schizophrenia, bipolar affective disorder, major depression, and panic disorder. For each of these illnesses, key pharmacological and psychosocial treatments have been identified and reviewed using the international evidence of effectiveness of these treatments. WHO-CHOICE has been used to evaluate the cost-effectiveness of interventions in seven countries; one low-income (the Federal Republic of Nigeria), two lower-middle-income (the Democratic Socialist Republic of Sri Lanka and the Kingdom of Thailand), three upper-middle-income (the Republic of Estonia, the United Mexican States, and the Republic of Chile), and one high-income (Spain) (World Health Organization 2006b).

Completed national-level studies on schizophrenia and depression in Nigeria, Sri Lanka, and Estonia indicated that the rank order of intervention cost-effectiveness differed across countries. For example, newer antipsychotic drugs ranked worse than the older ones in Nigeria and Sri Lanka for schizophrenia, but the opposite was observed in Estonia (e.g., newer antipsychotic drugs ranked better because of a small difference in drug price but a high differential in drug adherence). Combined pharmacological-psychosocial strategies ranked better than drug treatments alone in

Estonia and Nigeria but not in Sri Lanka. In depression, treatment with tricyclic antidepressants was most cost-effective in Nigeria but not in Sri Lanka or Estonia, where the small price differences between selective serotonin reuptake inhibitors (SSRIs) and tricyclic antidepressants, and the former's superior adherence profile, made SSRIs the drug of choice (World Health Organization 2006b).

IMPROVED ACCESS TO MENTAL HEALTH SERVICES THROUGH PRIMARY CARE IN LOW- AND MIDDLE-INCOME COUNTRIES

An increasing number of countries worldwide have implemented public health policies and plans for prevention, early recognition, and treatment of mental disorders in primary care (World Health Organization 2001b). This process has been facilitated since the mid-1990s by the ICD-10 and DSM-IV adaptations for primary care, which have made it feasible for general practitioners to diagnose and treat the most frequent and simple psychiatric conditions. The introduction of mental health in primary care has also been facilitated by prevalence studies using ICD-10 and DSM-IV diagnostic categories. These studies have highlighted the public health significance of mental disorders in primary care settings and have prompted governments in some countries to invest in new human resources, mental health training, and medication to treat mental disorders in these settings.

Mental disorders are highly prevalent in persons attending primary care in LAMI countries, but estimates vary by country. Prevalence of mental disorders can fluctuate from 9.8% in the People's Republic of China (Üstün and Sartorius 1995) to 17.46% in the Republic of India (Pothen et al. 2003; Üstün and Sartorius 1995); 21.3% in Nigeria (Abiodun 1993); 38.2% in China, Province of Taiwan (Liu et al. 2002); 47%–56% in the Federative Republic of Brazil (Mari et al. 1987); and 53.5% in Chile (Üstün and Sartorius 1995).

Approximately 80% of LAMI countries in the world have implemented mental health care in primary care. For example, India and the Islamic Republic of Iran (World Health Organization 2001b), most Pacific Islands (World Health Organization and University of Auckland 2005), South Africa (Peltzer et al. 2006), and Chile (Alvarado et al. 2005), among other LAMI countries, have been able to implement successful mental health services in primary care. A lower percentage of countries have carried out treatment for persons with severe mental disorders in primary care, with greater penetration in higher-middle- and high-income countries. Yet there is still a severe gap in mental health training for primary care workers, regardless of a country's level of income (World Health Organization 2001a, 2005a).

Constraints of Current Psychiatric Diagnosis and Classification for Public Health in Low- and Middle-Income Countries

Most persons with mental disorders worldwide live in LAMI countries. For example, the total disease burden for selected major psychiatric disorders in South Asia, East Asia, the Pacific, and Sub-Saharan African regions—in terms of thousands of DALY—was found to be three or four times higher than similar disease burdens in high-income countries (408,655; 346,941; 344,754; and 149,161, respectively) (World Health Organization 2006a). However, psychiatric diagnosis and classification are created in high-income Western countries, based mainly on research carried out with persons living in cultural and social environments very different from those in LAMI countries. This raises concerns relative to the importance of separate estimates of disease burden across high-income Western countries and LAMI countries.

CURRENT PSYCHIATRIC DIAGNOSIS DOES NOT ALWAYS WORK WELL IN THE REAL WORLD OF LOW- AND MIDDLE-INCOME COUNTRIES

In LAMI countries, where a lack of psychiatrists/mental health personnel and resources is common, general practitioners (GPs) play a crucial role in detection and treatment of mental illnesses (Udomratn 2007). However, GPs in these countries have a heavy workload and are under severe time constraints. For example, in Thailand, 40% of GPs see more than 70 patients per day, and a typical visit for each patient lasts about 3–5 minutes (Lotrakul and Saipanish 2006). As a consequence, it is extremely difficult for GPs to give a specific psychiatric diagnosis to a patient within current ICD-10 or ICD-10 primary health care frameworks. They usually give a broader diagnostic term, such as anxiety disorder (or anxiety) or depressive disorder (or depression), rather than a specific disorder.

Data from LAMI countries relative to type of psychiatric disorder seem to fall into two main categories. One group of studies showed that depressive disorders were more common than anxiety disorders in India (Üstün and Sartorius 1995), Nigeria (Abiodun 1993), Brazil (Mari et al. 1987), and Malaysia (Varma and Azhar 1995). Another group showed that anxiety disorders had a higher prevalence than depressive disorders in the Republic of Colombia, the Lebanese Republic, Mexico (Demyttenaere et al. 2004), and Thailand (Lotrakul and Saipanish 2006). The reason that anxiety disorders are generally diagnosed more frequently than depressive disorders by GPs in LAMI countries may come from less awareness and knowledge of depressive disorders compared with anxiety disorders. Another possible explanation is that a condition called "mixed anxiety and depressive disorder"

(MADD) is much more common than depressive disorders at the primary care level in these countries (Udomratn and Fog 2001).

MIXED ANXIETY AND DEPRESSIVE DISORDER IS A CONCEPTUAL CHALLENGE IN LOW- AND MIDDLE-INCOME COUNTRIES

ICD-10 introduced the concept of MADD in order to provide a clinical definition for patients who present with both anxiety and depressive symptoms of only limited number and/or intensity (World Health Organization 1992). In concert with ICD-10, the appendix of DSM-IV defines MADD as a clinical syndrome characterized by the equal presence of both anxiety and depressive symptoms, neither of which reaches the diagnostic threshold of an established disorder. However, in contrast with ICD-10, DSM-IV does not classify MADD as a separate disorder but within a group for further research (American Psychiatric Association 1994).

Most of the studies about MADD focus mainly on the symptomatology of this condition, and only a few provide epidemiological data. At least two papers have examined MADD in primary care settings: one from Thailand (Silpakit 1997) using ICD-10 criteria and the other from Canada (Stein et al. 1995) using DSM-III-R (American Psychiatric Association 1987) modified criteria. These researchers found that 10.9% and 12.8% of persons studied, respectively, met criteria for MADD.

Considering the time constraints of GPs, one alternative diagnostic strategy to providing specific diagnosis in primary care would be to use a broader term such as *anxiety-depression spectrum.* Persons who are referred to mental health specialists could have a more sophisticated evaluation and receive a diagnosis according to ICD-10 or DSM-IV once they have been designated as being on that spectrum. The diagnosis could group together various disorders, such as anxiety disorder, depressive episode, recurrent depressive episode, and MADD. The idea of grouping anxiety and depression together is concordant with the American Psychiatric Association project "Refining the Research Agenda: The Future of Psychiatric Diagnosis" (American Psychiatric Association 2005). This project, which was divided into 14 sections (or work areas), combined depression and generalized anxiety disorder into one section. This approach might allow GPs in LAMI countries to be relieved of the pressure of giving a specific diagnosis and allow them a few minutes for patient education. Informing persons on the anxiety-depression spectrum why psychosocial interventions and medications could help them is crucial in these countries, where stigma and mental health illiteracy are still significant problems.

Regarding drug treatment, GPs could also be taught how to use antidepressants for persons with this condition. The common practice in primary care in many LAMI countries is to prescribe anxiolytics for any psychological problem, especially benzodiazepines. For example, 48% of persons with anxiety-depression spectrum were prescribed benzodiazepines in Chile, 33% in China, 32% in India (Üstün and Sartorius 1995), and 40.6% in Thailand (Lotrakul and Saipanish 2006).

One study from Thailand (Srisurapanont et al. 2005) showed that 45.5% of GPs stated that part of their reasons for excessive use of benzodiazepines was a lack of time, as well as a lack of knowledge and skills, which is in line with results from a study in Brazil (Üstün and Sartorius 1995). GPs could be taught to prescribe an SSRI that has wide-range efficacy in various types of anxiety disorders and depression and has better tolerability than tricyclic antidepressants (Vaswani et al. 2003). A generic SSRI such as fluoxetine could be recommended as the first line of drug treatment for depressive disorders by the guideline from the National Institute for Clinical Excellence (2004), given than these agents are as effective as TCAs and are less likely to be discontinued because of side effects. Recently, a study from India has shown that fluoxetine can be used safely, and cost effectively, in primary care settings in low-income countries (Patel et al. 2003) to treat patients with anxiety or depression.

On the other hand, financial and institutional constraints in primary health care services need to be taken into account. The service delivery system should adapt in order to maintain adequate care for the many persons with mental disorders in LAMI countries (Cohen et al. 2002). In places where there is a shortage of GPs, a structured approach that encourages an increased role for non-medical staff, patients, and family members may be more appropriate (McKenzie et al. 2004). A broader term such as anxiety-depression spectrum can facilitate participation of these human resources in the diagnostic and treatment processes of mental health problems.

Lessons from good primary care practices in developing countries might provide appropriate models to improve the treatment of anxiety-depression spectrum. For example, a study from Chile demonstrated a successful program, using multicomponent interventions, that can be carried out by GPs and nonmedical health workers. This program included group psychoeducation about depression and a structured drug treatment for persons with severe depression (Araya et al. 2003). Many instruments, such as the Center for Epidemiological Studies Depression Scale or the Mini International Neuropsychiatric Interview, which have already been translated and validated in many languages, can be used in LAMI countries and administered by well-trained nurses or other mental health workers to help busy GPs make appropriate standardized diagnoses.

IS POSTTRAUMATIC STRESS DISORDER A VALID DIAGNOSIS IN LOW- AND MIDDLE-INCOME COUNTRIES?

Damage caused by natural disasters and other circumstances with traumatic effect on large populations—such as migrations, armed conflicts, and ethnic confrontations with discriminated minorities—demands, at times, the highest concerns and suitable responses from health care systems. Whereas these disasters more commonly occur in LAMI countries, most of the studies on psychological consequences have been conducted on populations from high-income countries. The universality of the Western construct of posttraumatic stress disorder (PTSD), one of the most specific and frequent mental disorders associated with disasters, has been questioned by several investigators (Batniji et al. 2006). According to those researchers, focusing on PTSD in LAMI countries would tend to personalize social distress and isolate individuals from the political, religious, or social struggle from which the suffering and symptoms arise. Although many persons in disaster situations in these countries would experience PTSD symptoms similar to the ones reported from rich populations, their main expressed concerns are related to poverty, unemployment, political situation, and other social issues.

Studies in different LAMI countries used ICD and DSM definitions for PTSD and applied research instruments created in high-income countries have shown prevalence estimates of PTSD fluctuating between 5.8% and 80.2% in populations exposed to different types of disasters. Six months after Hurricane Mitch hit Nicaragua, 5.8% of the population was identified as having PTSD, according to the Harvard Trauma Questionnaire and a clinical interview in which DSM-IV criteria were used (Caldera et al. 2001). de Jong et al. (2003) found a prevalence of PTSD of 15.8% in a community of Eritrean refugees living in temporary shelters in the Federal Democratic Republic of Ethiopia; 17.8% in a long-term refugee population exposed to ongoing violence in West Bank and Gaza Strip; 28.4% in Cambodian communities exposed to decades of violence, including autogenocide; and 37.4% in a periurban area exposed to large massacres in the People's Democratic Republic of Algeria. A literature review about mental health of war refugees in Africa (Njenga 2007) reported prevalence rates of PTSD of 24.8% 8 years after genocide in the Rwandese Republic; 32.0% among residents of a refugee camp in the Republic of the Sudan; and as high as 80.2% among heads of household internally displaced in the Republic of Kenya. In a study that used the PTSD Checklist—Civilian version, 53.4% of a household sample of the population of the Kingdom of Nepal, which has been affected by civil war, was identified as having PTSD symptomatology (Thapa and Hauff 2005).

Results from all these epidemiological studies suggest that PTSD is highly prevalent in populations exposed to disasters in LAMI countries. However, studies that have also determined the prevalence of other mental disorders in this type of population have shown that the combined prevalence of those disorders is higher than that of PTSD. For example, de Jong et al. (2003) found in Ethiopia, Algeria, the Kingdom of Cambodia, the West Bank, and Gaza Strip a prevalence of 5.2%–22.7% for mood disorder, 9.6%–40.0% for anxiety disorder, and 1.6%–8.3% for somatoform disorders. The Nepal survey (Thapa and Hauff 2005) found, on the other hand, that 80.7% of the population had anxiety symptoms and 80.3% had depressive symptoms.

The indiscriminate transfer of the PTSD concept from Western societies to other cultures may produce an unnecessary medicalization of normal distress and discourage use of other potentially effective public health approaches (van Ommeren et al. 2005). The utility of the PTSD construct has been questioned because of the type of interventions most often used in LAMI countries for the prevention or treatment of this condition—mainly psychological interventions and benzodiazepine medication, both of which have little evidence of effectiveness and might even be harmful if used indiscriminately (van Ommeren et al. 2005). Furthermore, the WHO approach to mental health in disaster situations in recent years has not been focused on PTSD but on social interventions based on local culture, mobilization of human and community resources, intersectoral collaboration, and care of people with preexisting mental disorders (World Health Organization 2003b).

Considering all the questioning about the value and validity of the diagnosis of PTSD in LAMI countries, it would be highly desirable to carry out more cross-cultural research about this diagnostic construct in these countries before its inclusion in future formulations of the ICD and DSM classifications. The complex and varied situations associated with disasters and the importance of socioenvironmental factors (de Jong et al. 2003; Kohn et al. 2005a; Naeem et al. 2005; Thapa et al. 2003) demand the development of a different diagnostic approach for victims of disasters, one suitable for a multisystemic understanding and for early and effective social and psychological interventions.

Qualities of Psychiatric Diagnosis and Classification That Support Public Health Usage

GENERAL FEATURES OF PSYCHIATRIC CLASSIFICATION THAT HELP PUBLIC HEALTH USAGE

Public health use of psychiatric diagnosis and classification has certain special features different from those that are necessary for clinical settings. Characteristics of a diagnostic system in public health that are mentioned in the literature include the following:

- Simplicity, especially in the provision of names for mental disorders, making it accessible to the general population and thus useful as a promotion and prevention tool (Berganza et al. 2002; Mezzich 2002)
- Universality (Berganza et al. 2002; Nakane and Nakane 2002; Regier et al. 2002), with one diagnostic classification for all countries, for both research and clinical practice, that is widely accepted by mental health professionals

- Transculturality (Berganza et al. 2002; Kastrup 2002; Otero-Ojeda 2002; Regier et al. 2002), with validation studies in different social environments and in countries with different income levels
- High reliability, sensitivity, and specificity for the principal mental disorders (Berganza et al. 2002; Regier et al. 2002)
- Diagnostic categories that respond to specific psychosocial and pharmacological interventions for prevention, treatment, and rehabilitation (Berganza et al. 2002; Bye and Partridge 2004; Moller 2005; Regier et al. 2002)
- Multiple dimensionalities (Berganza et al. 2002; First 2005; Kastrup 2002; Mezzich 2002; Regier et al. 2002), such as diagnoses of disability, distress, quality of life, comorbidity, and psychosocial and environmental problems
- Feasibility for use in different contexts, including primary care settings (Kastrup 2002)

Other characteristics of diagnostic systems that should be considered in public health, although no mention was found in the references reviewed, include minimizing the potential stigma produced by psychiatric labels and freedom from conflicts of interest related to professional organizations, the pharmaceutical industry, and other institutions.

RELATION BETWEEN PSYCHIATRIC DIAGNOSTIC CLASSIFICATION AND PUBLIC HEALTH FUNCTIONS

In order to be useful for public health functions, a psychiatric diagnostic classification should help public health professionals carry out their daily activities, such as needs assessment, estimation of population prevalences and treatment gaps, priority setting, resource allocation, epidemiological surveillance, and assessment of interventions and their effectiveness. The diagnostic system should also be able to be applied in contexts as different as primary and specialized care, general and vulnerable populations, and normal life and special circumstances (e.g., natural disasters, armed conflicts). Finally, the diagnostic classification should facilitate the elaboration of diagnostic tools that can help identify persons with the highest needs for mental health services to orient the population to help-seeking behaviors. Figure 8–1 illustrates the relation between psychiatric diagnosis and public health activities, contexts, tools, and help-seeking determinants.

Psychiatric Diagnosis and Estimation of Population Prevalences and Treatment Gaps

In public health, it is important to know both the global magnitude of mental illness and the specific magnitudes of certain types of disorders, as well as to obtain information about the distribution and severity of these disorders and their sensitivity to available interventions. All of this information is needed for developing mental health policies, planning interventions for reducing the social effects of mental disorders, prioritizing resources, and monitoring public health policies and plans. Tools derived from psychiatric classification systems have been applied to distinguish people having some mental disorders from those that do not (Bott et al. 2005; Coid et al. 2006; Fournier et al. 1997; Goldney et al. 2004; Grant et al. 2004; Hasin et al. 2005; Hunt et al. 2002; Jacobi et al. 2002; Kessler et al. 1994, 2005a, 2005b; Lepine et al. 2005; Mackinnon et al. 2004; Mathet et al. 2003; Moreno and Andrade 2005; Ohayon et al. 1999; Vicente et al. 2006). Most of these studies have been carried out in high-income countries. LAMI countries in which such studies have been performed include Brazil (Sao Paulo; Moreno and Andrade 2005), Chile (Vicente et al. 2006), Mexico (Medina-Mora et al. 2005), and Puerto Rico (Canino et al. 2004).

Prevalence surveys based on psychiatric classification systems can also contribute to the identification of risk factors associated with certain disorders (Bott et al. 2005; Coid et al. 2006; Hasin et al. 2005; Kessler et al. 2005a; Mathet et al. 2003; McAlpine and Mechanic 2000). This makes it possible to implement preventive and early treatment actions addressing the highest-risk groups (e.g., high-risk prodromal cases with early psychotic symptoms).

One of the findings derived from household prevalence surveys is that many individuals with a psychiatric diagnosis do not actually use mental health services and that a portion of the population that has consulted a physician do not meet the criteria for a psychiatric disorder (Canino et al. 2004; Demyttenaere et al. 2004; Kohn et al. 2005a; Medina-Mora et al. 2005; Vega et al. 1999).

The first hypothesis that has been formulated to explain this finding is that this treatment gap can be the result of an accessibility problem; hence, some studies have addressed conditions probably associated with access (e.g., income level, urban-rural condition, minorities, gender, service coverage). Second, hypotheses have looked into needs perception and subsequent help-seeking behaviors (Aoun et al. 2004; Sareen et al. 2005c; Wang et al. 2004; Zimmerman 2005). Other studies have attempted a third potential explanation for the treatment gap, focusing on the classification system capabilities for detection and its derivative tools (Aoun et al. 2004; Brugha et al. 2001; Erkinjuntti et al. 1997; Moreno and Andrade 2005; O'Connor 2006; Pioggiosi et al. 2004; Poulin et al. 2005; Vilalta-Franch et al. 2006). Finally, other hypotheses point to the delay in seeking help, showing that there is a significant period of time—more than 10 years on average—between onset of the illness and help seeking, which would account for cases with a positive diagnosis but no seeking of mental health services (Wang et al. 2004).

The fact is that when it comes to determining help-seeking behaviors, prevalence surveys based on the available classification systems are still insufficient to predict accurately how many people, and with what type of disorders, are going to demand mental health services. Nonetheless, inferences should be made with caution, because research in this field has been scarce, especially in LAMI countries.

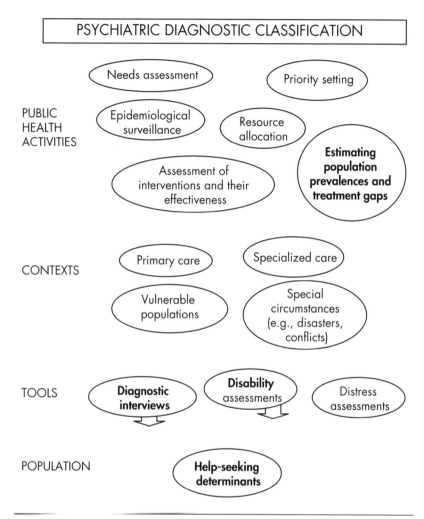

FIGURE 8–1. Relation between psychiatric diagnostic classification and public health functions.

Public health functions: 1) health situation monitoring and analysis; 2) epidemiological surveillance/disease prevention and control; 3) development of policies and planning in public health; 4) strategic management of health systems and services for population health.

Psychiatric Diagnosis and Priority Setting

Among public health activities, priority setting is one of the most essential for developing policies, planning interventions, and managing mental health systems and services. The number of individuals affected by mental disorders is not the only piece of information necessary to carry out this activity; different and more complex variables also need to be considered, including

- *Numbers of people with mental disorders.* It is obvious that the diagnostic classification systems should enable determination through prevalence surveys of the magnitude of the populations affected by these disorders.
- *Disability and distress.* Certain studies have set aside diagnostic classifications to focus on damage caused by the mental illness. In this respect, scales for measuring disability and distress due to mental disorders would seem more appropriate than symptoms interviews (Henderson et al. 2001; Kessler et al. 2002, 2003b; Poulin et al. 2005). These studies have shown that, in many cases, the disability or distress is not related only to a syndrome meeting the diagnostic criteria for a disorder in the ICD or DSM systems but that subthreshold cases also show considerable disability and distress. Data collected by using these scales may be more related to the real needs for mental health care, as is discussed in more detail in the next section, "Psychiatric Diagnosis and Needs Assessment."
- *Availability of effective interventions.* An important issue for public health is that psychiatric diagnosis be defined in terms of the availability of effective interventions to treat that particular condition. This subject was not considered sufficiently when the current diagnostic classification systems were created. Nevertheless, this criterion has been gradually adopted, with some of the modifications introduced to psychiatric diagnosis, in relation to the development of new, effective treatments.

Psychiatric Diagnosis and Needs Assessment

Public health and mental health care have shifted focus from an individual patient to the population, with a growing emphasis on community-based prevention and intervention at the public health level. In this changing environment, one of the objectives of public health is to provide estimates of the numbers of people who need mental health and substance abuse services. From this perspective, a psychiatric classification system should be able to contribute to

1. Evaluation of changes in the population, according to level of need.
2. Assessment of need estimates, by region, to help policy makers allocate available resources more efficiently.
3. Monitoring of the impact of services as an outcome measure, because this reflects the overall mental health status of the population.
4. Provision of useful information for service planning.

Traditionally, the definition of need for mental health services that is used most frequently to set policy and determine estimates for resource allocation has been constrained to one based on disease severity and functional impairment as measured by diagnostic criteria. For example, a 2002 report prepared by the Substance Abuse and Mental Health Services Administration (Epstein et al. 2004) stated that persons who are in need of treatment are defined as having at some time, in the past year, a diagnosable mental, behavioral, or emotional disorder that met criteria specified in DSM-IV (American Psychiatric Association 1994), resulting in a functional impairment that substantially interfered with, or limited, one or more major activities. The definition of need adopted by the U.S. Department of Health and Human Services (2001) is equated with prevalence of a psychiatric disorder. The appeal of using psychiatric diagnoses to define people in need of service is in the clarity of the criteria and the ability to use the information to compare prevalence uniformly across communities. Furthermore, the diagnoses capture the most severe cases and thus effectively meet the needs of payers in the system and ensure that funds are targeted to those with the most clear-cut need for care. However, this approach has been criticized for failing to predict who will actually use mental health services (Regier et al. 1993) and for not responding to the requirements of state planners (Ciarlo et al. 1992).

Spitzer (1998) has also cautioned against equating a psychiatric disorder diagnosis with treatment need. Diagnostically assessed need has limited correspondence to mental health service use (Lehtinen et al. 1990; Rogler and Cortes 1993), a finding that has recently been replicated internationally in the World Mental Health Surveys (Demyttenaere et al. 2004). In Chile, Araya et al. (2006b) found that among individuals with psychiatric disorders, only 20% had consulted a professional about these problems, resulting in a mismatch between need and provision of services. Whether someone uses mental health services has been found to be a function of the degree to which they perceive themselves to be impaired (Meadows et al. 2000, 2002) and is not necessarily correlated with objective severity, based on diagnostic measures (Demyttenaere et al. 2004). However, self-perceptions of need for mental health care, or subjective need, also appear to vary by place or culture (Katz et al. 1997), with higher rates of self-perceived need in the United States compared with, for example, Ontario, Canada, even after controlling for level of psychiatric disorders. Self-perceived need may therefore be subject to cultural, social, or contextual differences that may obscure the relationship between objective and subjective need for services.

An additional problem with narrow diagnostic definitions is that they fail to provide information that is useful from a community-prevention perspective (Aoun et al. 2004; Sareen et al. 2005c). Although they capture individual-level cases, these definitions may fail to capture the cases that are important to measure for estimates focused on prevention rather than on acute care. For example, Steele et al. (2005) showed a divergence between known levels of need for services and levels of psychiatric use in welfare-dependent neighborhoods in Canada. These investigators concluded that, where use of mental health services is not closely linked to need for services, utilization data may be unsuitable for evaluating programs or policies. In order to ensure that needs for services match consumer demand and use of these services, inclusion of the availability of mental health services should be considered as well as whether additional resources need to be made available.

Because of the need for public health monitoring of mental health needs, recent recommendations have been made to expand the criteria used to estimate mental health service need (Aoun et al. 2004) beyond current diagnostic measures. Recommendations include shifting from a dichotomous measure to a continuous approach for determining mental health need (Davis 2005) and expanding the definition of need for services to include more than just those who meet current diagnostic criteria (Sareen et al. 2005c). Particularly when considering issues of mental health service disparities for racial and ethnic minority populations, researchers and policy makers have expressed concern about whether the standard definition of need is accurate in providing estimates for resource allocations at the community level (U.S. Department of Health and Human Services 2001). Those concerned about providing more equitable care across social groups have stressed the importance of taking a population-level approach to defining need for mental health services in general, in order to identify and address different interactions between policies and mental health outcomes in different subgroups (Starfield 2006).

According to the evidence available, it seems convenient from the public health point of view to improve the DSM and ICD nosological classifications by incorporating need perspectives that go beyond symptomatic criteria. The use of a multiaxial diagnostic format can allow for inclusion of two or three axes that measure needs for mental health services.

Psychiatric Diagnosis and Resource Allocation

Precise estimates of the need for mental health services in the general population are also required for budget allocations, because governments and agencies confront budgetary constraints while being held accountable for meeting the needs of their target populations.

Diagnosis is an important component of a comprehensive approach to assessing the functional abilities and strengths of individuals. When combined with an understanding of treatment and support options available at the system level, diagnoses can provide public health officials with a "high-level" view of population health needs with respect to specific mental health conditions (Cargiulo 2007). However, at the individual and organizational level, diagnosis has tended to be less useful in predicting use of health resources.

Fetter et al. (1980) were among the first to attempt to model length of stay for psychiatry using diagnosis related groups (DRGs). In the 15 psychiatric DRGs identified by psychiatric diagnoses (e.g., depression), addiction and operating room procedures explained only about 3% of variance in length of stay. Taube et al. (1984) modeled length of stay using DRGs, supplemented by measures of age, marital status, legal status, and previous hospitalizations, but made only modest gains in variance reduction (to 12%). Similar observations were made by English et al. (1986), who reported gains of 2%–5% in explained variance when sex, age, comorbidity, and discharge against medical advice were considered. Sharfstein (1986) concluded that a DRG-based approach to prospective payment would not be appropriate for psychiatry, for reasons including low explanatory power. A later study by Wellock (1995) on an alternative coding scheme for DRGs found no substantial improvement in their predictive power and concluded that a payment system based on DRGs would result in funding inequities.

The limited utility of current psychiatric diagnosis as a predictor of resource utilization led most researchers to investigate clinical indicators (e.g., functional ability, behavior) as potential case-mix variables (Boot et al. 1997). Ashcraft et al. (1989) studied length of stay in all U.S. Veterans Administration discharges from psychiatric beds over a 13-year period, with a psychiatric or substance-abuse disorder as a principal diagnosis. The results were 12 psychiatric diagnostic groupings using DSM-III (American Psychiatric Association 1980) codes, along with disturbed state, first admission for a condition, admission to a PTSD unit, assistance with activities of daily living, and severity of symptoms on admission. However, the model was more successful in explaining variance in resource utilization for those with a substance abuse disorder (more than 31%) than for those with psychiatric disorders (about 11%). A United Kingdom of Great Britain and Northern Ireland study (Creed et al. 1997) reported substantial improvements in explained variance in length of stay from a baseline model of DRGs only when psychiatric symptoms, demographic variables, and behavioral indicators were included; however, this study was based on only 115 cases.

New research led by the Ontario Joint Policy and Planning Committee in collaboration with interRAI, a 26-country research network, focused on the development and application of assessment systems for vulnerable populations (including mental health) and has yielded promising new results related to psychiatric case-mix classification. The System for Classification of Inpatient Psychiatry (SCIPP) uses about 100 clinical variables (e.g., depressive symptoms, violence, suicidality, psychosis) and provisional diagnoses to classify patients into 47 distinct groups (Hirdes et al. 2002; Lave 2003). SCIPP explains about 26% of the variable portion of per-diem resource utilization for all psychiatric inpatients, and it has an 8.4-fold difference in resource use when the most and least resource-intensive SCIPP groups were compared. Plans are currently under way to implement SCIPP into Ontario's funding formula for psychiatry, and research related to SCIPP is under way in nine countries, including LAMI nations.

If this research approach proves that the interRAI is similarly useful in both high-income and LAMI countries, its results could contribute to improving psychiatric diagnosis and classification in the future. For example, diagnostic axes that can be added to measure needs for services may also include some variables that contribute to predicting use of mental health resources.

Psychiatric Diagnosis and Epidemiological Surveillance

One of the essential public health functions described earlier in this chapter is epidemiological surveillance for disease prevention and control. Even though this function was especially created and designed for communicable diseases, epidemiological transition in many countries has led to an increase in activities dealing with problems caused by noncommunicable diseases. In mental health, the range of surveyed problems has not been broad thus far, but there is no doubt that it will be broader in the future, especially regarding problems related to violence, substance abuse, and suicide, apart from the potential monitoring of severe and persistent mental disorders. A research study carried out in the Argentine Republic (Barrionuevo et al. 2008) has proved that the use of information provided by the existing health care system for epidemiological surveillance is feasible and highly useful. This country collects a significant amount of information that could be profitably utilized for improving recording, collecting, and analyzing of mental health conditions. In our literature review, we did not find any research on the implications of the psychiatric classification system on epidemiological surveillance. Probably the same considerations that have been analyzed in this chapter for diagnosis and prevalence surveys applied equally to epidemiological surveillance, but this is still an open field for research.

Psychiatric Diagnosis and Help-Seeking Behavior

One of the most significant pieces of information for use in public health is how the available mental health services are used. This involves determining the quantities and types of services used and the relations of these help-seeking behaviors with the diagnoses and other diverse associated conditions that can explain these behaviors. Most of the studies found in our review carried out household or telephone interviews (Fournier et al. 1997; Lefebre et al. 1998; Ohayon et al. 1999), and they inquired whether individuals felt the need to and actually did seek help. Among the studies reviewed, only one, in 1991 (Martinez et al. 1991), researched mental health services directly.

Research on the use of mental health services has explored different factors, other than diagnoses, that can influence help-seeking behavior, such as the relation of insurance availability with access to and quality of services (Landerman et al. 1994; McAlpine and Mechanic 2000); illness severity (Coid et al. 2006; Lefebre et al. 1998); comorbidity (Goldstein and Levitt 2006; Lefebre et al. 1998); urban-rural residence (Canino et al. 2004; Naganuma et al. 2006); presence of suicidal ideation (Essau 2005); dwelling and income level (Buckner and Bassuk 1997); and some characteristics of minority groups such as indigenous people and migrants (Beals et al. 2005a, 2005b; Lefebre et al. 1998; Vega et al. 1999). These factors have been correlated with frequency of the use of mental health services (McAlpine and Mechanic 2000; Naganuma et al. 2006; Shapiro et al. 1984) and with type of professional consulted.

Some of the factors found to have some influence on help-seeking behavior are type of health insurance; awareness of having a problem; self-reliance; cultural determinants (Beals et al. 2005a, 2005b); comorbidity (Bland et al. 1997); quality of life (Sareen et al. 2005c); suicidal ideation (Sareen et al. 2005c); and among children, gender, group position, and father's presence (Zimmerman 2005). Comorbidity and severity are the only factors associated with diagnostic characteristics that have been found to influence help-seeking behavior. The presence of a second diagnosis, as well as the severity of the mental disorder or level of impairment, increases the probabilities of consulting mental health services. This is a recurrent result in several studies (Bland et al. 1997; Cohen et al. 2007; Goldstein and Levitt 2006; Hasin et al. 2005; Vicente et al. 2006). When looking for other associations related to use of services, some studies found subthreshold disorders also increased the likelihood of seeking mental health services (Moreno and Andrade 2005).

Although all the factors mentioned seem to play roles in help-seeking behavior for mental health services, the strongest associations found with this type of research were with disability and distress. Studies applying specific scales for these factors have found that persons with high distress or high disability levels presented high frequencies of help-seeking behavior (Bland et al. 1997; Henderson et al. 2001; Kessler et al. 2002, 2003b; McAlpine and Mechanic 2000; Medina-Mora et al. 2005; Sareen et al. 2005c). From the public health point of view, these results suggest that, for assessing and predicting mental health service use, simple distress and disability scales might be more useful than psychiatric syndromes or diagnoses according to the current ICD and DSM classifications (Kessler et al. 2002).

How to Improve the Use of a Classification and Diagnostic System From a Public Health Perspective

We offer some recommendations on how best to improve the nosological classification system to better match service needs. Such recommendations include creating need measures that go beyond syndrome criteria as well as providing better training to those responsible for establishing diagnostic assessments.

DEFINITIONS OF MENTAL HEALTH NEEDS BEYOND THE TRADITIONAL PSYCHIATRIC DIAGNOSIS

Multidimensional definitions of need are more appealing because they can include measures of need that may be particularly relevant to specific communities but may fall outside traditional psychiatric diagnostic frameworks. Optimally, measures of need for treatment should be constructed as a continuum, rather than a dichotomy, because categorical measures with several levels of need allow for more variability. The measure of need should include elevated measures of subthreshold diagnoses, impairment, distress, severity, and dysfunction in role performance, along with measures of culture-bound syndromes as well as measures of suicidality and exposure to severe violence.

Elevated symptomatology (as defined by subthreshold criteria) should be considered in an expanded definition of need for mental health care when assessing immigrant populations, because such cases may reflect actual disorders that not measured by Western symptomatology. This is consistent with concerns that Kleinman (1987) has termed "category fallacy" in cross-cultural psychiatric diagnosis: the "reification of a nosological category developed for a particular cultural group applied to members of another culture for whom it lacks coherence and its validity has not been established" (p. 452). Individuals may have elevated psychiatric symptomatology that is impairing, even though the symptoms may fall short of narrow diagnostic thresholds, or people in treatment may have symptomatology that has been reduced, although they still require ongoing care; thus, the need of all these individuals for mental health services may not be recognized if standard definitions are applied (U.S. Department of Health and Human Services 2001). Subthreshold cases with impairment have been shown to have substantial negative consequences if left untreated (Helmchen and Linden 2000; Kessler et al. 2003a; Magruder and Calderone 2000; Saunders and Lee 2000). A high level of comorbidity among subthreshold conditions has been found, including comorbidity between subthreshold anxiety and subthreshold alcohol use disorder, conduct disorder, and attention-deficit/hyperactivity disorder (Lewinsohn et al. 2004). For depression in particular, evidence indicates that significant impairment occurs on a continuum rather than by crossing a diagnostic threshold (Fergusson et al. 2005; Lewinsohn et al. 2004). Omitting such cases from need definitions may have significant implications for policy and resource planning, given that both subthreshold cases of depression and those meeting diagnostic criteria have been shown in some cases to have comparable levels of service use and costs (Katon et al. 2003).

Level of risk should be evaluated in relation to self (i.e., suicide attempts or plans) as well as others (e.g., history of fighting, hitting a spouse, neglecting a child, using a weapon in fights) and considered in the definition of need. Including measures of attempting to kill someone else in the definition of need is also based on the public health research showing violence associated with mental disorders can be better treated in the mental health sector than in the legal or justice sector in terms of clinical outcomes and decreased societal costs (U.S. Department of Health and Human Services 2004; Wolff et al. 1995). The relation between intimate partner violence and psychiatric problems is well documented (Nicolaidis et al. 2004; Nixon et al. 2004). Assessing violence to others, and to self, might facilitate early identification and treatment of disorders that might be a serious public health concern.

Suicidality is also an important criterion because it is correlated with psychiatric morbidity (Friedman et al. 1999; Kim et al. 2003), and suicidal ideation increases the chance of subsequent suicide attempts (Kessler et al. 1999; Kuo et al. 2001). Including measures of suicidality and violence in the definition of need is important because disorders in community populations may not have the clinical significance, or the level of severity, of those identified with the same criteria in clinical populations (Narrow et al. 2002; Regier et al. 1998).

Self-perceived need for treatment, independent of meeting criteria for a mental disorder according to DSM or ICD, has been found to be associated with increased disability and distress (Sareen et al. 2005b). Disability has been included as Axis V in DSM-IV and as Axis II in ICD-10. DSM uses the Global Assessment of Functioning Scale, which rates the overall psychopathological status and social and occupational functioning from 1 to 100, whereas ICD assesses disablement in personal care and functioning in occupation, family, and society at large based on the International Classification of Impairments, Disabilities, and Handicaps (Kastrup 2002). However, the concept of distress has not been included in the current diagnostic systems.

Culture-bound syndromes, such as *ataque de nervios* and neurasthenia, are also important to consider when assessing need for mental health services among LAMI countries and ethnic minority groups (Berganza et al. 2002; Takeuchi and Kramer 2002). DSM-IV recognizes the existence of these culturally related syndromes as markers for individuals with problems but offers no diagnosable disorder. For example, even though Asians overall have low prevalence of psychiatric disorders (Abe-Kim et al. 2007), in a study of Chinese Americans in Los Angeles, California, nearly 7% of Asians were found to have neurasthenia and substantial impairment (Zheng et al. 1997), suggesting a need for care.

Demand for care should not be incorporated as a dimension of need for mental health care, because demand for care has also been shown to vary by socioeconomic status, in the absence of any psychiatric disorders (Alegría et al. 2000). Use of mental health care in the absence of any assessed past-year psychiatric diagnosis ranges between 40% and 45% in both the Epidemiologic Catchment Area study and the National Comorbidity Survey (Kessler et al. 1997; Regier et al. 1993). Given these findings, demand for care as an indicator of need may differ depending on the demographics and access characteristics of the study sample, biasing the estimates of need in favor of those with greater access or higher socioeconomic status. At the same time, these data have shown that the vast majority of users of mental health services without a past-year psychiatric diagnosis have either a lifetime psychiatric diagnosis or elevated psychiatric symptoms (Robins and Regier 1991; Wang et al. 2005), suggesting that an expanded definition for need that includes these components might map more accurately across actual use.

TRAINING OF CLINICIANS RESPONSIBLE
FOR DIAGNOSTIC ASSESSMENTS

Furthermore, to ensure that the classification systems operate effectively in public health, those dealing with mental disorders need to learn to use the nosological classification system and then use it conscientiously. Although the diagnostic interview in mental health is used frequently to establish need for care and is often the basis of clinical care, it has been subject to little empirical investigation and oversight (Wood et al. 2002). Such oversight is particularly important because the questions asked and observations made by providers during the interview have an impact on subsequent patient care. Effective models of conducting the initial diagnostic interview, emphasizing the role of good listening and responsiveness on the part of the provider in facilitating good rapport (Clark and Mishler 1992), should be taught and later supervised in public health practice as a way to collect optimum classification data.

There is no question that providers vary substantially in ways they use the classification systems for assigning psychiatric disorders (American Psychiatric Association 1994). DSM-IV uses a symptom approach that puts clinicians in the role of a statistician (Claxton et al. 2006; Craig 2005; Plante 1991) in which they are expected to use decisions to estimate the probability of the disorder while statistically quantifying uncertainties as subjective probabilities in the process of arriving at the correct diagnosis (Aspinall and Hill 1984; Reeve 2002; Stickle and Weems 2006). Some research suggests that reduced reliability of diagnoses is related to poor knowledge of the criteria, which is often connected with failure to obtain key information or to correctly interpret diagnostic criteria; this is particularly true when clinicians need to decide on clinical significance (Malt 1986). Given the complexity of such predictions, it is not surprising that clinicians and public health personnel are likely to encounter serious limitations in implementing diagnostic classification systems.

Systematic assessment procedures that employ semistructured interviews to improve clinical utility can increase reliability of measurements and predictive validity of assessments (Stickle and Weems 2006). A multidimensional measure of need with multiple criteria, including impairment, distress, culture-bound syndromes, subthreshold disorders, suicidality, and violence toward self and others, may capture a more accurate representation of the extent of need for public health planning purposes (Aoun et al. 2004). In this way, we may avoid a mismatch between public health needs for mental health care and the approach used by health care delivery systems largely designed for acute illness. Evidence of urgency to address changes in the definition of need that will improve the match to care is mounting. Future diagnostic classification work should be oriented toward a simplified continuous version of the need measure that could be administered through a semistructured interview. This measure could include a short diagnostic screener, like the Quick CIDI (Kessler et al. 2004); a rapid assessment of distress and impairment in role performance and daily functioning; a measure of lifetime severity of mental health problems that is not linked to any service use; a short but comprehensive measure of psychiatric symptomatology, such as the K-10 (Kessler et al. 2002); a brief assessment of substance use that is less subject to social desirability, such as the Dartmouth Assessment of Lifestyle Instrument (Rosenberg et al. 1998); and an assessment of risk (suicidality and violence items). This measure should be calibrated to function equivalently for different populations, such as the disadvantaged and those who may not be exposed to medical terminology or Western symptomatology.

Availability of scales for symptoms, disability, distress, and risk could significantly facilitate both case screening in populations and diagnostic processes in clinical settings. These types of tools could also identify psychiatric symptomatology that is not above the threshold determined by the traditional classification system, especially if it is associated with high levels of risk, distress, and/or disability. Considering the ease of use of these scales and the magnitude of information that they can provide from the public health point of view (Alvarado-Esquivel et al. 2006; Brugha et al. 2001; Davis and Fong 1996; Grothe et al. 2005; Hasin et al. 2005; Henderson 2002; Kessler et al. 2002, 2003b; Kojima et al. 2002; Medina-Mora et al. 2005; Moos et al. 2002; Poulin et al. 2005; Sareen et al. 2005c), these scales could be incorporated routinely for the strategic management of mental health systems and services.

Proposal of a Diagnostic Model for Public Health Usage

Considering the strengths and limitations of the current ICD and DSM classification systems for public health usage as described in this chapter, we propose a multiaxial diagnostic model that balances the weight of symptomatic diagnosis with other criteria that can facilitate its use in public health, allowing a better approximation to needs for mental health services and use of mental health resources. This diagnostic model could also be appealing to clinicians because it could give them a broader perspective of a patient's needs, rather than just a syndrome diagnosis, allowing them to formulate and carry out a more comprehensive individualized therapeutic plan.

The model proposed includes four axes based on the evidence available about factors that correlate with mental health service use: diagnosis of syndromes, diagnosis of the level of distress, diagnosis of the level of functionality/disability, and diagnosis of the level of risk in relation to self and others.

DIAGNOSIS OF SYNDROMES

These axes can be based on current ICD and DSM criteria but in a simplified version that merges both classifications into one and responds to public health and clinical needs. This simplified version should include only major diagnostic categories, mainly the headings of the diagnostic groups. Divisions of the main headings into two or more categories could be done when there is hard evidence that these categories require different psychotropic medication and/or psychosocial interventions. For example, mood disorders could be divided into depressive and bipolar disorders, whereas anxiety disorders could remain as a single category or be merged with depressive disorders into anxiety-depression spectrum. A special effort should be made to define clearly the criteria for these major categories and to develop semistructured interviews and training tools to improve screening, as well as reliability in their application, in different countries and settings.

A simplified diagnostic classification syndrome (Axis 1) could serve several purposes from the public health point of view. First, it could increase the possibility of the classification being learned and applied by general health clinicians, even in LAMI countries where a GP's workload only allows 3–5 minutes per patient. Second, it could facilitate a common language between consumers, primary health care teams, and mental health and psychiatric specialists. Third, the simplification can improve the reliability of diagnosis by specialists and general clinicians, and the incorporation of psychiatric diagnosis into health information systems would be made easier. Finally, having a few broad diagnostic categories would also facilitate the process of validation in different cultures and the adoption of a psychiatric classification that can be reliably applied worldwide.

A simplified diagnostic system does not preclude mental health and psychiatric specialists from making both diagnoses of major syndromes and diagnoses of subtypes, if that is considered useful for decision making in treatment. Diagnostic subtypes could also include culture-bound syndromes as well as the differences found in some syndromes from one country (or region) to another, according to local cultural and socioeconomic conditions. In other words, the syndromal diagnostic system could have two subsystems: one that is shared by the general population, primary care providers and specialists, and public health personnel and clinicians and another that would be used by mental health and psychiatric specialists to complement this simplified version.

Because persons who do not meet criteria for ICD or DSM diagnoses often demand mental health services, and they can also present disability, this axis should be continuous, including both threshold and subthreshold syndromes. In the diagnostic model proposed here, Axes II, III, and IV (distress, functionality/disability, and risk) would be more crucial than Axis I to determine the need for treatment and to set public health priorities. Axis I should also register comorbidity, utilizing the diagnosis of two or more syndromes when they coexist in a single person, including personality disorders.

DIAGNOSIS OF DISTRESS

Considering that the level of subjective suffering reported by persons with mental disorders has been shown to be directly associated with the frequency of help-seeking behavior, this variable should be considered in the diagnosis and probably deserves a specific diagnostic axis. Distress is also related to ethical issues because persons with the highest levels of distress and the most severe mental disorders should have prompt access to mental health interventions to relieve their suffering.

The intensity of distress has been determined with different scales, and the challenge for the future is to develop scales that can be brief, simple, transcultural, and time efficient. Such scales are more likely to be used in settings with severe time constraints, by health professionals and technicians other than physicians and clinical practitioners, and in countries and regions with different socioeconomic and cultural realities. Distress scales can also be useful to assess intervention outcomes, both from the clinicians' point of view, when they evaluate results in individual patients, and from the public health point of view, when the evaluation is for a specific population with specific disorders.

DIAGNOSIS OF FUNCTIONALITY OR DISABILITY

Most authors agree that functionality or disability should be an axis of any psychiatric classification. Functionality/disability, on the other hand, has strong financial implications that make its inclusion in a classification system imperative. Persons with disability require more health and social services than do those who are fully functional, their work performance is usually diminished, and they can need periods of sick leave or even permanent disability pensions. Actually, the level of disability is frequently used to measure the severity of a particular mental disorder in a person or in a population sample. The Global Assessment of Functioning Scale of DSM-IV has been a valuable contribution in the direction of the type of psychiatric classification system proposed in this chapter. It remains to be determined in future research if this scale, or a different one, is the most appropriate for use in a new diagnostic classification in terms of reliability and validity. Similar to what has been said about distress scales, functionality/disability scales should be brief, simple, and cross-cultural.

DIAGNOSIS OF RISK IN RELATION TO SELF AND OTHERS

Inclusion of a diagnostic axis about risk for violent and suicidal behaviors is based, similarly to the two previous axes, on evidence that this variable correlates with needs for mental health services and use of health resources. However, systematically assessing risk to self and others might also facilitate early identification of persons with mental disorders who require urgent and intensive treatment. There is also the need, in this axis, to develop brief, simple, and cross-cultural scales. The massive application of scales that can measure risk of violent and suicidal behaviors as part of a diagnostic process could also facilitate implementation of an epidemiological surveillance system. This system will be a valuable public health initiative that could contribute to controlling these important mental health problems.

Recommendations Related to Research on Psychiatric Diagnosis and Classification for Public Health Usage

From the literature reviewed for this chapter, it is clear that current knowledge about the implications of diagnostic classification systems for essential public health functions and activities is still insufficient. Most studies on this subject have been carried out in Western high-income countries, whereas most of the population affected by mental disorders lives in LAMI countries. Few studies have applied a cross-cultural approach, even though it is well known that, in mental health, the human environment has a very strong influence. There are many areas in which research about public health and psychiatric diagnosis will be welcomed; among them we would like to highlight the following:

- Reliability, sensitivity, and specificity of major diagnostic categories in the real world of primary health care in LAMI countries. This should be compared with the reliability, sensitivity, and specificity of diagnosis made by psychiatrists.
- Reliability, sensitivity, and specificity of diagnoses made by clinicians with different levels of training. This type of research can help to define the minimal level of training required by a clinician to obtain valid diagnoses.
- Stigma associated with different diagnostic categories and names of disorders in different cultures. This type of research could influence the choice of names for some psychiatric diagnoses.
- Feasibility of using a multiaxial diagnostic system in different countries, both in terms of clinicians actually making diagnoses in all the axes and clinicians and public health specialists using this information in the proper way.
- Prediction of the use of mental health resources based on diagnosis of syndromes, compared with prediction based on a multiaxial diagnostic system.
- Reliability, sensitivity, and specificity of some diagnostic categories that are critical from the public health point of view, such as anxiety-depression spectrum, PTSD, and culture-bound syndromes.

- Reliability, sensitivity, and specificity of some tools used to facilitate diagnosis, such as semistructured interviews and scales, in both high-income and LAMI countries. These studies should consider the use of these tools by different health technicians and professionals.

Conclusions

After analyzing different relations between public health and psychiatric diagnosis and classification, we can point out the following conclusions:

1. Both ICD and DSM diagnostic systems have proved that their major diagnostic categories and their tools for measuring prevalence are functional and useful, from the public health perspective, in countries with different income levels, especially when determining burden of disease and detecting treatment gaps and inequalities.
2. In the same way, these systems have determined that when these major diagnostic categories respond to specific treatments, they are useful for formulating and implementing national mental health policies and plans, including priority setting, identification of cost-effective interventions, and development of mental health programs in primary health care.
3. A universal mental health diagnostic system merging ICD and DSM classifications is needed. This system should be simple, transcultural, feasible in LAMI countries, reliable, related to available interventions, able to minimize stigma, and free of conflicts of interest.
4. A diagnostic model from a public health perspective is proposed. Rather than the usual standard diagnosis based mainly on syndromes, it incorporates other possible dimensions of diagnosis linked to need for care and use of mental health resources (distress, functionality/disability, and risk to self or others).
5. To ensure that the public health system provides appropriate feedback to those revising the classification systems, public health programs need to interact with the designers of the classification systems. At the same time, those establishing diagnostic systems need to always take into account a community- rather than an individual-based perspective, directed at need for services and embedded in the epidemiological and social context.
6. There is a strong need for more research on the implications of diagnostic classification systems for essential public health functions and activities. This research can contribute to development and implementation of mental health policies and plans and to the strategic management of mental health systems and services.

References

Abe-Kim J, Takeuchi DT, Hong S, et al: Use of mental health-related services among immigrant and US-born Asian Americans: results from the National Latino and Asian American Study. Am J Public Health 97:91–98, 2007

Abiodun OA: A study of mental morbidity among primary care patients in Nigeria. Compr Psychiatry 34:10–13, 1993

Alarcón RD, Aguilar-Gaxiola SA: Mental health policy developments in Latin America. Bull World Health Organ 78:483–490, 2000

Alegría M, Bijl RV, Lin E, et al: Income differences in persons seeking outpatient treatment for mental disorders: a comparison of the United States with Ontario and The Netherlands. Arch Gen Psychiatry 57:383–391, 2000

Alvarado R, Vega J, Sanhueza G, et al: [Evaluation of the program for depression detection, diagnosis, and comprehensive treatment in primary care in Chile.] Rev Panam Salud Publica 18:278–286, 2005

Alvarado-Esquivel C, Sifuentes-Alvarez A, Salas-Martinez C, et al: Validation of the Edinburgh postpartum depression scale in a population of puerperal women in Mexico. Clin Pract Epidemiol Ment Health 29:2–33, 2006

American Psychiatric Association: Diagnostic and Statistical Manual of Mental Disorders, 3rd Edition. Washington, DC, American Psychiatric Association, 1980

American Psychiatric Association: Diagnostic and Statistical Manual of Mental Disorders, 3rd Edition, Revised. Washington, DC, American Psychiatric Association, 1987

American Psychiatric Association: Diagnostic and Statistical Manual of Mental Disorders, 4th Edition. Washington, DC, American Psychiatric Association, 1994

American Psychiatric Association: Refining the Research Agenda. Washington, DC, American Psychiatric Association, 2005

Aoun S, Pennebaker D, Wood C: Assessing population need for mental health care: a review of approaches and predictors. Ment Health Serv Res 6:33–46, 2004

Araya R, Rojas G, Fritsch R, et al: Treating depression in primary care in low-income women in Santiago, Chile: a randomized controlled trial. Lancet 361:995–1000, 2003

Araya R, Flynn T, Rojas G, et al: Cost-effectiveness of a primary care treatment program for depression in low-income women in Santiago, Chile. Am J Psychiatry 163:1379–1387, 2006a

Araya R, Rojas G, Fritsch R, et al: Inequities in mental health care after health care system reform in Chile. Am J Public Health 96:109–113, 2006b

Ashcraft MLF, Fries BE, Nerenz DR, et al: A psychiatric patient classification system: an alternative to diagnosis-related groups. Med Care 27:543–557, 1989

Aspinall P, Hill A: Clinical inferences and decisions, III: utility assessment and the Bayesian Decision Model. Ophthalmic Physiol Opt 4:251–263, 1984

Barrionuevo H, Grana D, Silva C: Vigilancia epidemiológica en Salud Mental. Pautas para su implementación en Argentina. Serie de estudios Isalud No 6, 2008. Available at: http://www.isalud.org/htm/pdf/SE6-Gascon.pdf.

Batniji R, Van Ommeren M, Saraceno B: Mental and social health in disasters: relating qualitative social science and the Sphere Standard. Soc Sci Med 62:1853–1864, 2006

Beals J, Manson SM, Whitesell NR, et al: Prevalence of DSM-IV disorders and attendant help-seeking in 2 American Indian reservation populations. Arch Gen Psychiatry 62:99–108, 2005a

Beals J, Novins DK, Whitesell NR, et al: Prevalence of mental disorders and utilization of mental health services in two American Indian reservation populations: mental health disparities in a national context. Am J Psychiatry 162:1723–1732, 2005b

Berganza CE, Mezzich JE, Jorge MR: Latin American Guide for Psychiatric Diagnosis (GLDP). Psychopathology 35:185–190, 2002

Bland RC, Newman SC, Orn H: Help-seeking for psychiatric disorders. Can J Psychiatry 42:935–942, 1997

Boot B, Hall W, Andrews G: Disability, outcome and case-mix in acute psychiatric inpatient units. Br J Psychiatry 171:242–246, 1997

Bott K, Meyer C, Rumpf HJ, et al: Psychiatric disorders among at-risk consumers of alcohol in the general population. J Stud Alcohol 66:246–253, 2005

Brugha TS, Jenkins R, Taub N, et al: A general population comparison of the Composite International Diagnostic Interview (CIDI) and the Schedules for Clinical Assessment in Neuropsychiatry (SCAN). Psychol Med 31:1001–1013, 2001

Buckner JC, Bassuk EL: Mental disorders and service utilization among youths from homeless and low-income housed families. J Am Acad Child Adolesc Psychiatry 36:890–900, 1997

Bye L, Partridge J: State level classification of serious mental illness: a case for a more uniform standard. J Health Soc Policy 19:1–29, 2004

Caldera T, Palma L, Penayo U, et al: Psychological impact of the hurricane Mitch in Nicaragua in a one-year perspective. Soc Psychiatry Psychiatr Epidemiol 36:108–114, 2001

Canino G, Shrout PE, Rubio-Stipec M, et al: The DSM-IV rates of child and adolescent disorders in Puerto Rico: prevalence, correlates, service use, and the effects of impairment. Arch Gen Psychiatry 61:85–93, 2004

Cargiulo T: Understanding the health impact of alcohol dependence. Am J Health Syst Pharm 64 (suppl):S5–S11, 2007

Chien I, Chou YJ, Lin CH, et al: Prevalence of psychiatric disorders among National Health Insurance enrollees in Taiwan. Psychiatr Serv 55:691–697, 2004

Ciarlo JA, Tweed DL, Shern DL, et al: Validation of indirect methods to estimate need for mental health services: concepts, strategy, and general conclusions. Eval Program Plann 15:115–131, 1992

Clark JA, Mishler EG: Attending to patients' stories: reframing the clinical task. Sociol Health Illn 14:345–372, 1992

Claxton K, Fenwick E, Sculpher M: Decision making with uncertainty: the value of information, in The Elgar Companion to Health Economics. Edited by Jones A. Cheltenham, UK, Edward Elgar, 2006

Cohen A, Kleinman A, Saraceno B: Introduction, in World Mental Health Casebook: Social and Mental Programs in Low-Income Countries. Edited by Cohen A, Kleinman A, Saraceno B. New York, Springer, 2002, pp 1–26

Cohen E, Feinn R, Arias A, et al: Alcohol treatment utilization: findings from the National Epidemiologic Survey on Alcohol and Related Conditions. Drug Alcohol Depend 86:214–221, 2007

Coid J, Yang M, Tyrer P, et al: Prevalence and correlates of personality disorder in Great Britain. Br J Psychiatry 188:423–431, 2006

Craig RJ: Substance abuse, in Clinical and Diagnostic Interviewing, 2nd Edition. Edited by Craig RJ. Lanham, MD, Jason Aronson, 2005, pp 163–179

Creed F, Tomenson B, Anthony P, et al: Predicting length of stay in psychiatry. Psychol Med 27:961–966, 1997

Davis DE, Fong ML: Measuring outcomes in psychiatry: an inpatient model. Jt Comm J Qual Improv 22:125–133, 1996

Davis JA: Differences in the health care needs and service utilization of women in nursing homes: comparison by race/ethnicity. J Women Aging 17:57–71, 2005

de Jong JT, Komproe IH, Van Ommeren M: Common mental disorders in postconflict settings. 361:2128–2130, 2003

Demyttenaere K, Bruffaerts R, Posada-Villa J, et al: Prevalence, severity, and unmet need for treatment of mental disorders in the World Health Organization World Mental Health Surveys. JAMA 291:2581–2590, 2004

English JT, Sharfstein SS, Scherl DJ, et al: Diagnosis-related groups and general hospital psychiatry: the APA Study. Am J Psychiatry 143:131–139, 1986

Epstein J, Barker P, Vorburger M, et al: Serious Mental Illness and Its Co-Occurrence With Substance Use Disorders, 2002. Rockville, MD, U.S. Department of Health and Human Services, Substance Abuse and Mental Health Services Administration, Office of Applied Studies, 2004

Erkinjuntti T, Ostbye T, Steenhuis R, et al: The effect of different diagnostic criteria on the prevalence of dementia. N Engl J Med 337:1667–1674, 1997

Essau CA: Frequency and patterns of mental health services utilization among adolescents with anxiety and depressive disorders. Depress Anxiety 22:130–137, 2005

Fergusson DM, Horwood LJ, Ridder EM, et al: Subthreshold depression in adolescence and mental health outcomes in adulthood. Arch Gen Psychiatry 62:66–72, 2005

Fetter RB, Shin Y, Freeman JL, et al: Case mix definition by diagnosis-related groups. Med Care 18 (suppl):iii, 1–53, 1980

First MB: Clinical utility: a prerequisite for the adoption of a dimensional approach in DSM. J Abnorm Psychol 114:560–564, 2005

Forsell Y: The pathway to meeting need for mental health services in Sweden. Psychiatr Serv 57:114–119, 2006

Fournier L, Lesage AD, Toupin J, et al: Telephone surveys as an alternative for estimating prevalence of mental disorders and service utilization: a Montreal catchment area study. Can J Psychiatry 42:737–743, 1997

Friedman S, Smith L, Fogel A: Suicidality in panic disorder: a comparison with schizophrenic, depressed, and other anxiety disorder outpatients. J Anxiety Disord 13:447–461, 1999

Funk M, Minoletti A, Drew N, et al: Advocacy for mental health: roles for consumer and family organizations and governments. Health Promotion International, December 2005. Available at: http://heapro.oxfordjournals.org/content/21/1/70.full.pdf+html. Accessed December 17, 2009.

Goldney R, Hawthorne G, Fisher L: Is the Australian National Survey of Mental Health and Wellbeing a reliable guide for health planners? A methodological note on the prevalence of depression. Aust N Z J Psychiatry 38:635–638, 2004

Goldstein BI, Levitt AJ: A gender-focused perspective on health service utilization in comorbid bipolar I disorder and alcohol use disorders: results from the national epidemiologic survey on alcohol and related conditions. J Clin Psychiatry 67:925–932, 2006

Grant BF, Hasin DS, Stinson FS, et al: Prevalence, correlates, and disability of personality disorders in the United States: results from the national epidemiologic survey on alcohol and related conditions. J Clin Psychiatry 65:948–958, 2004

Grothe KB, Dutton GR, Jones GN, et al: Validation of the Beck Depression Inventory–II in a low-income African American sample of medical outpatients. Psychol Assess 17:110–114, 2005

Gureje O, Alem A: Mental health policy development in Africa. Bull World Health Organ 78:475–482, 2000

Hasin DS, Goodwin RD, Stinson FS, et al: Epidemiology of major depressive disorder: results from the National Epidemiologic Survey on Alcoholism and Related Conditions. Arch Gen Psychiatry 62:1097–1106, 2005. Comment in: Evid Based Ment Health 9:59, 2006

Helmchen H, Linden M: Subthreshold disorders in psychiatry: clinical reality, methodological artifact, and the double-threshold problem. Compr Psychiatry 41 (suppl):1–7, 2000

Henderson S: The National Survey of Mental Health and Well-Being in Australia: impact on policy. Can J Psychiatry 47:819–824, 2002

Henderson S, Korten A, Medway J: Non-disabled cases in a national survey. Psychol Med 31:769–777, 2001

Hirdes JP, Fries BE, Botz C, et al: The System for Classification of In-Patient Psychiatry (SCIPP): A New Case-M Methodology for Mental Health. Toronto, Ontario, Canada, Ontario Joint Policy and Planning Committee, 2002

Hough RL, Hazen AL, Soriano FI, et al: Mental health services for Latino adolescents with psychiatric disorders. Psychiatr Serv 53:1556–1562, 2002

Hunt C, Issakidis C, Andrews G: DSM-IV generalized anxiety disorder in the Australian National Survey of Mental Health and Well-Being. Psychol Med 32:649–659, 2002

Issakidis C, Andrews G: Who treats whom? An application of the Pathways to Care model in Australia. Aust N Z J Psychiatry 40:74–86, 2006

Jacobi F, Wittchen HU, Holting C, et al: Estimating the prevalence of mental and somatic disorders in the community: aims and methods of the German National Health Interview and Examination Survey. Int J Methods Psychiatr Res 11:1–18, 2002

James S, Chisholm D, Murthy RS, et al: Demand for, access to and use of community mental health care: lessons from a demonstration project in India and Pakistan. Int J Soc Psychiatry 48:163–176, 2002

Kastrup M: Experience with current multiaxial diagnostic systems: a critical review. Psychopathology 35:122–126, 2002

Katon W, Lin E, Russo J, et al: Increased medical costs of a population-based sample of depressed elderly patients. Arch Gen Psychiatry 60:897–903, 2003

Katz SJ, Kessler RC, Frank RG, et al: The use of outpatient mental health services in the United States and Ontario: the impact of mental morbidity and perceived need for care. Am J Public Health 87:1136–1143, 1997

Kessler RC, McGonagle KA, Zhao S, et al: Lifetime and 12-month prevalence of DSM-III-R psychiatric disorders in the United States: results from the National Comorbidity Survey. Arch Gen Psychiatry 51:8–19, 1994

Kessler RC, Frank RG, Edlund M, et al: Differences in the use of psychiatric outpatient services between the United States and Ontario. N Engl J Med 336:551–557, 1997

Kessler RC, Borges G, Walters EE: Prevalence of and risk factors for lifetime suicide attempts in the National Comorbidity Survey. Arch Gen Psychiatry 56:617–626, 1999

Kessler RC, Andrews G, Colpe LJ, et al: Short screening scales to monitor population prevalences and trends in non-specific psychological distress. Psychol Med 32:959–976, 2002

Kessler RC, Merikangas KR, Berglund P, et al: Mild disorders should not be eliminated from the DSM-V. Arch Gen Psychiatry 60:1117–1122, 2003a

Kessler RC, Barker PR, Colpe LJ, et al: Screening for serious mental illness in the general population. Arch Gen Psychiatry 60:184–189, 2003b

Kessler RC, Abelson J, Demler O, et al: Clinical calibration of DSM-IV diagnoses in the World Mental Health (WMH) version of the World Health Organization (WHO) Composite International Diagnostic Interview (WMHCIDI). Int J Methods Psychiatr Res 13:122–139, 2004

Kessler RC, Berglund P, Demler O, et al: Lifetime prevalence and age-of-onset distributions of DSM-IV disorders in the National Comorbidity Survey Replication. Arch Gen Psychiatry 62:593–602, 2005a

Kessler RC, Chiu WT, Demler O, et al: Prevalence, severity, and comorbidity of 12-month DSM-IV disorders in the National Comorbidity Survey Replication. Arch Gen Psychiatry 62:617–627, 2005b

Khaleghian P, Das Gupta M: Public Management and the Essential Public Health Functions. World Bank Policy Research Working Paper 3220. Washington, DC, World Bank, 2004

Kim C, Lesage A, Seguin M, et al: Patterns of co-morbidity in male suicide completers. Psychol Med 33:1299–1309, 2003

Kleinman A: Anthropology and psychiatry: the role of culture in cross-cultural research on illness. Br J Psychiatry 151:447–454, 1987

Kohn R, Levav I, de Almeida JM, et al: Mental disorders in Latin America and the Caribbean: a public health priority. Rev Panam Salud Publica 18:229–240, 2005a

Kohn R, Levav I, Donaire I, et al: Psychological and psychopathological reactions in Honduras following Hurricane Mitch: implications for service planning. Rev Panam Salud Publica 18:287–295, 2005b

Kojima M, Furukawa TA, Takahashi H, et al: Cross-cultural validation of the Beck Depression Inventory-II in Japan. Psychiatry Res 110:291–299, 2002

Kuo WH, Gallo JJ, Tien AY: Incidence of suicide ideation and attempts in adults: the 13-year follow-up of a community sample in Baltimore, Maryland. Psychol Med 31:1181–1191, 2001

Kutcher S, Chehil S, Roberts T: An integrated program to train local health care providers to meet post-disaster mental health needs. Rev Panam Salud Publica 18:338–345, 2005

Landerman LR, Burns BJ, Swartz MS, et al: The relationship between insurance coverage and psychiatric disorder in predicting use of mental health services. Am J Psychiatry 151:1785–1790, 1994

Lave JR: Developing a Medicare prospective payment system for inpatient psychiatric care. Health Aff (Millwood) 22:97–109, 2003

Lefebre J, Lesage A, Cyr M, et al: Factors related to utilization of services for mental health reasons in Montreal, Canada. Soc Psychiatry Psychiatr Epidemiol 33:291–298, 1998

Lehtinen V, Joukamaa M, Jyrkinen E, et al: Need for mental health services of the adult population in Finland: results from the Mini Finland Health Survey. Acta Psychiatr Scand 81:426–431, 1990

Lepine JP, Gasquet I, Kovess V, et al: [Prevalence and comorbidity of psychiatric disorders in the French general population.] Encephale 31:182–194, 2005

Lewczyk CM, Garland AF, Hurlburt MS, et al: Comparing DISC-IV and clinician diagnoses among youths receiving public mental health services. J Am Acad Child Adolesc Psychiatry 42:349–356, 2003

Lewinsohn PM, Shankman SA, Gau JM, et al: The prevalence and co-morbidity of subthreshold psychiatric conditions. Psychol Med 34:613–622, 2004

Liu SL, Prince M, Blizard B, et al: The prevalence of psychiatric morbidity and its associated factors in general health care in Taiwan. Psychol Med 32:629–637, 2002

Lopez AD, Mathers CD, Ezzati M, et al: Global and regional burden of disease and risk factors 2001: systematic analysis of population health data. Lancet 367:1747–1757, 2006

Lotrakul M, Saipanish R: Psychiatric services in primary care settings: a survey of general practitioners in Thailand. BMC Fam Pract 7:48, 2006

Loza N, Hasan N: Sudanese refugees: sufferings and suggested management. Int Psychiatry 4:5–7, 2007

Mackinnon A, Jorm AF, Hickie IB: A national depression index for Australia. Med J Aust 181 (suppl):S52–S56, 2004

Magruder KM, Calderone GE: Public health consequences of different thresholds for the diagnosis of mental disorders. Compr Psychiatry 41 (suppl):14–18, 2000

Malt UF: Teaching DSM-III to clinicians: some problems of the DSM-III system reducing reliability, using the diagnosis and classification of depressive disorders as an example. Acta Psychiatr Scand Suppl 328:68–75, 1986

Mari J de J, Iacoponi E, Williams P, et al: Detection of psychiatric morbidity in the primary medical care setting in Brazil. Rev Saúde Pública 21:501–507, 1987

Martinez RE, Sesman Rodríguez M, Bravo M, et al: [Use of health services in Puerto Rico by persons with mental disorders.] Acta Psiquiatr Psicol Am Lat 37:143–147, 1991

Mathet F, Martin-Guehl C, Maurice-Tison S, et al: [Prevalence of depressive disorders in children and adolescents attending primary care: a survey with the Aquitaine Sentinelle Network.] Encephale 29:391–400, 2003

McAlpine DD, Mechanic D: Utilization of specialty mental health care among persons with severe mental illness: the roles of demographics, need, insurance, and risk. Health Serv Res 35:277–292, 2000

McKenzie K, Patel V, Araya R: Learning from low income countries: mental health. BMJ 329:1138–1140, 2004

Meadows G, Burgess P, Fossey E, et al: Perceived need for mental health care, findings from the Australian National Survey of Mental Health and Well-Being. Psychol Med 30:645–656, 2000

Meadows G, Burgess P, Bobevski I, et al: Perceived need for mental health care: influences of diagnosis, demography and disability. Psychol Med 32:299–309, 2002

Medina-Mora ME, Borges G, Lara C, et al: Prevalence, service use, and demographic correlates of 12-month DSM-IV psychiatric disorders in Mexico: results from the Mexican National Comorbidity Survey. Psychol Med 35:1773–1783, 2005

Mezzich JE: Comprehensive diagnosis: a conceptual basis for future diagnostic systems. Psychopathology 35:162–165, 2002

Minoletti A, López C: Las Enfermedades Mentales en Chile: Magnitud y Consecuencias [Book in Spanish]. Santiago, Chile, Ministerio de Salud, 1999

Minoletti A, Saxena S: Informe WHO-AIMS sobre Sistema de Salud Mental en Chile [Book in Spanish]. Santiago, Chile, World Health Organization and Ministerio de Salud, 2006

Minoletti A, Zaccaria A: [The national mental health plan in Chile: 10 years of experience.] Rev Panam Salud Publica 18:347–358, 2005

Minoletti A, Narváez P, Sepúlveda R, et al: Chile: Lecciones aprendidas en la implementación de un modelo comunitario de atencion en salud mental [Learned lessons in the implementation of a community mental health care model], in Capitulo 26, Salud Mental en la Comunidad, Edited by Rodríguez J. Serie PALTEX. Washington, DC, Organización Panamericana de la Salud, pp 339–348

Mirza I, Mujtaba M, Chaudhry H, et al: Primary mental health care in rural Punjab, Pakistan: providers and user perspectives of the effectiveness of treatments. Soc Sci Med 63:593–597, 2006

Mojtabai R, Olfson M: Treatment seeking for depression in Canada and the United States. Psychiatr Serv 57:631–639, 2006

Moller HJ: Problems associated with the classification and diagnosis of psychiatric disorders. World J Biol Psychiatry 6:45–56, 2005

Moos RH, Nichol AC, Moos BS: Global Assessment of Functioning ratings and the allocation and outcomes of mental health services. Psychiatr Serv 53:730–737, 2002

Moreno DH, Andrade LH: The lifetime prevalence, health services utilization and risk of suicide of bipolar spectrum subjects, including subthreshold categories in the Sao Paulo ECA study. J Affect Disord 87:231–241, 2005

Mufti KA, Naeem F, Chaudhry HR, et al: Post-traumatic stress disorder among Afghan refugees following war. Int Psychiatry 4:7–9, 2007

Murray CJL, Lopez AD: Alternative projections of mortality and disability by cause 1990–2020: Global Burden of Disease Study. Lancet 349:1498–1504, 1997

Naeem F, Mufti KA, Ayub M, et al: Psychiatric morbidity among Afghan refugees in Peshawar, Pakistan. J Ayub Med Coll Abbottabad 17:23–25, 2005

Naganuma Y, Tachimori H, Kawakami N, et al: Twelve-month use of mental health services in four areas in Japan: findings from the World Mental Health Japan Survey 2002–2003. Psychiatry Clin Neurosci 60:240–248, 2006

Nakane Y, Nakane H: Classification systems for psychiatric diseases currently used in Japan. Psychopathology 35:191–194, 2002

Narrow WE, Rae DS, Robins LN, et al: Revised prevalence estimates of mental disorders in the United States: using a clinical significance criterion to reconcile 2 surveys' estimates. Arch Gen Psychiatry 59:115–123, 2002

National Institute for Clinical Excellence: Depression: Management of Depression in Primary and Secondary Care. Clinical Guideline 23. London, NICE, 2004

Negash A, Alem A, Kebede D, et al: Prevalence and clinical characteristic of bipolar I disorder in Butajira, Ethiopia: a community-based study. J Affect Disord 87:193–201, 2005

Nicolaidis C, Curry M, McFarland B, et al: Violence, mental health, and physical symptoms in an academic internal medicine practice. J Gen Intern Med 19:819–827, 2004

Nixon RD, Resick PA, Nishith P: An exploration of comorbid depression among female victims of intimate partner violence with posttraumatic stress disorder. J Affect Disord 82:315–320, 2004

Njenga FG: Refugee mental health challenges in Africa. Int Psychiatry 4:3–5, 2007

O'Connor DW: Do older Australians truly have low rates of anxiety and depression? A critique of the 1997 National Survey of Mental Health and Wellbeing. Aust N Z J Psychiatry 40:623–631, 2006

Ohayon MM, Priest RG, Guilleminault C, et al: The prevalence of depressive disorders in the United Kingdom. Biol Psychiatry 45:300–307, 1999

Otero-Ojeda AA: Third Cuban glossary of psychiatry (GC-3): key features and contributions. Psychopathology 35:181–184, 2002

Pan American Health Organization: Public Health in the Americas: Conceptual Renewal Performance Assessment and Bases for Action. Washington, DC, Pan American Health Organization, 2002

Patel V, Kleinman A: Poverty and common mental disorders in developing countries. Bull World Health Organ 81:609–615, 2003

Patel V, Todd C, Winston M, et al: Outcome of common mental disorders in Harare, Zimbabwe. Br J Psychiatry 172:53–57, 1998a

Patel V, Pereira J, Coutinho L, et al: Poverty, psychological disorder and disability in primary care attenders in Goa, India. Br J Psychiatry 172:533–536, 1998b

Patel V, Araya R, de Lima M, et al: Women, poverty and common mental disorders in four restructuring societies. Soc Sci Med 49:1461–1471, 1999

Patel V, Chisholm D, Rabe-Hesketh S, et al: Efficacy and cost-effectiveness of drug and psychological treatments for common mental disorders in general health care in Goa, India: a randomized, controlled trial. Lancet 361:33–39, 2003

Peltzer K, Seoka P, Babor T, et al: Training primary care nurses to conduct alcohol screening and brief interventions in South Africa. Curationis 29:16–21, 2006

Pioggiosi P, Forti P, Ravaglia G, et al: Different classification systems yield different dementia occurrence among nonagenarians and centenarians. Dement Geriatr Cogn Disord 17:35–41, 2004

Plante D: Quantitative diagnostic methods and decision analysis, in Neurology in Clinical Practice, Vol 1: The Neurological Disorders. Edited by Bradley WG, Daroff RB, Fenichel GM. Boston, MA, Butterworth Heinemann, 1991

Pothen M, Kuruvilla A, Philip K, et al: Common mental disorders among primary care attenders in Vellore, South India: nature, prevalence and risk factors. Int J Soc Psychiatry 49:119–125, 2003

Poulin C, Lemoine O, Poirier LR, et al: Validation study of a nonspecific psychological distress scale. Soc Psychiatry Psychiatr Epidemiol 40:1019–1024, 2005

Reeve BW: A guide to the assessment of psychiatric symptoms in the addictions treatment setting, in Managing the Dually Diagnosed Patient: Current Issues and Clinical Approaches, 2nd Edition. Edited by O'Connell DF, Beyer EP. Binghamton, NY, Haworth Press, 2002, pp 189–212

Regier DA, Narrow WE, Rae DS, et al: The de facto US mental and addictive disorders service system: Epidemiologic Catchment Area prospective 1-year prevalence rates of disorders and services. Arch Gen Psychiatry 50:85–94, 1993

Regier DA, Kaelber CT, Rae DS, et al: Limitations of diagnostic criteria and assessment instruments for mental disorders: implications for research and policy. Arch Gen Psychiatry 55:109–115, 1998

Regier DA, Narrow WE, First MB, et al: The APA classification of mental disorders: future perspectives. Psychopathology 35:166–170, 2002

Robins LN, Regier DA (eds): Psychiatric Disorders in America: The Epidemiologic Catchment Area Study. New York, Free Press, 1991

Rocha FL, Vorcaro CM, Uchoa E, et al: Comparing the prevalence rates of social phobia in a community according to ICD-10 and DSM-III-R. Rev Bras Psiquiatr 27:222–224, 2005

Rogler LH, Cortes DE: Help seeking pathways: a unifying concept in mental health care. Am J Psychiatry 50:554–561, 1993

Rosenberg S, Drake RE, Wolford GL, et al: Dartmouth Assessment of Lifestyle Instrument (DALI): a substance use disorder screen for people with severe mental illness. Am J Psychiatry 155:232–238, 1998

Saldivia S, Vicente B, Kohn R, et al: Use of mental health services in Chile. Psychiatr Serv 55:71–76, 2004

Salsberry PJ, Chipps E, Kennedy C: Use of general medical services among Medicaid patients with severe and persistent mental illness. Psychiatr Serv 56:458–462, 2005

Sareen J, Cox BJ, Afifi TO, et al: Mental health service use in a nationally representative Canadian survey. Can J Psychiatry 50:753–761, 2005a

Sareen J, Cox BJ, Afifi TO, et al: Perceived need for mental health treatment in a nationally representative Canadian sample. Can J Psychiatry 50:643–651, 2005b

Sareen J, Stein MB, Campbell DW, et al: The relation between perceived need for mental health treatment, DSM diagnosis, and quality of life: a Canadian population-based survey. Can J Psychiatry 50:87–94, 2005c

Saunders JB, Lee NK: Hazardous alcohol use: its delineation as a subthreshold disorder, and approaches to its diagnosis and management. Compr Psychiatry 41:95–103, 2000

Shapiro S, Skinner EA, Kessler LG, et al: Utilization of health and mental health services: three Epidemiologic Catchment Area sites. Arch Gen Psychiatry 41:971–978, 1984

Sharfstein SS: Commentary on "Prospective Payment for Outpatient Mental Health Services: Evaluation of Diagnosis Related Groups" by Wood and Beardmore. Community Ment Health J 22:292–293, 1986

Shibre T, Kebede D, Alem A, et al: An evaluation of two screening methods to identify cases with schizophrenia and affective disorders in a community survey in rural Ethiopia. Int J Soc Psychiatry 48:200–208, 2002

Sigman M, Hassan S: Benefits of long-term group therapy to individuals suffering schizophrenia: a prospective 7-year study. Bull Menninger Clin 70:273–282, 2006

Silpakit C: A Study of Common Mental Disorders in Primary Care in Thailand (PhD thesis). London, University of London, Faculty of Medicine, 1997

Spitzer RL: Diagnosis and need for treatment are not the same. Arch Gen Psychiatry 55:120, 1998

Srisurapanont M, Garner P, Critchley J, et al: Benzodiazepine prescribing behaviour and attitudes: a survey among general practitioners practicing in northern Thailand. BMC Fam Pract 6:27, 2005

Starfield B: State of the art in research on equity in health. J Health Polit Policy Law 31:11–32, 2006

Steele LS, Glazier RH, Lin E, et al: Measuring the effect of a large reduction in welfare payments on mental health service use in welfare-dependent neighborhoods. Med Care 43:885–891, 2005

Stein MB, Kirk P, Prabhu V, et al: Mixed anxiety-depression in a primary-care clinic. J Affect Disord 34:79–84, 1995

Stickle T, Weems C: Improving prediction from clinical assessment: the roles of measurement, psychometric theory, and decision theory, in Strengthening Research Methodology: Psychological Measurement and Evaluation. Edited by Bootzin RR, Mcknight PE. Washington, DC, American Psychological Association, 2006, pp 213–230

Takeuchi DT, Kramer EJ: Mental health services research in Asian Americans. West J Med 176:225–226, 2002

Taube C, Lee ES, Forthofer RN: Diagnosis-related groups for mental disorders, alcoholism and drug abuse: evaluation and alternatives. Hosp Community Psychiatry 35:452–455, 1984

Thapa SB, Hauff E: Psychological distress among displaced persons during an armed conflict in Nepal. Soc Psychiatry Psychiatr Epidemiol 40:672–679, 2005

Thapa SB, Van Ommeren M, Sharma B, et al: Psychiatric disability among tortured Bhutanese refugees in Nepal. Am J Psychiatry 160:2032–2037, 2003

U.S. Department of Health and Human Services: Mental Health: Culture, Race and Ethnicity. A Supplement to Mental Health: A Report of the Surgeon General. Rockville, MD, U.S. Department of Health and Human Services, Office of the Surgeon General, Substance Abuse and Mental Health Services Administration, 2001

U.S. Department of Health and Human Services: Community Based Participatory Research: Assessing the Evidence (AHRQ Publ No 04-E022-2). Rockville, MD, Agency for Healthcare Research and Quality, July 2004. Available at: http://www.ncbi.nlm.nih.gov/books/NBK37280/. Accessed January 24, 2012.

Udomratn P: Mental health and psychiatry in Thailand. Int Psychiatry 4:11–14, 2007

Udomratn P, Fog R (eds): Mixed Anxiety and Depressive Disorder: New Findings and Updating Evidence of Treatment. Copenhagen, Denmark, H Lundbeck A/S, 2001

Üstün TB, Sartorius N (eds): Mental Illness in General Health Care: An International Study. Chichester, UK, Wiley, 1995

van Ommeren M, Saxena S, Sarraceno B: Mental and social health during and after acute emergencies: emerging consensus? Bull World Health Organ 83:71–75, 2005

Varma SL, Azhar MZ: Psychiatric symptomatology in a primary health setting in Malaysia. Med J Malaysia 50:11–16, 1995

Vaswani M, Linda FK, Ramesh S: Role of selective serotonin reuptake inhibitors in psychiatric disorders: a comprehensive review. Prog Neuropsychopharmacol Biol Psychiatry 27:85–102, 2003

Vega WA, Kolody B, Aguilar-Gaxiola S, et al: Gaps in service utilization by Mexican Americans with mental health problems. Am J Psychiatry 156:928–934, 1999

Vicente B, Kohn R, Saldivia S, et al: [Service use patterns among adults with mental health problems in Chile.] Rev Panam Salud Publica 18:263–271, 2005

Vicente B, Kohn R, Rioseco P, et al: Lifetime and 12-month prevalence of DSM-III-R disorders in the Chile psychiatric prevalence study. Am J Psychiatry 163:1362–1370, 2006

Vilalta-Franch J, Garre-Olmo J, López-Pousa S, et al: Comparison of different clinical diagnostic criteria for depression in Alzheimer disease. Am J Geriatr Psychiatry 14:589–597, 2006

Wang PS, Berglund PA, Olfson M, et al: Delays in initial treatment contact after first onset of a mental disorder. Health Serv Res 39:393–415, 2004. Comment in Health Serv Res 39:221–224, 2004

Wang PS, Lane M, Olfson M, et al: Twelve-month use of mental health services in the United States: results from the National Comorbidity Survey Replication. Arch Gen Psychiatry 62:629–640, 2005

Wellock CM: Is a diagnosis-based classification system appropriate for funding psychiatric care in Alberta? Can J Psychiatry 40:507–513, 1995

Wolff N, Helminiak TW, Diamond RJ: Estimated societal costs of assertive community mental health care. Psychiatr Serv 46:898–906, 1995

Wood J, Garb HN, Lilienfeld SO, et al: Clinical assessment. Annu Rev Psychol 53:519–543, 2002

World Health Organization: The ICD-10 Classification of Mental and Behavioural Disorders: Clinical Descriptions and Diagnostic Guidelines. Geneva, World Health Organization, 1992

World Health Organization: Cross-national comparisons of the prevalences and correlates of mental disorders: WHO International Consortium in Psychiatric Epidemiology. Bull World Health Organ 78:413–426, 2000

World Health Organization: Atlas, Country Profiles on Mental Health Resources 2001. Geneva, World Health Organization, 2001a

World Health Organization: The Effectiveness of Mental Health Services in Primary Care: The View From the Developing World. Geneva, World Health Organization, 2001b

World Health Organization: The World Health Report 2001, Mental Health: New Understanding, New Hope. Geneva, World Health Organization, 2001c

World Health Organization: Advocacy for Mental Health: Mental Health Policy and Service Guidance Package, Nonserial Publication. Geneva, World Health Organization, 2003a

World Health Organization: Mental Health in Emergencies: Mental and Social Aspects of Health of Populations Exposed to Extreme Stressors. Geneva, World Health Organization, 2003b

World Health Organization: Planning and Budgeting to Deliver Services for Mental Health: Mental Health Policy and Service Guidance Package. Geneva, World Health Organization, 2003c

World Health Organization: Mental Health Atlas 2005. Geneva, World Health Organization, 2005a

World Health Organization: Mental Health Policy, Plans and Programmes—Updated Version: Mental Health Policy and Service Guidance Package. Geneva, World Health Organization, 2005b

World Health Organization: Disease Control Priorities Related to Mental, Neurological, Developmental and Substance Abuse Disorders. Geneva, World Health Organization, 2006a

World Health Organization: Dollars, DALYs and Decisions: Economic Aspects of the Mental Health System. Geneva, World Health Organization, 2006b

World Health Organization, University of Auckland: Situational Analysis of Mental Health Needs and Resources in Pacific Island Countries. Geneva, World Health Organization, 2005

World Health Organization Regional Office for the Western Pacific: Essential Public Health Functions: The Role of Ministries of Health. Geneva, World Health Organization, 2002

World Health Organization Regional Office for the Western Pacific: Essential Public Health Functions, A Three Country Study in the Western Pacific Region. Geneva, World Health Organization, 2003

Yach D: Redefining the scope of public health beyond the year 2000. Curr Issues Public Health 2:247–252, 1996

Zheng Y-P, Lin KM, Takeuchi D, et al: An epidemiological study of neurasthenia in Chinese Americans in Los Angeles. Compr Psychiatry 38:249–259, 1997

Zimmerman FJ: Social and economic determinants of disparities in professional help-seeking for child mental health problems: evidence from a national sample. Health Serv Res 40:1514–1533, 2005

9

FORMULATION OF FUNCTIONING, DISABILITY, AND CONTEXTUAL FACTORS IN THE DIAGNOSIS OF MENTAL DISORDERS IN DSM AND ICD

Bedirhan Üstün
Angelo Barbato
Tae-Yeon Hwang
Robert Jakob
Aleksandar Janca
Marianne Kastrup
Cille Kennedy
Nenad Kostanjek
Venos Mavreas
William E. Narrow
Martti Virtanen

This chapter was prepared at the invitation of the American Psychiatric Institute for Research and Education (APIRE) Public Health Conference Working Group

243

and presented at the World Health Organization/APIRE Conference on Public Health Aspects of Diagnosis and Classification in September 2007. Its purpose is to promote discussion on recommendations for revision of both ICD-10 (World Health Organization 1992) and DSM-IV-TR (American Psychiatric Association 2000). In this chapter, we basically explore two main issues:

1. *How does the environment contribute to the formulation of diagnoses of mental disorders? In this regard, how can DSM be linked with ICD Z codes? Also, in the ICD revision process, how could ICD Z codes be improved?* The ICD Z Codes are intended for identifying "contextual factors" that influence a person's health status but are not, in themselves, a current illness or injury. The original intent of these codes was to capture information about persons (who may or may not be sick) encountering health services for specific purposes that, in themselves, are not diseases or injuries: for example, to receive limited care or service for current conditions, to donate an organ or tissue, to receive prophylactic vaccinations, or to discuss problems. For use in mental health, these codes mainly refer to "contextual factors" indicating relevant psychosocial and environmental problems. Such problems may be related to the onset, exacerbation, or maintenance of a mental disorder or may, in themselves, be targets of clinical care. They also include personal problems that do not amount to a disorder proper but are of clinical significance (e.g., accentuated personality traits that are not personality disorders or hazardous, violent, abusive, or suicidal behaviors).

2. *How does disability contribute to formulation of diagnoses of mental disorders? In this regard, how could the ICD revision address the joint use of the International Classification of Functioning, Disability, and Health (ICF), and how could DSM be linked with ICF?* In this context, it is imperative to examine the effects of incorporation of disability criteria—termed *functional impairment* in DSM-IV (American Psychiatric Association 1994)—on formulating diagnoses of mental disorders. Disability criteria are not required for the diagnosis of physical disorders, such as diabetes mellitus or tuberculosis, in general health care. The World Health Organization's two classification systems of ICD and ICF World Health Organization 2001 advocate for separate assessments of disease and disability dimensions and then use of these constructs jointly in case formulation. Thus, the DSM-IV requirement for functional impairment in the diagnosis of mental disorders is not compatible with this scheme. This requirement can be seen as a remnant of the dualism between physical and mental disorders, and it works against the conceptual parity of mental disorders with other diseases. However, without the immediate clinical measures (such as temperature or blood pressure) or objective laboratory findings (such as electrolytes) of physical disorders, treatment planning for mental disorders may require such criteria to establish diagnostic thresholds. Perspectives gained from development and use of the ICF, jointly with ICD, could be used to inform thinking on DSM's use of functional impairment criteria.

Capturing Contextual Factors With ICD Z Codes in Formulation of Mental Disorder Diagnoses

Many mental health workers are cognizant of the fact that various psychosocial and environmental problems affect the diagnosis, treatment, and prognosis of mental disorders. Such contextual factors may be involved in initiation or exacerbation of a person's mental disorder, may be a consequence of the disorder, or may involve a situation that needs to be accounted for in development of a care plan. These contextual factors range from immediate family, housing, and education or work setting to broader economic, cultural, and environmental factors.

The ICD system attempts to capture such situations in Z codes: "Factors influencing health status and contact with health services." ICD Z codes were originally intended for identifying contextual factors that are not, in themselves, current illnesses or injuries but that influence a person's health status. The original intent of these codes was for capturing information about persons encountering health services for some specific purpose; these codes are not intended for primary mortality coding. For use in mental health, these codes mainly refer to "contextual factors" indicating relevant psychosocial and environmental problems; the basic rubrics of these codes are displayed in Table 9–1. These codes for contextual factors consist of all major relevant domains of psychosocial and environmental problems. Of particular significance to the mental health area, such problems may be related to the onset, exacerbation, or maintenance of a mental disorder or be, in themselves, targets of clinical care. These also include personal problems that do not amount to a disorder proper but are of clinical significance (e.g., hazardous, violent, abusive, or suicidal behaviors), similar to those listed in DSM-IV-TR (American Psychiatric Association 2000) as "Other Conditions That May Be a Focus of Clinical Attention."

Similarly, the DSM system captures such contextual factors on Axis IV, "psychosocial and environmental problems." Nine categories are given:

1. Problems with primary support group
2. Problems related to the social environment
3. Educational problems
4. Occupational problems
5. Housing problems
6. Economic problems
7. Problems with access to health care services
8. Problems related to interaction with the legal system/crime
9. Other psychosocial and environmental problems

On Axis IV, the environment is taken as the key factor bearing on the patient's condition. For the most part, the examples given for Axis IV problems are situations

TABLE 9–1.   Main ICD Z code blocks: factors influencing health status and contact with health services

Codes	Health status and services contact
Z00–Z13	Examination and investigation
Z20–Z29	Health hazards related to communicable diseases
Z30–Z39	Circumstances related to reproduction
Z40–Z54	Specific procedures and health care
Z55–Z65	Potential health hazards related to socioeconomic and psychosocial circumstances
Z70–Z76	Other circumstances
Z80–Z99	Potential health hazards related to family and personal history and certain conditions influencing health status

that cannot be changed by psychiatric treatments, such as medication or psychotherapy. These situations include death, divorce, job loss, extreme poverty, and inadequate health insurance—situations for which psychotherapy might help a patient gain insight or improve coping strategies. Examples of potentially mutable problems involve "discord" in relationships with family, friends, coworkers, and so on. Changes in a patient's behavior as a result of treatment may reduce discord.

Could these categories listed in ICD Z codes and DSM Axis IV be improved and render a useful international coding scheme? The revision processes of ICD and DSM both call for closer examinations of these categories and determination of whether they could possibly create a harmonious relevant set of codes useful for practice.

As noted in Axis Three of *Multiaxial Presentation of the ICD-10 for Use in Adult Psychiatry* (World Health Organization 1997), the ICD Z codes and DSM Axis IV problem categories are indeed relevant for clinical care of the current illness episode and useful in understanding the context of a mental disorder (Janca et al. 1996a, 1996b). The multiaxial presentation of ICD-10 includes brief definitions, based on those in the ICD Z00–Z99 codes. A clinician can use these codes to assess and record contextual factors that contribute significantly to the occurrence, presentation, course, outcome, or treatment of present mental and physical disorders. The Z codes are designed as global, or generic, factors to permit a clinician to denote the domain of the problem and add specificity, with regard to the individual patient, to the medical record. For example, Z56.2, "Threat of job loss," may indicate "events or situations which are threatening for the continuation of gainful employment." This is very useful information in understanding the personal job situation of a person. Similarly, Z61.3, "Events resulting in loss of self-esteem in childhood," indicates "events resulting in a negative self-reappraisal by the child such as failure in tasks with high personal investment; disclosure or discovery of a shameful or stigmatizing personal or family event; and other se-verely humiliating experiences." The high proportion of persons with mental disorders in prisons and among homeless populations has highlighted the need for a detailed capture of the nature of this type of contextual information in standard fashion.

PROPOSALS FOR FUTURE DEVELOPMENT FOR CONTEXTUAL FACTORS

The issue of contextual and environmental factors is indeed very important: cap-turing relevant dimensions for health conditions in a parsimonious fashion is a challenge for a classification. There seem to be three options for improving the coding of these factors:

1. *Use the ICF environmental factors codes.* These codes are relatively concise and relevant for health care. They are more detailed than is required on Axis IV of DSM-IV-TR. A crosswalk could be built for appropriate linkage between two coding systems, and simple checklist or assessment instruments would assist in operationalizing these factors for pragmatic assessment in clinical settings. ICD revision groups should also seek congruence between ICD Z codes and ICF environmental factors codes.
2. *Use the ICD Z codes within DSM Axis IV.* ICD Z codes in their present config-uration are not fully applied internationally and are not built as a jointly ex-haustive list that may serve to cover all the possible contextual factors required from a mental health reporting point of view. The ICD revision process, how-ever, could be used to address the shortcomings of this approach and build a more comprehensive classification that is fit for this purpose.
3. *Merge the multiaxial systems of ICD and DSM.* This option proposes to harmo-nize existing ICD and DSM multiaxial systems in a bridged formulation. Given the evidence accumulated through use of the multiaxial versions of ICD and DSM, a potential workgroup could examine the possible harmonization and pro-pose a common solution for field testing.

To evaluate the coverage and possible utility of these three options, a crosswalk between DSM-IV-TR, the ICD-10 multiaxial presentation, and the ICF environ-mental factors codes should be completed. Such a crosswalk could show the joint coverage areas as well as possible missing dimensions. This may be useful in future decisions as to what factors to report in a possible future Axis IV of DSM-5.

As a potential research area, the scope of contextual factors could be explored by computerized search techniques, using a large sample of patient health records with standardized health care terminology (e.g., SNOMED-CT or similar coding systems) and by using the ICD Z codes and ICF environmental factor codes as possible targets for lexical and semantic matches. This exploration would create an "item pool" that covers the universe of commonly used contextual factors. The concordance rates of empirical records with proposed schemes would serve as "relevance ratings" and would provide evidence of specific factors that should be taken into account. As a second step of the research, the role of these factors in identifying the possible predictive validity of a classification scheme could be explored.

Functioning, Disability, and Linking of Diagnostic Criteria for Mental Disorders With Further Operationalizations From ICF

Individuals with mental disorders have various functional limitations in terms of body functions, personal activities, or participation in society that are due to the very nature of their mental illnesses. In a way, these limitations may be part of the mental disease process (e.g., reduced attention, problems with mood regulation or motivation) or may be a consequence of the disorder itself (e.g., activity limitations in self-care, daily life activities). Because these two dimensions of functions are relatively distinct, the World Health Organization scheme of classifications has generated two sets of classifications: ICD for identifying diseases or disorders as entities that relate to pathophysiological deficits in the human body and ICF for identifying the dysfunctions in terms of body, person, or societal functions. This perspective advocates for separate assessments of disease and disability dimensions and use of these constructs jointly in case formulation. ICD Chapter V has therefore purposefully avoided formulating the disability criterion in the mental disorder diagnosis. Various remnants of functional aspects need to be addressed in the ICD-11 revision process, and a workgroup has been identified to deal with these issues.

It is widely recognized that a major difference between the ICD and the DSM classifications of mental disorders is the inclusion of "disability" (also termed *functional impairment*) within the diagnostic system of DSM. Functioning and disability constructs are used in different ways throughout DSM-IV and DSM-IV-TR, integrated into four Axes (I, II, IV, and V). The use of functioning and disability constructs in DSM is discussed in the following paragraph.

In Axes I and II, concepts of *functioning* and *disability* are used basically for two different purposes: 1) to establish a threshold for diagnosis through the "clinical significance criterion" and 2) to establish the severity of a diagnosis. On Axis IV, these concepts are used to report psychosocial and environmental problems (as explained earlier in the section "Capturing Contextual Factors With ICD Z Codes in Formulation of Mental Disorder Diagnosis" and on page 31 of DSM-IV-TR). On Axis V, they are used to assess the overall level of functioning (i.e., Global Assessment of Functioning) for use in planning, measuring the impact of, and predicting the outcome of treatment.

DSM-IV-TR does not, however, provide a clarifying overview with sufficient information to permit an efficient, clear method to put these concepts and their relationships into operation. It will be useful to rethink and operationalize functioning and disability in the revision process, as indicated in the recommendations of the workgroup on mental disorders and disability for *A Research Agenda for DSM-V* (Kupfer et al. 2002).

CLINICAL SIGNIFICANCE, SYMPTOMS, FUNCTIONING, AND DISTRESS

Each edition of the DSM since DSM-III (American Psychiatric Association 1980) has defined a *mental disorder* as

> a clinically significant behavioral or psychological syndrome or pattern that occurs in an individual and that is associated with present distress (e.g., a painful symptom) or disability (i.e., limitations in one or more important areas of functioning), or with a significantly increased risk of suffering death, pain, disability, or an important loss of freedom. (American Psychiatric Association 2000, p. xxxi)

Taken alone, this definition of mental disorder does not define clinical significance. Further guidance, not entirely consistent with this definition, is provided elsewhere, in the DSM-IV-TR explanation of the "clinical significance criterion":

> The definition of *mental disorder* in the introduction to DSM-IV requires that there be clinically significant impairment or distress. To highlight the importance of considering this issue, the criteria sets for most disorders include a clinical significance criterion (usually worded "…causes clinically significant distress or impairment in social, occupational, or other important areas of functioning"). This criterion helps establish the threshold for the diagnosis of a disorder in those situations in which the symptomatic presentation by itself (particularly in its milder forms) is not inherently pathological and may be encountered in individuals for whom a diagnosis of "mental disorder" would be inappropriate. Assessing whether this criterion is met, especially in terms of role function, is an inherently difficult clinical judgment. (American Psychiatric Association 2000, p. 8)

Criteria for most disorders include this clinical significance criterion: namely, that the symptoms/syndrome "causes clinically significant distress or impairment in social, occupational, or other areas of functioning." Although it has been inferred that the clinical significance criterion indicates that the presence of functional impairment or distress increases the probability of some underlying pathology, it is equally possible to infer that the criterion indicates that this distress or impairment increases the probability of a need for clinical attention in a person meeting symptom criteria for a disorder. The ambiguity of the DSM text regarding this issue has led to considerable confusion and controversy related to the definition of *caseness,* particularly in epidemiological studies (Kessler et al. 2003; Narrow et al. 2002; Spitzer and Wakefield 1999; Wakefield and Spitzer 2002).

Whatever the past intent of the clinical significance criterion, it is clear that its inclusion in the criterion sets of DSM blurs the construct of functioning with symptomatology. A suggestion to separate these constructs (Lehman et al. 2002) has considerable merit, given the multiple uses of DSM diagnoses in clinical, research, and disability evaluation settings, where the relative importance of the symptom constellation and the associated functional impairments may vary considerably. Efforts to promote early provision of care may also be enhanced; it has been established that considerable functional impairment can occur in persons with "subsyndromal" symptomatology and that these cases respond to treatment. This separation would also be consistent with diagnosis in the rest of medicine. For so-called physical disorders (e.g., diabetes, tuberculosis, or cancers), clinical significance (in the form of distress or functional impairment) is not required for diagnosis. One can be diagnosed with any of these "physical" disorders and still have a full level of functioning. The fact remains, however, that the DSM concepts of "distress" and "impairment in functioning" are not operationalized or independently assessed (Üstün et al. 1998).

SEVERITY

Severity of a mental disorder is not always clearly and operationally defined in DSM, and severity is confounded with a combination of the symptomatic constellation of a disorder and impairment in social or occupational functioning. Usually, there is a correlation between the level of symptoms and subsequent disability, but this is not always the case. The three levels of severity, defined in DSM-IV-TR, are

1. *Mild.* Few, if any, symptoms in excess of those required to make the diagnosis are present, and symptoms result in no more than minor impairment in social or occupational functioning.
2. *Moderate.* Symptoms or functional impairment between "mild" and "severe" are present.
3. *Severe.* Many symptoms in excess of those required to make the diagnosis, or several symptoms that are particularly severe, are present, or the symptoms result in marked impairment in social or occupational functioning.

Specific criteria for defining these three levels of severity have been provided for mental retardation (coded on Axis II), conduct disorder, manic episode, and major depressive episode, among other disorders.

To compare, severity of a physical disease or disorder is conceived as

- Various thresholds on indicators (e.g., mild, moderate, severe hypertension, based on blood pressure levels).

- Staging of the progress or dissemination of a disease (e.g., Stage 1, 2, 3 of syphilis; primary infection with tuberculosis, secondary tuberculosis, or miliary tuberculosis); this model is also used in the TNM classification of tumors to stage the extent of the cancers.
- With degree of complications (e.g., latent, manifest, and complicated diabetes mellitus).

There may be other or mixed models of severity of a disease. However, functional consequences, in terms of what a patient cannot do, is a different construct than severity of the disease itself and has to be evaluated in its own right. The extent of disability may have some correlation, because, for example, severe forms of diseases usually cause more disability; however, disability itself is an interaction between the person and the environment, and depending on the context, it is perfectly possible that there are examples of no disability in severe diseases or some disability with very mild forms of mental disorders. To address this association, this confounding relation has to be operationalized as distinct constructs of disorder/disease and disability.

ASSESSMENT OF DISABILITY AS A SEPARATE CONSTRUCT

DSM-IV includes in its multiaxial approach an additional axis directly relevant to functioning and disability—that is, Axis V for Global Assessment of Functioning, as noted earlier. This axis is included because it is useful for planning for treatment, measuring effect of treatment, and predicting outcome of treatment. Although the Global Assessment of Functioning provides a gauge for overall severity, it mixes symptomatology with disability.

The ICD tradition of mental disorder classification has purposefully omitted the "disability" dimension in description of the illness. This is in line with general medical thinking, and it independently addresses aspects of disability that are more context dependent. For this purpose, the World Health Organization (2001) has published ICF (Üstün et al. 2001).

ICF gives standard definitions of functioning and disability: *functioning* refers to general aspects of a person's body functions, activities, and social participation in a neutral and positive way, and *disability* indicates problems in any one of these dimensions. This system can be summarized in more detail as shown in Table 9–2.

Body Functions, Body Structures, and Impairments

Body functions are the physiological or psychological functions of body systems. *Body structures* are anatomical parts of the body, such as organs, limbs, and their components. *Impairments* are problems in body function or structure, such as a significant deviation or loss. Body functions and body structures refer to the human organism

TABLE 9–2.   ICF system of functioning and disability

Level	Functioning	Disability
Body	Functions	Impairments
Person	Activities	Activity limitations
Society	Participation	Participation restrictions

Note.   ICF = *International Classification of Functioning, Disability, and Health.*

as a whole; hence, they include the brain and its functions (i.e., the mind). Therefore, mental (or psychological) functions are subsumed under *body functions.*

Body functions and structure are classified along body systems; accordingly, mental disorders are all considered within the central nervous system. Impairments can involve anomalies, defects, losses, or other significant deviations in central nervous system structures or functions. Impairments can be temporary or permanent; progressive, regressive, or static; and intermittent or continuous. The deviation from the norm may be slight or severe and may fluctuate over time. These characteristics are captured in further descriptions, mainly in the codes, by means of qualifiers. The symptoms listed in the DSM diagnostic criteria roughly correspond to impairments in the ICF system.

Activities and Participation

An *activity* is the execution of a task or action by an individual, and *participation* is involvement in a life situation. *Activity limitations and participation restrictions* are difficulties an individual may have in these areas. The activity and participation domains are listed in a single common list that covers a full range of life areas:

- Learning and applying knowledge
- General tasks and demands
- Communication
- Mobility
- Self-care
- Domestic life
- Interpersonal interactions
- Major life
- Community, social, and civic life

These nine domains are divided into two basic qualifiers of *performance* and *capacity.* The performance qualifier describes what an individual does in his or her current environment. The capacity qualifier describes what an individual could possibly do.

Using the concepts of disability definitions in different domains of life (i.e., impairments of body functions, limitations in capacity, and restrictions in performance), a person's disability can be described better and can be disentangled from the description of the disease. The separation of signs/symptoms and consequences, in return, permits better understanding of the disease pathophysiology.

Therefore, we need to focus on "operationalization" of disability as a separate construct with multiple dimensions that are relatively congruent within themselves. For example, activities of a person can be grouped as understanding and communication, moving around, self-care, interpersonal relationships, work relationships, and societal participation. These dimensions have appeared in a large qualitative study—involving 15 different countries—that used empirical measurements and factor-analytic techniques (Üstün et al. 2010). These measurements included

- Understanding and communicating with the world *(cognition)*
- Moving and getting around *(mobility)*
- Self-care *(attending to one's hygiene, dressing, eating, and staying alone)*
- Getting along with people *(interpersonal interactions)*
- Life activities *(domestic responsibilities, leisure, and work)*
- Participation in society *(joining in community activities)*

In this way, we can develop improved assessment strategies that are more specific and more comprehensive at the same time, which may be more useful in some situations than a simple measure of overall functioning. Using the disability construct, we may then generate relevant information that is useful for evaluation of health needs and outcomes of interventions.

Conclusions and Proposals for Formulating Disability and Linking to DSM Criteria

Terminology used throughout DSM-IV does not sufficiently distinguish the relations of different dimensions of functioning and disability, symptoms, and disorders. Our group proposes that DSM-5 adopt an unambiguous and internationally harmonious terminology (e.g., congruent with the ICF) to allow better operationalization of physiological and other personal functioning components. In this way, thresholds for each impaired functioning could be better defined; cultural contexts could be better addressed; and flexibility in the use of the disability construct can occur for research, clinical, or other settings.

Diagnosis of a mental disorder should be uncoupled from disability, as in the case of physical disorders. Each DSM diagnostic entity should be defined only by its disease characteristics, apart from disability, such as 1) specific phenomenology;

2) signs and symptoms (some of which may be defined as body-function impairments, as defined in ICF); and 3) rules that exclude the diagnosis being made in certain circumstances. Assessment and classification of the disability should then be made separately. In particular,

- No functioning or disability phenomena should appear as criteria for diagnosis on Axis I or II of DSM (e.g., phenomena that refer to functional impairment in social, occupational, academic, and other life areas).
- A separate rating of the disorder severity (i.e., mild, moderate, or severe) after a diagnosis has been made should rely on the individual's symptom count or nature of symptoms (e.g., suicidal ideation or any significant symptom), rather than disability (functional impairment).
- Former "functional impairment" criteria should be operationalized, using common domains such as self-care, domestic responsibilities, work, school, or joining community activities.
- Some clinicians may prefer pragmatic formulations that combine symptomatology with clinical significance measures. DSM may explicitly operationalize clinical significance, based on both symptomatology and disability.

In addition, in DSM, "disability" (or functioning) could be formulated as a redefined axis replacing current Axis V. To this end, we recommend the replacement of the existing Global Assessment of Functioning Scale with a new scale that would serve to document only disabilities (excluding any signs or symptoms). The content of the new scale should be based on existing research on disabilities associated with mental disorders. It is desirable that this new measure have clinically meaningful anchor points, depending on the extent of functioning, and be sensitive to change by clinical interventions. It is also desirable that the measure have a correspondence to ICF.

Crosswalks between DSM and ICD and ICF should be developed, and these should be built better on operational definitions. These steps will be useful to put mental health in parity with the rest of health care and integrate mental health information systems to the general health information systems.

The mental health classifications of both ICD and DSM should include common models and elements such as

- *Common terminology,* indicating the span of universe from genes, molecules, cells, diagnostic methods, signs, symptoms, interventions, and other entities
- *Common ontological structure* of disease models, including the etiology, pathogenesis, clinical manifestations, course, and outcome
- *Common reporting methods,* such as case-mix groupings or resource groupings and outcome measurement systems

References

American Psychiatric Association: Diagnostic and Statistical Manual of Mental Disorders, 3rd Edition. Washington, DC, American Psychiatric Association, 1980

American Psychiatric Association: Diagnostic and Statistical Manual of Mental Disorders, 4th Edition. Washington, DC, American Psychiatric Association, 1994

American Psychiatric Association: Diagnostic and Statistical Manual of Mental Disorders, 4th Edition, Text Revision. Washington, DC, American Psychiatric Association, 2000

Janca A, Kastrup MC, Katschnig H, et al: The ICD-10 multiaxial system for use in adult psychiatry: structure and applications. J Nerv Ment Dis 184:191–192, 1996a

Janca A, Kastrup M, Katschnig H, et al: Contextual aspects of mental disorders: a proposal for axis III of the ICD-10 multiaxial system. Acta Psychiatr Scand 94:31–36, 1996b

Kessler RC, Merikangas KR, Berglund P, et al: Mild disorders should not be eliminated from the DSM-V. Arch Gen Psychiatry 60:1117–1122, 2003

Kupfer DJ, First MB, Regier DA (eds): A Research Agenda for DSM-V. Washington, DC, American Psychiatric Association, 2002

Lehman AF, Goldberg R, Dixon LB, et al: Improving employment outcomes for persons with severe mental illnesses. Arch Gen Psychiatry 59:165–172, 2002

Narrow WE, Rae DS, Robins LN, et al: Revised prevalence estimates of mental disorders in the United States: using a clinical significance criterion to reconcile 2 surveys' estimates. Arch Gen Psychiatry 59:115–123, 2002

Spitzer RL, Wakefield JC: DSM-IV diagnostic criterion for clinical significance: does it help solve the false positives problem? Am J Psychiatry 156:1856–1864, 1999

Spitzer RL, Wakefield JC: Why requiring clinical significance does not solve epidemiology's and DSM's validity problem, in Defining Psychopathology in the 21st Century: DSM-V and Beyond. Edited by Helzer JE, Hudziak JJ. Washington, DC, American Psychiatric Publishing, 2002, pp 31–40

Üstün TB, Chatterji S, Rehm J: Limitations of diagnostic paradigm: it doesn't explain "need." Arch Gen Psychiatry 55:1145–1146, 1998

Üstün TB, Chatterji S, Rehm J, et al (eds): Disability and Culture: Universalism and Diversity. Seattle, WA, Hogrefe & Huber, 2001

Üstün TB, Kostanjsek N, Chatterji S, et al (eds): Measuring Health and Disability: Manual for WHO Disability Assessment Schedule WHODAS 2.0. Geneva, World Health Organization, 2010

Wakefield JC, Spitzer RL: Lowered estimates—but of what? Arch Gen Psychiatry 59:129–130, 2002

World Health Organization: International Statistical Classification of Diseases and Related Health Problems, 10th Revision. Geneva, World Health Organization, 1992

World Health Organization: Multiaxial Presentation of the ICD-10 for Use in Adult Psychiatry. Cambridge, UK, Cambridge University Press, 1997

World Health Organization: International Classification of Functioning, Disability and Health (ICF). Geneva, World Health Organization, 2001

INDEX

Page numbers printed in **boldface** *type refer to tables or figures. Page numbers followed by an* n *refer to note numbers.*